FISH

THE COMPLETE GUIDE TO
BUYING AND COOKING

FISH

THE COMPLETE GUIDE TO BUYING AND COOKING

MARK BITTMAN

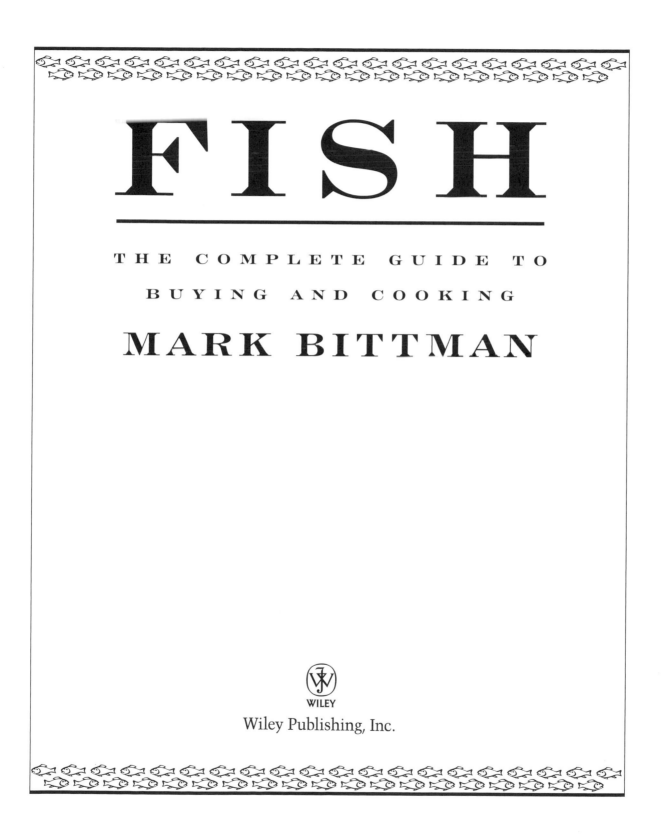

WILEY

Wiley Publishing, Inc.

Library of Congress Cataloging-in-Publication Data
Bittman, Mark.
    Fish / Mark Bittman.
        p.   cm.
    Includes index.
    ISBN-13 978-0-02-863152-3
    ISBN-10 0-02-863152-8
    1. Cookery (Fish)   I. Title.
TX747.B47   1994   93-38092
641.6'92—dc20   CIP

Manufactured in the United States of America
16   15   14   13   12   11   10

In memory of Max and Helen Art
and Charlie and Sarah Bittman

CONTENTS

ACKNOWLEDGMENTS

First of all, I'd like to thank Murray and Gertrude Bittman, for teaching me to enjoy life in general and eating in particular. Twenty years after they began that process, I was lucky enough to meet Ellen Furstenberg, Judy Lieberman, and Karen Baar, who showed me that time spent in the kitchen could be sublime. Ten years later, I became a food writer.

There are countless people in the fish business who have been kind to me. Chief among them were Andrew Gambardella and Joe Acabbo, two great fishmongers whose stores I haunted for hours throughout the 1980s. I learned a great deal from Jim Wallace, Richard Lord, and Ken Coons, who were patient enough to answer my questions, no matter how trivial. The folks at the National Fisheries Institute, especially Clare Vanderbeek, were supportive throughout this process; Dixie Blake was especially helpful in teaching me about shrimp, Marion Kaiser about salmon, Pat Shanahan about things West. Rod Mitchell and Denny Durante were two early fans who gave me encouragement and even fish.

There is not enough room here to adequately thank all the people in the "food world" who contributed, directly or indirectly, to this book. I hope that seeing their names here will let some of them know how much I have appreciated their help: Pam Anderson, Fern Berman, Jack Bishop, Jane Freiman, Dorie Greenspan, Maria Guarnaschelli, Barbara Kafka, Nora Kerr, Carole Lalli, Stefanie Lyness, Priscilla Martel, Hal McGee, Pamela Mitchell, Scott Mowbray, Jacques Pepin, Charlie Van Over, and Nach Waxman.

I fortunately have met scores of good chefs in my career, and would like to single out Eberhard Mueller, who has an unparalleled love of fish and talent at cooking it; Jean-Louis Gerin, whom I count among my friends and who has created several of the greatest fish dishes I have ever tasted; and Chris Schlesinger, another friend, whose approach to cooking should serve as a role model for all of us who sometimes take ourselves too seriously. I am also an admirer of Rick Stein of Padstow, an uncompromising fish lover.

I received help and support from Pam Hoenig and Justin Schwartz, my talented and energetic editors at Macmillan.

The contribution of Mary Flower, a supremely competent copyeditor, may not be as readily apparent; but she has left her mark throughout the book, and it is better for it.

Among the many books which served as inspiration, Alan Davidson's *North Atlantic Seafood* was the most important; it is read and admired by every cook, chef, and food writer who loves fish, and is not only brilliant but fun. Elizabeth Schneider's *Uncommon Vegetables—A Commonsense Guide* gave me a clue, after many years of struggling, as to how best to organize my own book. Ian Dore's more technical work, *Fresh Seafood—The Commercial Buyer's Companion*, has been helpful for years.

Several people believed in my abilities as a cook and writer long before I did, and they are all not only colleagues but good friends: Linda Giuca and Louise Kennedy, two of the world's great editors; Chris Kimball, a first-rate thinker and someone with whom I will never tire of brainstorming; and Angela Miller, my generous, intelligent, sympathetic, and considerate agent.

Four of my friends have been especially encouraging over the yeras: Pamela Hort, David Paskin, Sally Connolly, and Semeon Tsalbins. Both David and Semeon spent hours helping me figure out seemingly absurd cooking tasks; at least they were rewarded with generally decent food (and plenty of wine).

Finally, I want to express my love and gratitude to John Willoughby, a fine friend who I am lucky enough to have as a colleague as well; Kate and Emma Baar-Bittman, who will tell their children stories of eating octopus and shark while their friends were at McDonald's; and especially Karen Baar, without whose encouragement, patience, love, and intelligence I would not be writing these words.

New Haven
Thanksgiving, 1993

PREFACE

The fact that you are reading this page probably means that, like most Americans, you fall into one of three categories when it comes to cooking fish: The very thought of it intimidates you; you've cooked the same fish according to the same recipes, over and over, since you began cooking, and want some new ideas; or you like cooking fish, and have played around with it some, but want a definitive source for information and recipes.

To the first group, I say "Don't worry about it." To the second, I say, "There is no obstacle to taking your fish cooking to the next level." And to the third, I say, "You've come to the right place."

This is not a collection of chef's recipes adapted for the home cook. Nor is it a description of exotic fish cooked with esoteric ingredients. Although I have spent much time in the company of chefs—as a reporter and as a student—I am and always have been a home cook. These recipes were developed with supermarket ingredients, which fortunately are far better than they were ten years ago. Indoors, they were cooked on my woefully inadequate kitchen stove with its average oven and broiler and my not-very-special kitchenware. Out-

doors, I relied on my antiquated charcoal grill, my beat-up $149 gas grill, and a series of rather poorly built wood fires. There is nothing here you cannot master.

I don't need to sell you on fish. Like other mass-distributed foods, of course, fish has problems: What you find in water, you find in fish; its distribution system is far from ideal; and, when it is raised on "farms," its flavor is usually a pale shadow of that of its wild cousins. But the fact that fish is healthy food is a given, as is the fact that it is the last major wild food available to us. There is no animal group with as much variety and flavor, nor—for my money—is there any food at all that offers as much enjoyment. Only fruits and vegetables compete with fish for variety of texture, appearance, and flavor.

And it seems to me that if you combine all current nutritional "wisdom," one ideal daily diet could consist of five servings each of grains, fruit, and vegetables, a minimum of dairy, and a serving of fish. This is not, however, a book about eating fish to be healthy, but one about cooking fish to enjoy eating it. The fact that most fish is low in fat, and lends itself to low-fat preparations—of which there are literally hundreds in the following pages—is, as far as I'm concerned, a very happy coincidence.

Equally fortuitous is the fact that fish cooks quickly; except for large whole fish, or big cuts from tuna, swordfish, and other giants of the sea, fish is done in twenty minutes or less. That fish is intrinsically tender means that most recipes involve building a sauce or other coating before or after cooking the fish; that's about as complicated as it gets.

Why, then, have we had so many problems with fish? More because it is difficult to buy than because it presents cooking challenges. The question I'm most frequently asked is, "Where do you get good fish?" These days, usually, I buy it at the supermarket. It's not my favorite place to shop, but the fish there is at least as good, generally speaking, as the vegetables, and often better than the beef, veal, pork, or chicken, some of which can be quite nasty. It is all a matter of knowing what species will work for you on any given day, and of becoming a competent judge of fish quality. None of this involves magic or intensive training, and it's all right here.

A word about nomenclature: You'll note that I don't often distinguish between "fish" and "seafood." For simplicity's sake, I have chosen to use the word "fish" to include all the animals of the sea covered in this book. I don't know whether a squid is technically a fish or not, and I'm sure that snails are not; but I don't care. There are specific instances in which I talk about fish with shells, and then I may use the term "shellfish"; I also use the term "finfish" occasionally, for the sake of precision. But this is a book about "fish," and every animal in it qualifies (luckily, I omitted frogs' legs and caviar).

Naming individual fish is one of the great challenges facing not only consumers but the entire industry. There are so many fish called sole, rockfish, and snapper—just to name some of the most outrageous examples—that almost no one can keep track of them all. Using Latin would help (and I have included Latin names in a limited fashion), but we don't use Latin, do we? I have opted, then, to follow what should be the standard text on fish nomenclature, The Retail Seafood Identity System, produced by the National Fisheries Institute with the cooperation of the FDA. For added help, I turned to the *Multilingual Dictionary of Fish and Fish Products*, an international standard.

Unfortunately, even if we all used the same common names for the same fish—pollock, for example, instead of Boston bluefish—there remain common names that can be correctly applied to more than one species. Sometimes it doesn't make much difference, but often it does. There are objectively inferior species of halibut, turbot, salmon, rockfish, flatfish, and so on. Buying pink salmon instead of sockeye is much like buying chuck steak instead of sirloin; the differences are very real, even though both are "salmon" or "steak," and there's a good reason one costs more than the other: It is better.

What's a consumer to do? Read, ask, and learn. I have tried to walk a fine line in these pages, pointing out the not-so-subtle differences among similar (and not-so-similar) species with the same common names, without being a stickler for precision. Armed with imperfect knowledge, limited space, and a strong desire to stick to the basics, there is no doubt that at times my judgment has been faulty. For this I apologize, and trust that you will learn from this book, enjoy it, and value it, despite its weaknesses.

FISH

THE COMPLETE GUIDE TO
BUYING AND COOKING

INTRODUCTION

Despite its size, the goal of this book is really quite simple: to teach you how to buy good, commonly available fish, and cook it quickly in a variety of basic and delicious ways.

My aim is not to tell you about the life history of fish, how to catch them, or even how anyone else catches them. I won't tell you much about fish farming, fish transport, or the fish business. Nor will I tell you how to make Marinated Shrimp Wrapped in Ham Over a Red Peppercorn Passionfruit Sauce, Topped with a Spinach-Basil Pesto, or any other restaurant nightmare, the type of which we see all too often.

When it comes to fish, the goal is pure: Buy it right, cook it simply.

Americans like fish—consumption has risen fairly steadily during the course of the last decade—but we have trouble buying it right and cooking it simply. This explains why nearly three quarters of all the seafood in this country is eaten away from home. Yet one survey after another shows that people would cook more fish if only it were "less complicated."

Again, that's the goal of this book: Making the buying and cooking of fish less complicated. If you read the following few chapters, you'll gain an overview of the world of fish that will probably be new to you. If you turn straight to the recipe section, you'll find brief but fairly comprehensive descriptions of the most commonly found fish, and straightforward, delicious ways to prepare them.

When I first began cooking fish, I learned a great deal from *James Beard's New Fish Cookery*, first published in 1954. Beard's most important statement remains supremely valid: "I suggest only one general rule: Don't overcook fish."

But many other aspects of the world of fish cuisine have changed since the dean of American cooking tackled the subject. We have seen the decline in popularity of heavy, cream-based sauces, countered by the surge of Mediterranean and Asian influences. Perhaps even more importantly, the supply of fish has been radically altered. Many changes have been wrought by fish farming (which literally cut the price of salmon in half and more than doubled its sales during the 1980s); air freight (more than half the fish in a typical fish store or supermarket case spent some time in an airplane);

and factory fishing vessels (almost all the fish destined for processing into sandwiches, frozen dinners, and restaurant fish-and-chips plates is cleaned and frozen at sea, as is much of the fish sold at retail counters).

Furthermore, although the supply of fish has always been cyclical, the population of many "standard" fish—halibut, for example, as well as cod, haddock, and regional species like redfish—is way down. The Atlantic salmon, once so plentiful that colonial servants demanded contracts limiting how many times a week they'd be forced to eat it, is now an endangered species. Similarly, lobster, though still widely available, now average two pounds rather than three and a half (or five, if the Pilgrims' accounts are to be believed).

Until just over a decade ago, no one had witnessed the impact of a modern food craze upon a single species. It was then that Paul Prudhomme (via Craig Claiborne) taught the country how to blacken redfish. Within three years, redfish—long a trash fish of the Gulf Coast which literally could not be given away in New York or Los Angeles—could be bought almost anywhere. The year after that it became scarce. Now its catch is limited by law.

Although subsequent crazes have not been as intense, our cravings for fish have decimated certain species and elevated others. Monkfish soared from eighty-nine cents to six dollars a pound in five years, and is now in short supply at any price; once labeled "poor man's lobster," it now costs almost as much as the real thing. Flounder, cod, and haddock, once staples in the Northeast, are increasingly hard to find. Halibut numbers are at a record low, and pollock—just five years ago an "underutilized" fish—is considered overfished.

Internationally, there is no shortage of fish; the market works to ensure that when one fish becomes scarce, another takes its place. The dwindling supply of haddock, for example, has meant that grouper, once sold strictly in the South, can be found in Massachusetts fish markets. New Zealand fishermen found a ready market for their orange roughy in the millions of Americans who couldn't care less that it wasn't cod; it was close enough. Even catfish, the lowly river-dweller that has supplanted cotton as Mississippi's major crop, is sold everywhere, and fetches pretty prices, too.

Now a New Englander can wander into a fish store or, more likely, a supermarket, and see Florida pompano but no flounder. A Gulf Coast cook might find Norwegian salmon or Thai shrimp, but no redfish or pompano. In California, there may be scallops from Chile or grouper from Florida, but no petrale sole from the nearby Pacific. Walk into a good supermarket today anywhere in the country and you are likely to find squid and skate, red snapper and ocean perch, mackerel and whiting, pompano, tuna, and swordfish. These may come from the Gulf of Maine, the Mediterranean, the Caribbean, the Indian Ocean . . . anywhere.

The net result of overfishing and the internationalization of the fish market is this: "Standard" fish are no longer standard, few fish remain regional, and we must now choose among fish with which we may be unfamiliar.

If you wish to enjoy fish on a regular basis, you must learn to be flexible. You must learn to handle fish other than those you or your parents grew up eating. This book will help you develop that flexibility, equip you to face the ever-changing seafood counter, and show you that buying fish is half the battle—or more. So armed, you will find that the quality of your eating will soar.

I have made no attempt to cover every species caught off our shores. Such a task would not only be virtually impossible, but would leave little room for recipes. Instead, I have included the roughly seventy species—and their relatives—that are routinely available in many parts of the country for part or most of the year. I have then, omitted entries on abalone, for example, which is delicious but almost extinct; sea urchin, the spiny ball with the creamy interior that is best reserved for restaurants, ribbonfish or needlefish, which you may see in your local Chinatown but nowhere else; or sea squab, a wonderful fish whose day may come (but not, I think, before I need to rewrite this book).

On the other hand, I have included many species with which you may not be familiar. To name just three: tilefish, a superb mid-Atlantic white fish more widely distributed than ever before; octopus, readily available almost everywhere, increasingly popular, and destined to become more so; and fresh sardines, practically a staple in much of Europe and too tasty to ignore.

Needless to say, fish are quite different from one another, but I have put much of my energy into discovering and describing their similarities, especially in the kitchen. When you begin to think of general categories of fish as opposed to individual species, you will enter the market with more confidence and leave with more success (see Buying Fish, pages 5–12). I have detailed these kinds of cross-references and potential substitutions in several ways in this book, but this general rule may be just as helpful: If the meat of two fish looks about the same, and if the cut is about the same, they can probably stand in for one another.

Although I maintain that the fish store or supermarket presents home cooks with their greatest piscatorial challenge, many people are equally intimidated by cooking fish in their own kitchen. I hear it all the time: Fish sticks to the grill. Fish stinks up the house. Fish is too dry. Fish is too tough.

But cooking fish ranks with cooking vegetables as among the simplest and most delightful of kitchen tasks. In many ways, fish are more like vegetables than like meat: Both are astonishing in their variety, and both are best cooked simply and quickly.

Basic fish cooking, like almost anything else in the kitchen, can be summed up by a few easy-to-follow rules, and the pairing of correct technique and appropriate fish solves most problems. A little experience—combined with the knowledge that the subtle flavors of most fish are better complemented by a drizzle of vinaigrette than a mass of elaborate sauce, and that, as Mr. Beard implied, undercooking fish is virtually always preferable to overcooking it—dispenses with the rest.

If this book helps you to relish cooking and eating fish at home, I've done what I set out to do. And you will find your life in the kitchen and at the table immeasurably enriched.

HOW TO READ AN ENTRY

Name: TUNA—**the single most commonly used name to describe this species or group of species.**

Latin name(s): *Thunnus thynnus* **(bluefin);** *T. albacares* **(yellowfin), etc.** *One or more Latin names describing this species or members of a group of species.*

Other common names: Albacore, tunny, bonito, ahi, bigeye, bluefin, yellowfin, skipjack—A short list of regional names for the fish or its close relatives.

Common forms: **Almost exclusively steaks, although some smaller skipjack may be filleted.** **Freezes well**—*The form or forms in which you are most likely to encounter this fish in the market.*

General description: Pale pink (albacore) to deep red (bluefin and yellowfin) meat, the most beeflike of all fish. Almost always sold without the skin, which is inedibly tough—A summary of the kind of fish this is, what its meat is like, whether its skin is edible, how it cooks.

For other recipes see: Blackfish, bluefish, eel, grouper, mackerel, mahi-mahi, mako shark, monkfish, pompano, salmon, red snapper, striped bass, swordfish—Other entries which include one or more recipes that are suitable for this fish.

Buying tips: Things to look for before purchase—what does this fish look like when it starts to go bad? Should you buy it whole or filleted?

My recipes are more or less standard. Serving sizes are usually for four to six ounces of fish per person. Preparation time includes marinating and other "down" time and assumes a certain level of basic kitchen skills—chopping, peeling, and dicing. If you are tackling onions with a butter knife, figure a bit more time.

In order to save space while providing more alternatives, I offer variations when they rely heavily on the same technique and include many of the same ingredients as the "master" recipe.

Finally, there is the line "Alternative fish for this recipe." By this I mean other fish that can be used in this recipe with little or no adjustment. In some recipes, I omit this line, because the recipe is too specific to the fish to make substituting easy; but this is rare.

Quite frequently, additional substitutions also can be made, but, generally speaking, these are the ones with which I feel most comfortable. Be aware that changing fish also may mean adjusting the cooking time. And sometimes, changes will necessitate following certain procedures necessary for the alternative fish, such as peeling shrimp when substituting it for squid; most of these changes are self-evident.

BUYING FISH

THE RIGHT FISH

I'm entirely serious when I say that buying fish is more challenging than cooking it. The perfect specimen requires little more than a blast of heat, a dash of salt, a sprinkling of lemon. It's finding that perfect specimen—without catching it yourself—that takes knowledge and patience.

There are times when entering a fish market overwhelms me with choices. The smell is of the sea, the fish looks alive, the selection is wonderful, the staff knowledgeable and enthusiastic. In these instances I buy more fish than I can possibly use; I can't help myself.

Not quite as often, there are times I walk into fish markets and am repelled. The smell is of ammonia or bad fish, the floor and counters are dirty, the fish looks very, very dead, and the answers to my question are nonsense. I leave and think about eating rice and beans.

The most important single element in buying fish is trust. If you can make friends with a fishmonger, you've established a relationship that will improve your chances of buying consistently good fish. Fair or not, regulars get the best fish in most stores. Go in three days in a row and be picky; return fish if it's bad; ask a lot of questions. By the fourth day, a good fishmonger will be steering you away from the fish that's not to his or her liking.

There was a time not too long ago when buying fish was a more personal experience than it is now. Two of my great mentors in the world of fish were older men who had been catching, buying, and selling fish here in New Haven since they were boys in the early part of this century. Some days, I'd ask, "What's good?" and be told "Everything." I could believe it, too. Other times, I'd ask, "What's good?" and be told, "It's not a great day, but the whiting came in last night and is gorgeous." With that information, I knew it was eat whiting or go elsewhere.

I don't have that option anymore; my favorite fish markets closed down, and the ones I like almost as well are out of my driving range except for special occasions. Now, like almost everyone else, I buy most of my fish in the supermarket. But it's not as bad as I first thought. There are two supermarkets within a couple of miles of my house and, at first glance, the fish counters are not dissimilar. Both are clean, with plenty of fish and plenty of ice.

One, however, specializes in precut fillets, bought centrally and shipped to the store; the staff turns over frequently, and none of them stays long enough to learn anything. Here, I'm almost always told that the obviously farm-raised salmon is Alaskan king, almost none of which reaches the East Coast. The tiny calico scallops are always labeled "bay," a travesty of gigantic proportions. Almost all the flatfish is "sole," an impossibility. And there are lots of sales, always on the fish that sells most quickly and can be bought at a favorable price in huge quantity by the Boston-based buyer. If I want one of these, and I'm in the neighborhood, I'll buy it here; often, the quality is quite good. But the other fish, the squid, sardines, octopus, mussels, tuna, mackerel, and so on—the fish that doesn't sell instantly—almost always looks horrible. I don't think it's even there to be sold, but rather to give the impression that this is indeed a "full-service" seafood counter.

Things are much different at the other supermarket. The manager has run the department for five years, and is there every day, including Sunday. She orders directly from her suppliers, and gets deliveries daily. She buys small quantities of fish that she knows doesn't sell very well—she might take three skate, for example, or ten pounds of sardines—because she knows that certain customers crave those fish, and will buy them if she tells them they're good. She brings in local fish when they're available; in May, when the other supermarket is running a sale on swordfish from the South Pacific, she's selling fresh shad from the Connecticut River. In January, when the first store is pushing Ecuadorian shrimp, she has mackerel from the Long Island Sound. She also buys "headfish"—fish that must be cleaned before sale—and trains her staff to scale, gut, and fillet. Yes, this operation is in a supermarket; but it's a real fish store.

At the first of these stores, there are no "regulars." There are only people lining up to buy fillets and shrimp. At the second, people of every ethnic group in New Haven stand and chat, swapping recommendations and recipes ("How do you cook that?"), buying their favorite fish or experimenting with something new. It's a pleasant and usually rewarding experience.

In the introduction to this book, I pointed out that the fish we buy now comes from everywhere. I prefer eating local fish when I can get it—and I am lucky enough to live near one of the world's richest fishing grounds, the North Atlantic—but I'm very happy that I can buy Florida pompano, Alaskan sable, Dover sole, and Louisiana shrimp. And, with air freight and good freezing techniques, I'll consider buying fish from anywhere. That is, as long as it looks and smells good.

Buying high-quality fish is not that difficult: You have to be able to distinguish between different degrees of good and bad, to be willing to say no, to be assertive, and to haggle—our grandmothers did it, why shouldn't we?

Looking at Fish

What follows is enough to get you through the sometimes harrowing experience of confronting a seafood counter. Your ultimate goal should be to find a store you like and gain experience in buying fish there. That, combined with the information about and recipes for individual fish found later in this book, should be enough to make you comfortable buying and cooking fish forever.

Overcoming this obstacle requires dedication, but anyone who can tell Savoy from regular cabbage can buy fish intelligently. To start with, the cut and color of finfish are often more important than the species. Nearly all pearly white fish is mild tasting and tender; it matters less whether it is haddock, flounder, tilefish, rockfish, orange roughy, or cod than whether it is a thick or thin fillet, whole fish, or steak. Similarly, many steaks and fillets of darker fish can be freely substituted for one another.

Seen this way, there are just a few categories of popular finfish: thin fillets, almost all of which are white or light; thick fillets, which break down into white, light, and dark; and white, light, and dark steaks. Some fish, of course, are unique, such as monkfish and the salmon-trout family. And it's more difficult to substitute for whole fish.

So many of the best-selling cuts are mislabeled anyway—out of ignorance, tradition, or greed—that setting your heart on cod and turning down tilefish doesn't make much sense. If you want to cook a thick white fillet, buy the best-looking one you see. Of course, you should also use this book as a reference; in every section, I've listed other entries to see for more recipes for each fish. And under most recipes, I list alternative fish that can be used (see How to Read an Entry, pages 3–4).

Shellfish are not as readily interchangeable, but there are far fewer of them. Since the supply is more consistent, and most shellfish freeze quite well, knowing how to substitute one for another is not that important. If you go to the store looking for shrimp, you will find it; if you go in search of weakfish or mahi-mahi, you'd better have alternatives in mind. See the chart on page 11 for more information about grouping fish in categories.

It's fortunate that many fish are freely interchangeable, because we get little help from most retailers in knowing just what we're buying. There is a tower of Babel of fish names, and informing consumers is not in the interest of those retailers who mislabel seafood in hope of increasing sales and profits. I often see flounder labeled as sole, rockfish or perch labeled as red snapper, Chilean salmon marked Norwegian, skipjack tuna called yellowfin. There may be times you stand at the fish counter feeling the way a nineteenth-century Russian peasant would in the breakfast-cereal aisle.

None of this is surprising: With hundreds of species of edible fish swimming off our coasts and thousands worldwide, nobody knows every popular name of every fish. And I am not sure that there's much that can be done about price gouging; if you buy "red snapper" that's actually perch, you've paid too much for it. The only solution here is to learn to identify red snapper—not easy—or, once again, buy fish from a trustworthy fishmonger who can tell the difference and buys and prices the fish accordingly.

If, at least, you know that fillets of perch can pretty much be cooked as red snapper, the result is hardly tragic. And if you know how to recognize top-quality fish, at least the perch you're paying two dollars too much for will be in good shape. You're still getting a decent piece of fish, just not the piece of fish you thought you were getting.

Checking Out the Fish Store

Before you even get to a fish counter, you may be turned off. Is there grime? Does it smell fishy? Is there enough ice, is the fish on it, and is the drainage adequate? If the answer to any of these questions is no, I'd go elsewhere. Most fish keep best on ice—whole fish can be buried, but fillets and steaks do best on ice, not in it—and the melting ice must be drained away and replenished frequently. For every degree in temperature that fish is stored over 32°F, there is a loss in quality. Fish held at 50°F deteriorates about four times faster than that held at 32°F.

It's possible to get good prewrapped fish—there's nothing intrinsically wrong with it—but I wouldn't touch it unless I really trusted the store, and felt that a knowledgeable buyer stood behind it. You can smell *really* bad fish right through the wrapper, but you can't smell just-off fish. And you can only see one side of the fish.

Once you're face to face with a fishmonger, you

must be willing to assert your right to high-quality food. Again, this job becomes easier if you can establish a relationship with the salesperson. Try, for example, distinguishing yourself to the fishmonger by returning any fish that you find unsatisfactory once you bring it home. Do this once or twice—even on the basis of appearance—and you'll be rewarded with better service. Praise, of course, works even better—provided it is warranted.

Generally speaking, good fish looks and smells good and has firm, unmarred flesh. The smell is important, and, until you trust the seller, I'd insist on taking a whiff. Most high-quality fish smells like fresh seawater. If it smells bad, it can't taste good. Some fishmongers at supermarket seafood counters may not allow you to smell fish before buying it. If that's the case, and the fish passes the appearance tests, you might consider buying it, opening the package on the spot, and—if the smell is at all off—handing it right back.

There are differences in how different fish—and different cuts of the same fish—should be handled. Here are some general guidelines; see specific fish entries for more information.

Shellfish

Whole clams, oysters, mussels, and certain other mollusks must be alive when sold; their viscera contaminates the meat shortly after death. If they are shucked and separated from their guts, as scallops routinely are, and oysters frequently are, shelf life is extended considerably. It's easy to tell whether whole mollusks are alive: Their muscles make it difficult to pry their shells apart, they usually respond to a light tap by closing their shells, and they should smell sweet. Mollusks should be iced or refrigerated; they remain alive and healthy at temperatures up to 40°F, about the temperature of your home refrigerator.

Mollusks should also be allowed to breathe; never store bivalves in a closed plastic bag, where they will suffocate. Prewrapped mollusks should be in nets or other porous wrappers. (Occasionally an ignorant clerk will wrap mussels or clams in plastic without poking holes in it; what you have then is a sack of dead, stinky shellfish.) At home, store them, dry and uncovered, in a pot or bowl.

Snails and conch may be alive or precooked and removed from the shell before sale. Frozen precooked conch is often of high quality and a good buy.

Shrimp are almost always frozen at sea or at the farm and defrosted before sale. If you can buy them still frozen, usually in five-pound blocks, you can get a better price and more control over how they are defrosted; see A Note About Frozen Fish, page 9, as well as the shrimp entry, page 260. When you're buying any shrimp, look for a full shell and firm meat. Except for black tiger shrimp, reject those with black spots or rings, or a dark area around the abdomen. The meat should not be dead white, which indicates freezer burn, or pink, which means it has been defrosted at too high a temperature.

Lobsters and crabs should be alive or frozen when sold; soft-shell crabs can be killed and cleaned before sale, but have a very short shelf life after death and are usually frozen. And remember this: Alive doesn't mean fresh. If a lobster has been swimming in a tank for two weeks, chances are good it will be tasteless. Ask. Lobsters and crabs should be very lively when you buy them.

Steaks and Fillets

Although it is happening with less and less frequency, steaks and fillets are best cut to order, from whole fish. Whole fish keep better than precut steaks and fillets. In addition, cutting to order allows you to dictate the size and thickness of a steak, and to request fillets from the best-looking fish. If you find a store that provides this service, you've probably found a store where quality is a priority.

Increasingly, fillets and even steaks are cut from fish before they reach the fish counter. There are, of course, differences in appearance from one fish to another, but there are some basic rules you should keep in mind in order to get the highest quality possible:

- Use your eyes. The surface of the fish should glisten; it should be bright, clear, reflective, and almost translucent. The color should be consistent with the type of fish; pearly white fish should not have spots of pink (which are usually bruises) or gray or brown (which indicates spoilage). Creamy or ivory-colored fish should have no areas of deep red or brown. Dark-fleshed fish, such as tuna, should have no surface "rainbows." Get to know the ideal appearance of your favorite fish, and reject any that don't meet your standard. Generally, you don't want any fish whose surface appears brown, dull, opaque, and/or muddy. Remember, fillets and steaks should be set on—not in—ice, and there should be no puddles of water.
- Use your fingers. Most fishmongers won't let you touch fish—it's usually against local health standards, and reasonably so. But you can ask the counterperson to press his or her finger into the fish's flesh; it should appear firm and elastic. If it looks mushy, if the finger leaves a lasting impression, move on.
- Use your nose. If it doesn't smell sweet, if it doesn't smell like the sea, turn your nose up.

Whole Fish

Whole fish give you more signals than fillets or steaks. First off, they should be buried in ice, or at least layered in it; piles of fish atop ice can develop hot spots where the fish touch each other. Then look for red gills, bright, reflective skin, firm flesh, an undamaged layer of scales, and no browning anywhere. The smell—even in the body cavity—should be sweet. Ignore the common wisdom about clear eyes; those of some fish cloud up immediately after death, and those of others remain clear after the rest of the fish is rotten. In general, though, the best whole fish look alive, as if they just came out of the water.

A NOTE ABOUT FROZEN FISH

All of the above pointers are more important than whether a given fish is labeled "fresh" or "previously frozen." Recent technological advances have allowed modern fishing fleets to clean and flash-freeze fish—at -60°F, or even colder—within minutes of its capture. When thawed, such fish is frequently in better shape than that which spent several days sitting in a hold before reaching the dock, at which point it was sold as "fresh." Much of the fish that you eat in restaurants—swordfish, salmon, tuna, mahi-mahi, cod, almost all sushi and sashimi, and other fish that you might assume was never frozen—has been treated this way. That's in addition to about 98 percent of all shrimp sold in this country; soft-shell crabs almost any time but midsummer; and large amounts of squid, whiting, smelts, and fillets from a variety of white fish.

That's one of the problems with the way many merchandisers—and consumers—view freshness when it comes to seafood: "Fresh" fish, we believe, is fish that has never been frozen; according to this axiom, frozen fish can never be fresh.

Yet many of us cannot afford to think this way. If you routinely buy fish straight off the boat or from a reliable market, you should continue to do so; generally speaking, such top-quality fish is fresh and not frozen. But many of us occasionally must make compromises in our definitions of freshness. Both frozen and chilled (never-frozen) fish vary in quality.

There is a lot of second-rate chilled fish in the market, and it's up to us to identify it and reject it at fish counters, using the techniques I've described above. Meanwhile, there can be advantages to buying high-quality frozen fish.

Much frozen fish makes good eating; its advocates in the industry like to say that their procedure "captures a moment in quality." Indeed, well-frozen fish has good color, texture, and flavor. When fish is frozen quickly, the ice crystals that form are tiny. When it is thawed properly, the liquid from those ice crystals remains in the flesh, and the fish is nearly as moist and flavorful as it was when it was first frozen.

Problems arise when fish is frozen slowly, forming larger ice crystals which may rupture cell walls. When this fish is defrosted, two problems arise: The ice crystals contain too much liquid to be reabsorbed into the flesh, and additional liquid is lost from the broken cells. This "drip loss" not only affects the weight of the fish, but its flavor and texture. The flavor elements of fish are tied up in the cells' liquids, and drip out right along with the moist quality of the fillet or steak. The result is dry, tasteless fish.

Drip loss is most often a problem with fish that was frozen by faulty equipment, or fish that's frozen at home—something only rarely worth doing. But it can also result from faulty defrosting. Frozen fish should be thawed slowly, in the refrigerator, for twenty-four hours or more. Defrosting fish at room temperature, in a microwave, or under warm water can alter the cell structure, again allowing fluids—and flavor—to escape from the cells. Furthermore, slowly melting ice crystals are more likely to be reabsorbed into the cell structure than those that thaw rapidly. If you are in a hurry to thaw fish, do so under cold running water—make sure the fish is wrapped tightly, so that it doesn't come in contact with the water—and cook it as soon as possible after thawing to minimize drip loss.

Two other factors affect the quality of frozen fish. First, the species. Some fish simply freeze better than others: Shrimp, squid, and other small-celled, flexible fish generally do well. And small cuts of fish, because they freeze quickly, retain their quality better: Flounder takes to freezing better than cod, for example.

Second, the quality of the fish when it was frozen. It's just as easy to freeze lousy fish as good fish, and more difficult for you to tell the difference. Fortunately, most frozen fish is sold under a brand name; if you get stuck once, forget that brand from then on—*after* writing a letter telling the company of your experience, *and* bringing the defective product back to the market.

How do you know when a fish has been frozen well? Frozen fish should be somewhat shiny, not flat-looking, and it should have none of the white spots that indicate freezer burn. It should also be as hard as a rock and have no evidence of prior defrosting. Thawing and refreezing fish is a virtual guarantee of bad quality, so look for even color and texture. Finally, frozen fish should be well wrapped. Some supermarkets buy fish in bulk and freeze it loosely in plastic bags; unless the fish was frozen when they bought it, this causes freezer burn.

Storing Fish at Home

High-quality fish has been frozen or continually iced from shortly after the catch until it reaches your hands. Your job is to keep its quality from deteriorating from the time you buy it until you cook it. Most refrigerators hold a temperature of around 40°F—not cold enough. In fact, fish held at 32°F keeps twice as well as that held at 42°F. Fish held in a hot car—where temperatures are roughly equivalent to those of a low oven—can spoil in thirty minutes. When I shop on a hot day and know I won't be coming home directly, I bring a cooler along for the ride and put the fish in there as soon as I come out of the store.

Keeping fish cold in the refrigerator is easy. You can fill the vegetable bin or a baking dish with ice and bury the still-wrapped fish in there. Make sure fillets, especially, are well wrapped (whole fish can be unwrapped or wrapped), and drain and replenish the ice once or twice a day.

I find it easier and just as effective to sandwich the fish between two or three ice packs, of the kind used to ship cold foods. I keep a half dozen or so of these in my freezer all the time. When I bring home some fish, I lay a couple of ice packs on a platter, put the fish on top of them, and throw a couple more ice packs on top. The platter goes on the bottom shelf of the refrigerator, where it is coldest, and the ice packs are replaced with fresh ones from the freezer about once a day. Keep fish well wrapped when using this technique—a couple layers of paper towels are sufficient—because ice packs are cold enough to freeze the surface of fish if they come in direct contact with it.

It's literally impossible to say how long fish will retain its quality in your refrigerator; if it was caught yesterday, you can count on four days or even more. If it was caught last week, you only have a day or two. It's important, then, to buy fish as you're going to use it.

If fish is really fresh, you can freeze it. Act quickly, wrap it well in a couple layers of plastic wrap, and put it in the coldest place you can find; the bottom of a chest or upright freezer turned to its coldest gives pretty good results. Freezing a good piece of fish at home and eating it two weeks later is preferable to keeping it refrigerated for five or six days before you get around to cooking it, and certainly preferable to letting it sit in the refrigerator until it goes bad.

Substituting One Fish for Another

If you go to the market looking for a specific cut and type of finfish, you may be disappointed. Armed with these charts, however, and the more specific information under the listing for each fish, you will usually be able to find a suitable substitute. No substition is perfect—even haddock and cod have differences—but many recipes work equally well for a wide variety of fish.

SOME NOTES:
- Certain fish appear in more than one chart, because words such as "firm," "tender," "thick," "thin" are relative.
- Certain fish, such as salmon, do not appear at all, even though they broadly fit one or more of the descriptions; these fish are too unusual to substitute for, more often than not.
- Shellfish substitutions can be made, but not broadly; see the individual entries and recipes.
- Only fairly common fish are considered here.
- Try other substitutions as they seem fit to you; the whole point is that many fish have more similarities than differences.

Firm, Thick, White-fleshed Fillets
  (mild-flavored)
  Blackfish
  Carp
  Grouper
  Monkfish (usually suitable in recipes for other members of this group)
  Atlantic pollock
  Sablefish (usually suitable in recipes for other members of this group)
  Red snapper
  Striped bass
  Tilefish

Tender, Thick, White-fleshed Fillets
  (mild-flavored)
  Carp
  Cod
  Haddock
  Pacific pollock

Red snapper
Tilefish
Turbot
Weakfish
Whiting

Firm, Thin, White-fleshed Fillets
(mild-flavored)
Catfish
Dogfish
Monkfish (can be cut to be used in recipes for
 other members of this group)
Rockfish
Red snapper
Wolffish

Tender, Thin, White-fleshed Fillets
(mild-flavored)
Flatfish
Haddock
Ocean perch
Sea bass
Weakfish
Whiting

Light- to Dark-fleshed Fillets
(strongly flavored)
Bluefish
Mackerel
Mahi-mahi
Mako shark
Pompano
Striped bass
Tuna (small species are occasionally filleted)

Tender, White-fleshed Steaks
(mild-flavored)
Cod
Halibut
Tilefish
Turbot

Light- to Dark-fleshed Steaks
(strongly flavored)
Bluefish
Mackerel
Mahi-mahi
Mako shark
Sturgeon
Swordfish
Tuna

Small Whole Fish with Tender White Flesh
(medium-flavored)
Butterfish
Croaker
Porgy
Spot

Small to Medium Whole Fish with Firm White Flesh
(mild-flavored)
Rockfish
Sea bass
Red snapper

Medium to Large Whole Fish with Dark, Oily Flesh
(strongly flavored)
Bluefish
Mackerel
Pompano
Small tuna

Medium to Large Whole Fish with Firm White Flesh
(mild- to medium-flavored)
Blackfish
Grouper
Sea bass
Red snapper
Tilefish
Wolffish

IS FISH GOOD FOR YOU?

Fish phobia comes and goes. In the best of times—if you're a fishmonger—people believe that a serving of fish a day guarantees long life. In the worst of times, they believe that each serving shortens their life span by a measurable amount.

There is little question that fish is a healthy, sound part of an overall diet. But fish, and the waters in which they live, need to be safeguarded more vigorously than they have been in the past. After all, most fish are still wild, and their environment—the oceans, seas, rivers, and lakes of the world—has been severely compromised.

I have studied and written about both the health-giving properties and dangers of seafood for years, and I have no intention of covering either of these topics in detail here; this is a cookbook. You bought it because you wanted to know how to cook fish, not because you needed to be convinced to eat it or to be made wary of it.

Yet I feel obligated to include a certain amount of health and safety information, if only because few conversations about fish—or any other food, for that matter—are strictly limited to a culinary perspective anymore. It isn't just "Wasn't that sautéed swordfish with capers wonderful?" but "Wasn't it wonderful? Too bad swordfish has so much mercury." And the question, "Did you love that grilled tuna?" is likely to receive an answer such as, "Yes, and it was so high in Omega-3s!"

I like to think that I avoid oat-bran trendiness, but in fact I'm quick to jump on stories about fish health or safety, and I can't count the number of times I've stressed in recent articles that—regardless of everything else—fish is essentially low in fat, and lean white fish is lower in fat than any other source of animal protein. I'm glad fish is better for my health than red meat—this, at least, is fairly safe to assume, although there are some who will take issue with it—but I would continue to eat more fish than meat even if the situation were reversed. Fish offers more variety of flavor and texture; in addition, I can eat more of it, even late at night, without feeling uncomfortably stuffed.

But that's a personal prejudice, one I hope you will soon share with me, if you don't already. There are also the facts. These are, quite basically, two:

1. Fish can be a sound part of a basic diet.
2. Fish is not as pure as we would like it to be.

The fact that either of these statements could be made about vegetables and grains does not make them any more or less true.

Fish Is a Sound Part of a Basic Diet

Almost all fish is relatively low fat, but flatfish such flounder and sole, cod, haddock, and many shellfish (especially lobster, scallops, and clams) are especially so. Generally, these fish contain less than 1 percent fat, and only about 10 percent of that fat is saturated. Compare this to skinless white meat chicken, generally considered the paragon of low-fat animal protein, which contains about 1.25 percent fat, approximately a quarter of which is saturated. And most fish, including shellfish, are quite low in cholesterol.

Furthermore, as you are undoubtedly aware, some of the fat in fish appears to be health-promoting. Although Danish researchers first linked Eskimo diets high in fish oils to low rates of heart disease and cancer in the early 1970s, no one really began raving about the Omega-3 fatty acids in fish until about ten years later. Studies continue, and belief in the benefits of fish oil in the diet is not universal; nothing is simple in nutrition. Overall, however, there are strong indications that Omega-3 lowers blood levels of the "bad" low-density lipoproteins (LDL), which are believed to contribute to arterial plaque buildup, while leaving undisturbed and sometimes raising levels of the "good" high-density lipoproteins (HDL).

There is also some evidence that Omega-3s increase the efficacy of antipain medication given to sufferers of rheumatoid arthritis; aid in the treatment of ulcerative colitis and psoriasis; and retard the growth and development of tumors, at least in animals.

Generally speaking, fatty fish living in deep waters, such as tuna, mackerel, and salmon, are highest in Omega-3s. Bluefish, striped bass, smelt, and shark are also good sources, as are many shellfish, especially mussels, oysters, shrimp, and squid.

Minimizing Risks

Fish phobics had a field day when medical waste washed up on New England beaches in the summer of 1988; that year, fish consumption, which had been rising steadily for a decade, actually fell by a pound per capita. The furor died down for a couple of years, but almost everyone agrees that the quality of fish is less than ideal, and many people believe that the federal seafood inspection program could be much more thorough. (I can't resist pointing out that many people are finally acknowledging that our meat and poultry inspection system needs to be reformed as well.) Ideally, we need a comprehensive inspection program, one that monitors waters, vessels, processing facilities, trucks, and everything else, right down to the retail counter. And early in 1994 the FDA took steps to initiate such a program.

Even without that, though, there are far fewer reported illnesses associated with fish than with chicken. And when you exclude those bivalve mollusks which are commonly eaten raw—clams and oysters, primarily—fish is as safe to eat as any other animal protein.

Eating raw shellfish, though, involves a certain amount of daring. Although exact numbers are hard to come by, reliable estimates indicate that somewhere around one per thousand servings of raw shellfish causes illness, and, although the illness is almost inevitably a mild gastric disturbance, it doesn't feel mild while it's happening. Due to underreporting, the odds are probably even worse.

The first person to eat a raw oyster ran a risk from naturally occurring bacteria and, every year, the USDA makes stricter and stricter recommendations concerning the foods that can be eaten raw or even rare (soft-boiled eggs, for example, are to be avoided, according to the food police). Cooking kills bacteria; that's one of the reasons we do it. But let's remember that we eat not only to live but because it brings us great pleasure.

Shellfish filter the water in which they live through their gills to remove particulates, including bacteria and viruses. And that's fine, as long as those bacteria and viruses aren't pathogens. But when waters become contaminated by domestic sewage or contain harmful viruses, raw shellfish become dangerous. That's why shellfish beds are closed when bacteria levels rise; beaches are closed, too.

Unfortunately, this method of control is an imperfect one. Even if we never ate shellfish from contaminated beds, not all viruses can be tested for. Even depurated shellfish, which have been moved to clean beds to take advantage of the animals' ability to self-cleanse, may not be free of pathogens. And there's nothing to guarantee that our shellfish come from clean beds. Because shellfish are high-priced and scarce, poachers take and sell fish from closed beds, which, because they are closed, contain lots of fish. Those fish are sold to knowing or unknowing distributors and retailers in what is at best a difficult-to-police cash business.

What can be done to make eating raw shellfish safer? In much of Europe, shellfish is bought and sold by brand and grower name. Retailers specialize in certain brands, and consumers develop preferences. When producers put their name on their package, they can't afford to fool around.

It's difficult to know the actual risk from eating raw shellfish, because no one knows just how much of it is eaten, and not everyone who eats it and gets sick associates the illness with the fish. But the lion's share of illnesses related to raw shellfish are of the gastroenteritis sort, are often attributed to illegally harvested shellfish, and are almost never life-threatening. The national Seafood Sanitation Program, which licenses growers and harvesters of shellfish, routinely closes shellfish beds during peri-

ods of red tide and other naturally occurring toxins, and its record on marine toxins is very good. The bacterial danger is very real, however, and some people advise against eating raw shellfish in warmer months. Unless you're certain of the source, this isn't a bad idea. (I try to buy clams and oysters I intend to eat raw directly from the harvester during the summer, and avoid them in restaurants I don't know.)

I do not wish to belittle illness, but the vast majority of fish-related ailments are far from life-threatening, and affect very small numbers of people. According to FDA figures, shellfish-related deaths from the naturally occurring bacteria *Vibrio vulnificus* rarely reach double figures in a given year, and are usually fewer than half that; furthermore, these deaths are almost always among people with liver dysfunction. It's safe to say that anyone with a compromised immune system—alcoholics, people who are HIV positive, and the elderly—should shun raw shellfish. I wouldn't eat raw oysters if I were pregnant, or feed them to a young child, either.

If you listen to me, a devourer of raw shellfish, you'll hear that it's a personal decision; I don't bungee jump or ride a motorcycle, which I imagine are also fun. If you listen to a health professional, especially one who never liked raw oysters anyway, you'll hear that eating raw shellfish is about as dumb as crossing a busy street with a blindfold, playing Russian roulette, or, I guess, bungee jumping or riding a motorcycle.

What about raw finfish, such as that you eat in sushi or sashimi, and the acid-"cooked" fish dishes like seviche? Health officials say that, to be safe, fish eaten raw should be commercially frozen at -20°F or colder to protect against parasites such as round-worms and tapeworms. Most good Japanese restaurants do just that. Top-quality tuna destined for sushi bars is often sold frozen. This leads to some interesting twists: George Hoskin, a seafood expert at the FDA, walks into sushi bars and says "Has this fish been frozen?" If the answer is "No," he walks back out. Freezing will also kill off many potentially harmful bacteria, although the acidity of seviche preparations also seems to do a good job of that.

Since almost all seafood-related illnesses can be traced to raw fish or recontamination of cooked seafood, it makes sense to follow the same procedure in handling fish as you do in handling meat or poultry: Wash your hands, all surfaces, and all utensils that come in contact with raw fish before bringing them in contact with other food.

The USDA recommends that you cook fish "thoroughly," which—from a culinary perspective—is overdone. For best flavor, fish should be slightly underdone when it leaves the stove; it will finish cooking before it reaches the table.

There are also rarely occurring but real safety concerns associated with cooked fish, most notably ciguatoxin and scombrotoxin. Ciguatera, generated in algaelike organisms in tropical waters, works its way up the food chain in fish such as grouper, barracuda, and amberjack. It is concentrated in the tropics—according to my sources, there have been no reported occurrences of ciguatoxin involving Florida or Gulf Coast grouper—where there have been periods during which local authorities banned the sale of some of these fish. I'd recommend that travelers to the Caribbean avoid eating repeated servings of barracuda, amberjack, red snapper—again, only from tropical waters—and grouper, especially from large fish, which are more likely to have elevated levels. In all there are probably a couple hundred cases of ciguatera poisoning annually. The symptoms, which are similar to those of an intense flu, can be long-lasting and recurring.

Unfortunately, at the moment there is no quick way to detect ciguatera in fish, and, since it is a naturally occurring toxin, no way of cutting down on its presence in tropical fish. Scombrotoxin, however, is a direct result of time and temperature abuse; it develops when certain fish are left to sit at high temperatures for long periods, and theoretically could be eliminated by better handling. Scombrotoxin develops in scombroids and related fish; tuna, mackerel, bluefish, and mahi-mahi are the prime examples. There are perhaps a couple hundred cases of scombrotoxin poisoning each year, none of which is fatal. The poison is a histamine, and symptoms begin with tingling of lips and shortness of breath. Antihistamines effectively treat scombrotoxin poisoning.

To avoid scombrotoxin altogether, shun bad-smelling or bad-looking scombroids (or any other fish, for that matter; see Buying Fish, pages 5–12), and be wary about accepting scombroids from recreational fishermen whose icing habits are questionable. Any fishing boat with an inadequate ice or refrigeration supply can become a breeding ground for scombrotoxins, yet another argument in favor of national standards for and monitoring of all links of the seafood supply chain.

Finally there are environmental pollutants, such as polychlorinated biphenyl, or PCB, pesticides, dioxin, and heavy metals such as mercury. Many of these problems are spotty; PCBs, for example, are primarily a concern with bluefish and striped bass in the Northeast. But mercury remains a problem in tuna, swordfish, shark, and other long-lived fish. When bacteria digest mercury, which can be naturally occurring or an industrial pollutant, and in turn are eaten by plankton, which in turn make their way up the food chain, the result can be deposits in the flesh of fish. The FDA sets "action levels" for mercury and other pollutants, and theoretically prevents fish with high levels from reaching market. But the FDA's power is limited, and the levels it sets are the subject of debate. The agency, for example, has set an action level of one part per million for mercury in fish; Canada's level is half that. Regardless of the action level, however, those who fish for subsistence are the most likely to be affected by pollutants in fish: Most problems occur when people eat large amounts of the same fish from the same area, an almost impossible practice for those people who buy fish in a store.

Here are my basic recommendations about fish and safety; they are hardly carefree but less strict than those of some. Bear in mind that I am first and foremost a cook and food lover who enjoys raw fish and even—on occasion—raw meat (gasp).

- Know your source. The more you know about the fish you're eating, the better. This is especially true when eating raw shellfish.
- Consider avoiding raw shellfish in the summer months; for optimal safety, don't eat it at all.
- Eat a variety of seafood. The chances of your accumulating mercury in your system are virtually nil unless you eat the same tainted fish over and over. Don't eat shark, swordfish, or tuna regularly if you are pregnant or nursing.
- Freeze finfish at -20°F before eating it raw or making seviche.
- Avoid fish taken from tropical waters, especially large specimens of grouper, barracuda, jack, and red snapper. Do not eat the roe of these fish.
- Avoid dark-fleshed fish of questionable quality. When in doubt, move on to another fish.
- Support a more vigorous national program of seafood, beef, and poultry inspection (while you're at it, support efforts to promote sustainable agriculture).

PREPARING AND COOKING FISH

With increasing frequency, we buy our fish cut to order. If we want a fillet, we buy one; if we want a whole fish, scaled and gutted, we ask for that. But there are times when you may want to "butcher" a fish yourself; a friend may give you a just-caught fish, or the cleaning line at the store may be too long. Or, as I often do, you may buy a whole fish, uncleaned, figuring you'll decide what to do with it when you get home. Although it's difficult to do as good a job of filleting as someone who practices all day long, there is no aspect of fish cutting that you can't do adequately with some practice.

What follows here are general rules for most finfish. I discuss techniques for certain unique finfish, along with shellfish, which vary greatly from one genus to the next, in the individual entries.

Assuming you have a sharp eight- or ten-inch chef's knife, a paring knife, and a boning knife, the only tool you need for cutting up fish that you may not already have is a fillet knife. Like boning knives, fillet knives have narrow, extremely thin blades, six or eight inches long. But many fillet knives feature flexible blades, which give you a little more margin for error; it's easier to manipulate them once you're

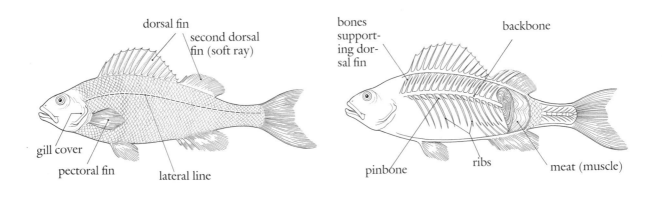

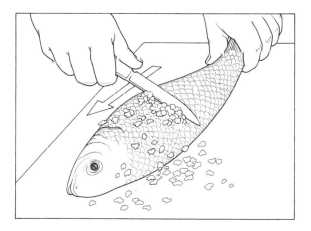

Scaling: To scale a fish, use a spoon or the back of a knife to scrape the scales off, moving in the direction of tail to head.

inside the fish. Rigid blades are better if you're filleting lots of big fish, such as a few six-pounders. I have a flexible-blade fillet knife and, when it isn't quite tough enough, I just put a good edge on my regular meat-boning knife and turn to that. You can actually fillet with anything as long as it's sharp and you're careful; many Asian chefs and fishmongers do beautiful work with thin cleavers.

Scaling

It's rare that a fish with scales doesn't need to be scaled before you cook it. (It isn't unheard of, though—see Pan-grilled Char on page 77.) Scaling is easy, but it can be messy; scales have a tendency to fly all over the place. If you're scaling a number of fish, you have a couple of alternatives: Move the operation outside, or put down a bunch of newspaper and be prepared to find scales in odd places for a couple of days.

If you only need to scale one or two fish, and they're not too big, put them, one at a time, in a clear plastic bag. Put the bag in the sink, and scale them by putting your hand, along with your scaler, into the bag. It's a bit awkward, but not difficult.

I scale with the back of a knife, but you can use a spoon or a fish scaler. Wet the fish—some people scale under a stream of running water—and grip the fish as best you can; the tail is best for most fish, although there are times you'll want to hold the head. If the fish is very slippery, sprinkle it with salt, wear a rough-surfaced glove, or hold it with a kitchen towel. Begin scraping up from the tail toward the head (see illustration), with short, authoritative strokes. Scale the whole fish, including the belly and the back. Within minutes, you'll be an expert.

Gutting

Messy but simple. With a sharp, small knife, cut a slit from the fish's anal opening, usually called the "vent," to the gill openings (you might call this the neck). If there are roe, you can remove these carefully and cook them with the fish, separately, or in a sauce. Pull out the guts with your fingers, then

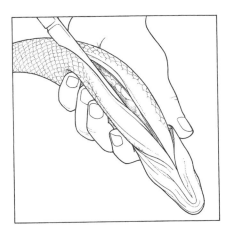

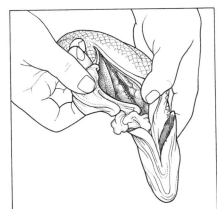

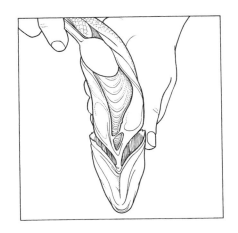

Gutting: Slit the fish from the jaw to the vent, open it up, and remove all the internal organs. Remove the kidneys by scraping against the backbone with a spoon.

scrape out the red kidneys that remain attached to the backbone. Use a spoon or dull knife to scrape out any viscera that remain, then rinse the fish. Discard the guts—they are not good in stock.

Gilling

Gills are bitter-tasting, and must be removed from any fish that will be served whole, or from any head to be used in stock. To do so, lift the gill covers and cut the gills out with a knife or scissors. Discard them.

Beheading and Removing the Tail

Reasons *not* to remove the head and tail:
- The head contains delicious meat (especially the cheeks).
- Assuming the eaters are not squeamish, whole fish makes a wonderful presentation.
- They give you something to hold on to if you intend to fillet the fish.
- The more intact the fish, the easier it is to turn, and the more difficult to overcook.

Reasons *to* remove the head and tail:
- The head is great for stock (once you remove the gills).
- The fish won't fit in your cooking pot unless you do.
- You will be serving the fish to a squeamish eater.

To behead a fish, use a fairly heavy knife to cut right behind the gill covers. If the backbone is thick, it might be easier to make the initial cut, then bend the fish sideways to break the backbone before cutting all the way through. To remove the tail, simply cut it off where it meets the body. Both head and tail should be reserved for stock.

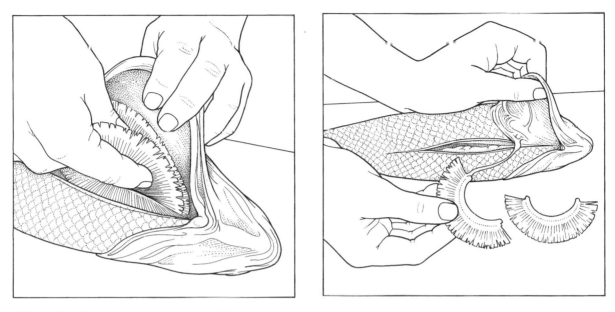

Gilling: The gills can be sharp, so be careful. Use a knife or scissors to detach them, then remove with your fingers.

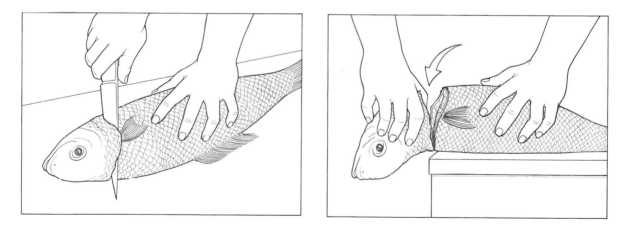

Beheading: Make a cut on either side of the fish's head just ahead of the pectoral fin. Holding the fish on the table and snapping down on the head can make removal easier if you cannot cut through the bone.

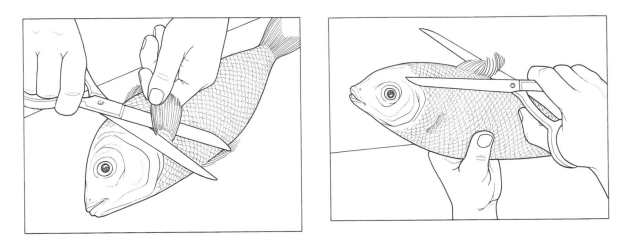

Removing fins: The easiest way to remove the fins is with a sharp, heavy scissors.

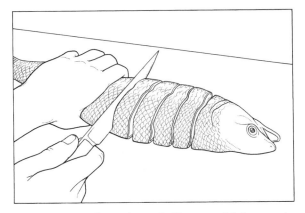

Steaking: Use a large, heavy knife to cut fish into steaks. If the backbone gives you trouble, rest the knife on the bone and hit the back of the kife with a wooden or rubber mallet.

Removing the Fins

Fins may be cut off with a scissors, which is the common and quick way to accomplish the job. And it's the way most fishmongers and home cooks do it. The most particular chefs, however, use another technique, which is marginally more effective and somewhat more time-consuming; you might try it on the dorsal (top) fin. Using a boning or paring knife, make a cut into the fish about ⅛ inch long on each side of the fin, on an angle, so that you form a "V," with the fin in the middle. Pull out the fin, along with the bones that attach it to the fish, using your hands (you may need a towel to get a good grip) or a pair of pliers. Fins should be reserved for the stockpot.

Cutting Steaks

You can cut steaks from almost any fish that weighs three pounds or more, although the technique is usually reserved for larger fish—say, six-pounders and up.

Start by scaling and gutting the fish; remove its head and fins. Using a sharp, heavy knife or cleaver, cut through the fish to make steaks of the desired thickness, usually about an inch or so. If the central bone gives you trouble, rest the knife against it and whack the back of the knife with a wooden or rubber mallet.

Try to make the cuts even and clean. Always leave the skin on steaks for cooking, even if it is inedible; it helps hold the steak together during cooking. If you like, you may trim off uneven belly flaps for a nicer presentation. Save the head, tail, fins, and all scraps for stock.

Filleting

In the hands of a skilled knife-wielder, filleting is an art. For most of us, however, it's an occasional chore. But common "roundfish"—the vast majority of finfish—have an uncomplicated bone structure, illustrated on page 24, and can be filleted with a good degree of success, even on the first try. If you want to really learn filleting skills, buy a dozen mackerel the next time they're cheap; they are the easiest fish to fillet, but are representative of many other species.

To begin, scale the fish if you will not be skinning it. Then remove its fins with a scissors, just to get them out of the way; gutting is unnecessary (if the guts were removed before you bought the fish, that's fine, too). Lay the fish on its side and make a top-to-bottom cut behind the gill cover. With the back of the fish facing you, make a long cut along the back from gill cover to tail, following the line of the central bone; lift the flesh as you cut to reveal the central bone and make the job easier. Turn the fish so that the belly is facing you and, again, make a long cut from gill to tail; the tip of the knife should meet the first cut at the backbone, and the fillet will be released.

The thin belly flap may contain a row of bones. Use your fillet knife to cut underneath and remove them. Alternatively, remove the belly flap entirely and use it for stock.

In addition, there may be a row of bones ("pin bones") running down the center of the fillet. You have three alternatives for dealing with these:

1. Ignore them until the fish is cooked, then pull them out before serving or at the table.
2. Remove them with a needlenose or similar pliers.
3. Remove them by cutting a "zip-strip," making a V-shaped cut on either side of the bones and pulling out the V with your fingers. Use this for stock.

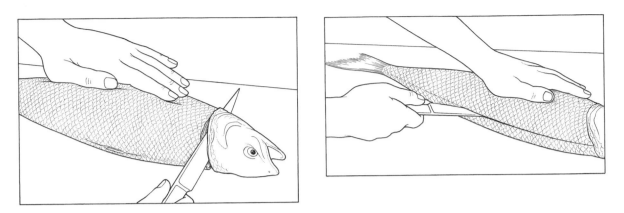

1. Filleting a roundfish: Remove the fins. Make a cut from the top to the bottom of the fish behind the gill cover.

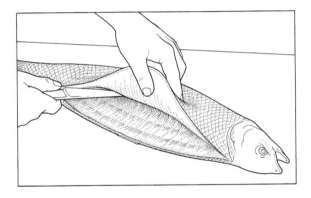

2. Cut on one side of the backbone right into the fish. Feel with the blade of the knife for the central bone and keep the knife right on top of it as you move down the length of the fish.

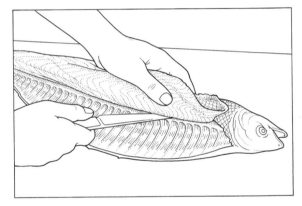

3. Peel back the meat so you can see the ribs beneath the backbone, keeping the knife on top of them. Turn the fish over and repeat the technique on the other side.

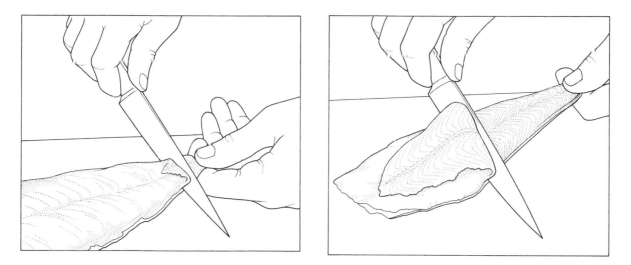

Skinning fillets: Make a small cut at the narrow end of the fillet and grab the skin. Use a sharp knife, held parallel to the skin, to run between the skin and flesh.

Skinning

Skinning is much easier than it looks, although I urge you to leave the skin on your fillets in most cases. Even when the skin is inedible or not appetizing—I note whether this is the case in the individual entries—it helps hold fillets together during cooking (it isn't needed in really tough fish like grouper and blackfish). And bear in mind that skin—even skin with scales left on—can be removed from most cooked fish with a minimum of effort.

To skin fillets, make a small cut just above the tail end—through the meat but not through the skin—as shown. Then, holding on to the small flap of skin, work your fillet knife up through the fillet, holding it at a slight angle to the cutting surface and cutting as close to the skin as possible. This, too, is easier than it sounds.

COOKING WITH DRY HEAT: GRILLING, BROILING, ROASTING, AND SMOKING FISH

Because it is intrinsically moist, fish takes extremely well to all methods of dry cooking. That is, as long as it is not overcooked. It's all too easy to remove all the moisture from fish when you cook it without liquid; avoid this single pitfall, and your dry cooking will be successful.

Grilling

Grilling is the most challenging method of fish cooking to master, but thanks to its bold flavor and uncomplicated preparation, grilled fish has universal appeal. You add little or even no fat to grilled fish, and you avoid turning the summer kitchen into an inferno. Yet when the fish sticks to the grill and makes a mess, or half of it falls through the grates, or it winds up dry and tough, you might wonder if it's worth it.

The first thing to learn is that certain fish—fillets of flatfish such as flounder and sole and many skinless fillets—should almost never be grilled. Even these, however, can be broiled without any trouble, with similarly satisfying results; see below.

But you can grill many fillets, especially those with skin, which helps the flesh maintain its shape and integrity and protects it from burning and drying out. Some fillets, such as those of monkfish and grouper, can be grilled without their skin. These tough fillets, along with steaks of swordfish, tuna, and other meaty fish, are the best to grill; they won't fall apart and stick to the grill any more than a chicken breast.

Keeping more tender fillets, steaks, and whole fish from sticking is more challenging. The common wisdom, repeated in many cookbooks and countless magazine articles, includes these steps:

1. Don't build a super hot fire; if, when you're ready to cook, you can't hold your hand above the grate for two or three seconds, let the fire cool down a bit. Gas grills should be preheated at the highest setting for at least ten minutes; it's difficult if not impossible to get most of these too hot.
2. Clean grill racks are important: Set the grill rack on the grill as it heats, then use a wire brush to scrape off any debris from your last grilling session.
3. Oil the fish lightly if you did not use an oil-based marinade. Too much oil will cause an instant flare-up, so be careful.
4. Place the fish on the grill (skin side down, if you have the option) and let it sit (in most cases) for at least two minutes before turning. This allows the fish to build up a firm crust, which helps it release from the grill rack.

All of this makes sense and, generally speaking, works. But try grilling a whole flounder or red snapper or a haddock fillet, and you will get some sticking no matter what you do.

Which brings us to the fish basket, a piece of equipment that is essential if you want to grill fish frequently. The best baskets are made of tough nonstick or at least stick-resistant material, have long, removable handles that make turning a breeze, and are adjustable, allowing them to hold the fish tightly. Even if you overcook your fish to the point of flaking, the basket will keep it from falling apart; it will, of course, fall apart when you remove it from the basket, but at least that will be onto a plate.

If you keep grilling times short and remove the fish from the grill before it overcooks, you'll have less trouble with sticking. Checking for doneness on the grill is simple—just take a thin-bladed knife and peek into the thickest part of the meat. Use a flashlight if you need one to get a sense of that internal color.

Doneness is a matter of taste, but to me fish is finished cooking just before the center loses its raw look (the heat of the surrounding flesh will take care of that last bit of cooking on the way to the table). If you cook fish until it is completely opaque throughout, especially on the grill, you run the risk of eating dry fish. If you remove the fish just when that last bit of translucence disappears, however, you'll be in good shape. Some fish—salmon, tuna, and scallops, for example—are best when fairly rare; again, however, this is a matter of taste.

Regardless of how done you like your fish, though, my point is this: Eventually, you will learn to judge doneness by a combination of touch and sixth sense; cook fish three times a week for a month and you'll see. In the meantime, it's best to take a look inside. Don't worry about releasing any precious moisture; your fish will be fine. You can also use an instant-read thermometer if you like— somewhere between 120° and 130°F is about right—but I don't find them reliable enough, especially for fillets.

Believe me: You will develop timing with experience. If you figure six to ten minutes per inch of thickness when grilling, you're on the right track, as long as you remember that a one-inch-thick scallop cooks much more quickly than a one-inch-thick swordfish steak, and that other such exceptions to the rule are quite common. In practice, turn one-inch-thick steaks after three or four minutes and check them after seven or eight. Whole fish should not be turned too often, and are best cooked on a covered grill to speed things along. Unless you are both skilled and practiced, a three-inch-thick, six-pound striped bass is going to drive you nuts. Take it to the oven or broiler, where you have more control.

There remains the question of marinades. Marinating fish is not a bad idea; it is just one that has been overplayed. Most fish have extremely subtle flavors, and grilling alone overwhelms many of them. A six-hour soak in a strong bath of garlic, lemon juice, and cayenne will produce a good-tasting monkfish fillet, but it will be virtually indistinguishable in flavor from a similarly marinated chicken breast. In general, I prefer mild marinades and short marinating times. To me, the best fish is fresh, perfectly grilled, sprinkled with salt, and drizzled with lemon. More exotic recipes should accent rather than smother the fish's intrinsic flavors.

In sum, most fish takes well to grilling, but each type requires slightly different handling. Here are some general guidelines.

SHELLFISH
Bivalve mollusks such as hard-shell clams, mussels, and oysters can be grilled in the shell or shucked and skewered. To grill them whole, scrub the shells well and place them directly on the grate above a hot fire; use the grill cover if there is one. The shells will pop open when cooked, usually in five to ten minutes. Discard any that don't open; for a more detailed recipe, see Grilled Mixed Mollusks, page 82.

Stick to large scallops for grilling. They can be skewered, as for Grilled Scallops and Shrimp on page 245, or grilled as if they were medallions of meat or fish. As in all scallop preparations, be especially careful not to overcook.

Other shellfish, such as shrimp, lobster, squid, and crab, can take a very hot fire and are easy to grill, but may take some preparation. Only shrimp are foolproof: Grill them in or out of their shells, and plan on less than five minutes total cooking time.

Whole lobster *can* be grilled; see the illustrations on pages 152–153 for preparing a lobster for grilling. But unless your grill is enormous, it is difficult to cook more than two or three at a time; consider grilling tails and claws only, saving the bodies for stock or bisque.

Blue crabs are best boiled, but grilled soft-shell crabs are incomparable. They're fast, too; just a couple of minutes per side does the trick.

STEAKS
Some steaks—such as those of cod—start to disintegrate almost the moment they are done. This doesn't mean you shouldn't grill cod steaks, but it does mean you should consider a basket and be extremely attentive.

On the other hand, steaks of tuna, swordfish, salmon, grouper, and other firm-fleshed fish hold up well to direct heat. Leave the skin on if possible, even if it is inedible, as it is on tuna, mako, swordfish, and many others; you can always take it off at the table. If you are in doubt about the ability of a given steak to maintain its shape during grilling, use a grilling basket; it's saved my dinner many times.

You can cut kebabs from steaks of muscular fish such as tuna, swordfish, salmon, monkfish, grouper, rockfish, shrimp, or scallops. If at all possible, include some skin on each chunk to help it stay together, and make the chunks large—two-inch cubes are fine—so they do not overcook. Baskets are helpful, or use skewers; two per kebab make turning easier. My favorite way to grill kebabs is to skewer them, then put the skewers in a basket. This allows you to turn the whole mess at once and still serve on the skewers.

FILLETS

With few exceptions, grilled fillets have little chance of holding together without the aid of a fish basket. Generally, do not attempt to grill skinless fillets. You can grill fillets of oily fish, such as salmon and mackerel, with little adornment. Their skin and melting fat provide protection and lubrication. But when attempting to grill white-fleshed fillets, you need additional protection. See, for example, Grilled Haddock "Sandwich" with Pickled Onions, page 140.

WHOLE FISH

The trick to grilling whole fish is to pick the right fish to begin with; the best are red snapper, pompano, small bluefish, rockfish, mackerel, salmon, and sea bass, in the one- to three-pound range; tackle larger fish as you gain experience. Because you have the skin, skeleton, and head to provide stability, it's not as hard as you might think. Oil the skin before grilling and let the fish grill for at least five minutes before you try turning it (use two spatulas to do this). Don't be upset if the skin falls off; although fish with skin is more attractive, and although the skin of many fish is delicious, the main purpose of the skin in grilling is to protect the flesh and keep it moist.

Broiling

There are four basic differences between broiling and grilling:

1. The position of the heat source: In grilling it is usually below, in broiling above.
2. The fuel for the heat source: In grilling it may be wood, charcoal briquets, or gas; in broiling it is either gas or electricity.

3. The flavor, determined primarily by the fuel and what is placed on top of it: Wood-grilled food has a distinctive and almost universally enjoyed flavor. All other fuels have either a neutral or (in the case of some briquets) slightly negative impact on flavor. Gas grills and briquets can be helped along by the addition of herbs or wood chips during grilling.
4. The location of your broiler and grill: The first inside, the second outside. This inclines us to associate broiling with winter rather than summer; remember, however, that most fish can be broiled in ten minutes, so the accumulated heat is rarely unbearable except on the hottest days.

Broiling is also less fussy than grilling, and, because it is usually easier to adjust the distance from the heat source to the food, it gives you greater control. You can broil thin fillets just two inches from the heat source, allowing them to brown before they overcook. Whole fish can be moved six inches or more from the broiling element, so that the interior cooks through before the skin burns, which is difficult to accomplish on a grill, especially with large fish. Finally, you can broil in a nonstick pan or on a nonstick cookie sheet, so there are fewer problems with sticking. You can even broil a flounder fillet, whereas you might as well throw it directly in the trash as try to grill it.

In general, when you broil, you need not bother to turn the fish; the ambient temperature is high enough so that the bottom and interior cook as the top browns. I turn only the thickest fillets and steaks and, of course, whole fish.

Broiling produces some of the purest and most wonderful fish dishes. If you have a really fresh whole flounder, a nice piece of swordfish or tuna, or a plain white fillet, just brush it with olive oil, melted butter, or a bit of soy sauce before broiling. Figure about eight minutes per inch of thickness, which means that a thin fillet will be done in three or four minutes, a thick steak in about ten to twelve. Check for doneness, as always, by peeking inside of the fish, using a thin-bladed knife; generally, when just a touch of translucence remains, the fish is done—it will finish cooking on the way to the table. A squeeze of lemon and you're done.

Guidelines for Broiling Specific Fish

SHELLFISH

I usually broil bivalves, such as hard-shell clams, mussels, and oysters, on the half shell and extremely quickly. This is a risky procedure, because they can overcook and toughen in an instant. Skewered mollusks also broil well, especially if there is other food on the skewer to temper the heat. If you want to cook mollusks in the oven, leave them whole and roast them until they pop open.

The major exception is scallops, which are wonderful when broiled; see Grilled or Broiled Scallops and Shrimp on page 245 for a basic recipe. Scallops can also be skewered before broiling.

Other shellfish, such as shrimp, lobster, and crab, can be broiled as easily as they can be grilled. Get them close to the heat source and try to brown them as they cook.

STEAKS

Swordfish, tuna, and other firm steaks are as good in the broiler as on the grill; steaks of tender fish, such as cod, can be broiled with far greater success than they can be grilled. As in grilling, leave the skin on if possible. Only steaks thicker than an inch or so need to be turned during broiling.

To broil kebabs, skewer them and lay them in a baking pan or on a broiling pan. As in grilling, try to include some skin on each chunk to help them stay together, and make the chunks large—two-inch cubes are fine—so they do not overcook. You can also broil chunks of fish without skewering, of course.

FILLETS

The broiler also does a great job with fillets. Broil thin fillets close to the heat and thicker ones farther away; the goal is to achieve a nicely browned top simultaneously with a cooked interior. Broil fillets of oily fish, such as salmon and mackerel, with little or no fat; white-fleshed fillets benefit from the addition of butter or oil. It's rare that a fillet needs to be turned during broiling; generally, if the top is browning too fast, it's easier to turn down the oven temperature and finish the cooking by roasting than it is to turn the fillet.

WHOLE FISH

Before broiling whole fish, make three or four vertical slashes on each side of the fish to allow both heat and flavorings to penetrate to the interior. Broil the fish far enough from the heat source so that the skin does not burn before the interior cooks; the gashes help you tell at a glance how fast the cooking is proceeding. Turn the fish only once. You can broil on a rack, although I like to use a nonstick baking pan; there's no harm in letting the fish sit in its juices.

Roasting

Quite simply, roasting is the ideal way to cook whole fish. The high, even heat crisps up the skin without much danger of burning while it cooks the interior relatively slowly, helping you avoid overcooking. As in broiling, cut a few vertical gashes on each side of the fish before you begin. Roast at high heat, 450°F or more, and baste the fish with liquid and/or fat as it roasts. Fish is usually roasted with herbs and aromatic vegetables.

You can roast any bivalve mollusks, dry, until they pop open. Generally, steaming is the better technique, because it retains the juices of the shellfish better. Once again, the exception is the scallop, which roasts beautifully, with or without a touch of liquid (see Roasted Sea Scallops Galician Style, page 246).

There isn't much reason to roast other shellfish, however. If you want them unadorned—or scantily seasoned—use the broiler or the grill. For more complicated dishes, you're better off braising or sautéing. Steaks and fillets are also better when broiled or cooked with liquid than roasted.

Hot-smoking

Smoking fish is only slightly more time-consuming than grilling it, and not much more complicated. You can use a charcoal or gas grill, or even the stovetop; smoking requires no special equipment. The gas grill, with its good control, steady, no-fuss heat source, and outdoor location—after all, smoking is smoky—is the ideal appliance.

I'm not talking here about the long, slow process of cold-smoking, in which food is brined for hours or even days before being placed in a chamber into which cool smoke is pumped from a remote location. That venerable process, which preserves foods (not just fish, but bacon, corned beef, and dozens of other favorites) through the combined action of salt and smoke, is too much hassle for most home cooks.

Hot-smoking, however, is quite another matter, well within the reach of anyone who has good fish, salt, and sugar. The most basic technique (see page 31) requires little more than a quick rub with a mixture of salt and sugar, a wait of thirty minutes or so, and a fifteen- to thirty-minute period on a grill next to—not over—a source of low heat covered with wood chips. It can also be done in an improvised stovetop smoker. The result is moist seafood with a mild, smoky flavor that seems to appeal to everyone, even fish-resistant children.

Start with a firm, flavorful fillet or steak, such as salmon, swordfish, sturgeon, blackfish, sablefish, bluefish, or mackerel, or with shrimp or other shellfish. Sprinkle the fish with equal parts salt and sugar and let it stand for thirty to sixty minutes; refrigerate it only if the room is very warm. This dry brine not only flavors the fish, but allows it to form a pellicle, the characteristic thin, shiny layer found on most smoked foods.

Turning your grill into a smoker is the work of a moment. If you have a covered charcoal grill, remove the racks and build a small pyramid of briquets on the bottom. When the coals are hot, move them to one side, top them with soaked wood chips or some twigs of any hardwood, place the fish on the opposite side, and cover the grill.

Gas grills are even easier: Remove the top rack and light only one burner, and that as low as possible. Immediately place soaked wood chips over that burner, either on the lava rocks or the heat plate. Replace the rack and you're ready to go.

If your stove or kitchen has a good exhaust fan, you can smoke fish on top of the stove. Place soaked wood chips on the bottom of an old pot (or use a good one, lined with heavy-duty aluminum foil). Put the fish on a rack on top of the chips, cover the pot, and turn the heat to medium; when it begins to smoke, reduce the heat to low and smoke until done, usually no more than twenty minutes or so.

All of these methods cook the fish as it smokes. And although it takes longer than direct grilling or broiling, almost all fillets and shellfish are fully cooked in fifteen to thirty minutes. (Unless you are using a gas grill, it's difficult to smoke anything more than an inch or so thick without adding more coals.) When it is done, the fish will have a characteristic sheen—that's the pellicle—and be firm to the touch. If you're in doubt, use a thin-bladed knife to cut into the thickest part of the fish; it should be opaque throughout, or nearly so.

Be aware that this brief salting and smoking does not extend the shelf life of seafood. Treat fish cooked this way as you would any cooked food, and consume it within a couple of days.

Here is a basic recipe for smoking fish; see the index for variations.

BASIC SMOKED FISH

Makes 4 to 8 servings
Time: 90 minutes

2 salmon, sturgeon, or any other firm finfish fillets, 2 pounds medium or large peeled shrimp, or 2 pounds sea scallops
¼ cup coarse salt
¼ cup sugar
2 handfuls hardwood chips (about 1 ½ cups)

Mix together the salt and sugar and sprinkle the fish on both sides. Let sit for at least 30 minutes but for no more than 60; refrigerate if the room is very warm. Meanwhile, soak the wood chips in water to cover.

If you are using a charcoal grill, remove the racks and build a small fire. When the coals are hot, move them to one side, top with the chips, and replace the racks. Drain the fish of its accumulated liquid, brush off any of the rub that has not dissolved, and place the fish on a sheet of aluminum foil. Put the foil on the side of the grill away from the coals. Poke some holes in the foil and cover the grill, closing all the vents but one. Check the fish for doneness after 15 minutes.

If you are using a gas grill, remove the racks, turn the heat of one burner to low, and top the lava rocks or heat plate over that burner with the soaked chips. Replace the rack. Place the fish on a sheet of aluminum foil; put the foil on the side of the grill away from the lit burner. Poke some holes in the foil and cover the grill. Check the fish for

doneness after 25 minutes; it should be firm, with a shiny crust, and opaque but not dry inside.

See above for instructions for smoking on top of your stove.

COOKING WITH FAT: SAUTÉING, STIR-FRYING, AND DEEP-FRYING FISH

Cooking in fat gives fish a delicious, crisp crust and, because the heat is high and the cooking medium in direct contact with the food, it is incomparably fast. In addition, sautéing—and its cousin, stir-frying—is quite easy, once you know a few basic rules.

Deep-frying is also easy, but the cleanup can be quite a hassle. And all of these methods add fat and, of course, calories, something you may or may not be concerned about.

Sautéing is among the most useful methods for cooking fish and many other foods. And it has become considerably easier in the recent past, thanks to the constant improvement of nonstick skillets. In fact, the first rule of sautéing fish is: Go Buy a Nonstick Skillet. I use inexpensive cast-aluminum, coated with Silverstone 2, or whatever the latest development happens to be, but I don't think it matters especially what material the skillet itself is made of. What is important is the coating and the size. You will need a twelve-inch nonstick skillet, and it helps to have a ten-inch one around also, for smaller portions.

Now that you need not worry about sticking, you can usually measure fat in teaspoons and tablespoons, rather than in cups, using only the amount you need to crisp up the food, give it a nice color, and improve its flavor. Sometimes it's still desirable to use a half cup fat in a recipe to duplicate the wonderful crust that results from what you might call pan-frying—sautéing in a good amount of fat. But other times you can use a teaspoon of butter or oil, just to add its flavor to the fish. In fact, nonstick skillets work so well now that you can actually dry sauté, that is, cook with no fat at all. But because of the irregular surface of fish and most other foods, sautéing without fat is, in effect, "steam-grilling"— the parts that touch the surface of the pan cook with dry heat, and that above steams in the moisture released by the fish. The result is a hybrid that serves little purpose; you tend to get some spots that are scorched and others that are a little mushy. If you want to cook without fat, try steaming, broiling, or grilling.

The other key to sautéing fish—or anything else, for that matter—is to get the skillet good and hot before adding anything to it. In restaurants, many chefs preheat the sauté pan before the first use of the evening, after which there is little chance that the skillet will cool off in the heat of service. I recommend you do the same thing; when you begin to prepare your meal, put your skillet on the stove over low heat and let it sit there for a while. Or, four or five minutes before you are ready to begin sautéing, preheat the pan over medium to high heat, depending on the power of your burner. Only just before sautéing should you add the fat, then wait a minute or so, during which you can begin dredging the fish in flour or other coating. When the fat is hot—oil will shimmer, butter foam will subside, and a pinch of flour will sizzle in either—you can add the fish.

On most home stoves, this should be done rather slowly, because our burners are not powerful enough to maintain a steady high heat in a skillet. If the temperature plummets too quickly, the fish will not brown properly. So, just after adding the first piece of fish, I like to turn the heat up to full blast as I add the other pieces. The idea is to regulate the heat so that the fat is sizzling nicely but not burning.

Most fish sauté so quickly that as soon as one side is nicely browned, you can turn the fish, brown the other side, and be assured that the fish is done. If you like, you can check by peeking into the interior, using a thin-bladed knife. With thick steaks or fish thicker than an inch or so, you may have to lower the heat at some point to prevent burning the outside while the inside continues to cook.

You need not use any coating whatsoever when you sauté fish. But if you like some crunch—most of us do—dredge the fish in flour, cornmeal, or bread crumbs just before sautéing it. If you want to flavor the coating, do so, adding a good amount of ground black or cayenne pepper, curry, chili, or five-spice powder, dried herbs, or whatever you like. If you want to coat the fish in batter, you can do that, too, although I do not. If the fish has edible skin, leave it on for extra crispness and flavor; if not, of course, it should be removed.

After sautéing, you may want to make a pan reduction. (The one drawback of nonstick pans is that there are no "little brown bits"—pieces of browned coating and fish—to stir into the reduction. This is unfortunate, but I don't know anyone, including professional chefs, who has gone back to traditional skillets after trying the nonstick variety.) This is the simplest method of sauce-making there is: After removing the fish, just add some liquid—stock, wine, or a combination is usually best, but water is perfectly acceptable—to the skillet. When that has cooked down a bit to a saucelike consistency, add seasonings such as herbs, spices, and/or aromatics. The texture of the sauce can be enhanced by the addition of a bit of butter or oil at the last moment, but this isn't necessary. Usually, you're just looking for a bit of a flavor kick and some moisture; sauces containing substantial amounts of butter or cream often overwhelm fish.

A NOTE ABOUT STIR-FRYING
Stir-frying is very similar to sautéing. The differences:

- Stir-fried food is usually cut up before cooking; preparation time, therefore, is a bit longer, and cooking time a bit shorter.
- Stir-fried food is only rarely coated, and is therefore not quite so crisp as sautéed.
- Stir-fried food tends to be seasoned with Asian spices rather than European ones. This tradition need not be followed in your kitchen.
- Similarly, stir-fries are usually made in a wok. But you can use a skillet if you prefer, with no difference in results.

As in sautéing, it is critically important to maintain a hot surface during stir-frying. Preheat that wok or skillet almost to the smoking point before you begin. Because stir-fries usually contain vegetables in addition to fish, consistently high heat is the norm to prevent temperature loss and subsequent steaming. My colleague and friend Pam Anderson stir-fries in small batches so that each morsel of food is subject to equally intense heat. This works well, but it defeats one of the purposes of stir-frying, which is to prepare a good-tasting fish-and-vegetable dish in one pot in very little time.

Generally speaking, it's difficult if not impossible to stir-fry delicate fish. Cut into small pieces, they cook incredibly quickly, and begin to degenerate into tiny flakes almost before you can do anything about it. My advice is to reserve stir-frying for any kind of shellfish or chunks of firm, meaty fish.

Sautéing and stir-frying produce wonderful fish dishes. Here are some general guidelines for specific types of fish.

SHELLFISH

Bivalve mollusks such as hard-shell clams, mussels, and oysters are not often sautéed, mostly because it's easier to steam them open and add desired flavors in the form of a reduced steaming liquid or sauce. But there are exceptions. Whole hard-shell clams and mussels are wonderful when sautéed until they open; see Sautéed Clams with Pasta on page 80, for example, for the best and easiest pasta with clams you've ever made. And scallops are among the best fish to sauté; see pages 247–248 for a slew of sautéed scallop recipes. In addition, all of these are great in stir-fries.

Other shellfish, especially shrimp and soft-shell crab, are also great candidates for sautéing. Lobster and hard-shell crab can also be sautéed in the shell; it's best to crack the shells a bit first to speed cooking and make eating easier.

STEAKS

Because they are so wonderful grilled or broiled, steaks are not sautéed as often as they might be. But delicate steaks, such as those of halibut or cod, are perfect for the stovetop, and sautéing swordfish or even tuna is far from a waste of time and effort; see, for example, Spice-crusted Pan-fried Tuna, page 334. Sautéing often gives you results that are somewhat moister than when you grill or broil the same fish. Firm steaks are also perfect for cutting into chunks and stir-frying.

FILLETS

The most commonly sautéed fish are fillets which, as noted above, are generally too delicate to cut up and stir-fry. Dredged in flour, cornmeal, bread crumbs, or something more complicated, this is the beginning of a meal that can take less than twenty minutes to prepare. By varying the coating, fish, and reduction sauces, you could sauté fish every night of the year without repeating yourself. Master this technique and you'll never be at a loss with a fish fillet.

WHOLE FISH

You can sauté whole fish as long as it fits in your skillet. If the fish is just a bit too large, you might cut off the head and/or tail. I'm usually reluctant to do this, because I like to present whole fish, and I also like to pick at the meat on the head, so I prefer roasting or broiling when I can't fit the whole fish in the pan.

Fish that are best for sautéing whole are called panfish, and include small individuals of usually larger fish—mackerel, salmon, bluefish, flounder, red snapper, and so on—as well as those fish that rarely exceed a pound or so in size, such as croaker, spot, and porgy. All should be sautéed with care so that the interior cooks before the skin or crust burns. With most, the color of the body cavity gives a good indication that the fish is done; when redness disappears, stop cooking. But to be sure, use a thin-bladed knife to cut down to the central bone; the fish should be nearly opaque.

Deep-frying

I love deep-fried fish, but I'm tempted to tell people not to try deep-frying at home. It has challenges and pitfalls galore and, even if you conquer the one and avoid the other, the results may be disappointing compared to fried fish you've had in restaurants.

Why? To start with, the sheer quantity of oil needed to do a good job of deep-frying a pound of food is more than most home kitchens can handle. (And do you really want a couple gallons of boiling hot fat in your kitchen?) Maintaining the proper temperature of that oil is tricky unless your fryer is equipped with a thermostat. And the spattering factor, which is very real, means that you'll be cleaning up much longer than it took you to eat the delicious tidbits you created. Not to mention the smell.

If you're not convinced, I don't blame you. Frying fish at home allows you to start with perfect fish, make the coating you like best, and cook it in top-quality oil. That's exactly what the best restaurants do, but it's not the treatment you can count on at the "clam shacks" or the giant restaurant chains of the world, where the oil and fish may be past their prime or weren't that good to begin with.

If you do decide to tackle fried fish at home, I have only one ironclad rule: Keep the quantities small. If you're not too ambitious, you can fry a meal of fish for two or an appetizer for four or even eight without much trouble. But if you try to deep-fry the kind of monstrous "fisherman's platter" you see in so many restaurants, you'll be disappointed.

You can deep-fry almost anything, including whole fish if they're small enough, clams or mussels on the half shell, and chunks of lobster. But shucked mollusks, shrimp, and small fillets are your best bet, because they cook in about the same amount of time it takes to brown them. The result, when things go well, is crisp, light fish that is tender and moist, and which retains its original flavor.

There's no point in frying fish without some kind of coating; the whole idea is to crisp up the outside, and the outside of fish is far too moist to become crisp on its own. Many different coatings work well; the standards are a light or heavy dusting of flour or cornmeal, which can be flavored with herbs and/or spices; a light batter made of flour and water; or a heavier batter thick enough to produce waffles or even fritters. I prefer dry coatings or light, tempuralike batters of flour and water; in my view, heavy batters completely overwhelm fish. When I use flour, I sometimes add a bit of baking soda to the mixture, which helps the flour brown.

Because most fish contains a great deal of moisture, it spatters when it is placed in hot oil; squid is notorious for being the most troublesome. This makes it important to get the surface of the fish as dry as possible before frying; batters also reduce spattering somewhat. Rinse the fish, then dry it between towels, repeatedly, until the surface is really dry. I pat fillets, which are not so troublesome, between paper towels, and I roll up squid, clams and oysters in a couple of kitchen towels; they can sit like that, wrapped and refrigerated, for a few hours. See Deep-fried Calamari with Three Dipping Sauces, page 295, for details on drying.

I usually use light, inexpensive vegetable oil for frying, and toss it when I'm done. Sometimes, for a treat, I use olive oil to fry flavorful fish such as shrimp or pieces of light tuna; it's quite delicious. Generally speaking, your oil should be at 350°F, or even a little bit higher. Use a frying thermometer, invest in a fryer with a thermostat (the DeLonghi, which also has a cover, is nice, although it is a complete nuisance to clean), or drop a small cube of bread into the oil; it should bounce to the top and start sizzling away when the oil is hot enough. Don't allow the oil to smoke.

Another of the great challenges about frying fish at home is that the relatively small quantity of oil used does not have enough volume to maintain its heat when you add cold fish to it. Again, electric fryers with automatic thermostats are helpful here, as is turning up the heat as you put the fish in the oil. But the only real solution is to keep your batches small; a quart of oil can handle just about one or at most one and a half cups of food at once. This means that, even for two servings, you will often have to fry more than one batch.

Deep-frying is very, very fast; it doesn't take anything long to cook when it is immersed in 350°F oil. Any piece of fish one half inch thick or less will cook in the time it takes the coating to turn golden. There are two ways to deal with fish that's much thicker than that: You can cut it into chunks, which is a good solution, or you can fry it normally at first, then lower the heat a bit until it cooks through, hopefully before the outside begins to scorch.

At home, fried food is never going to be elegant. It's best eaten in the kitchen; eat one batch while you fry the next. Sprinkle the fish with salt, drizzle it with lemon, or dip it in seasoned soy sauce or a tomato-based salsa. Anything more elaborate is a waste of time.

GENERAL GUIDELINES FOR DEEP-FRYING

SHELLFISH

As I mentioned earlier, you can deep-fry clams or mussels on the half shell; just remove the top shell, leave the critter attached to the bottom, coat—I prefer a dusting of flour with a bit of baking soda to help in browning—and fry. But it's far more common to deep-fry shucked clams, oysters, scallops, and mussels. Since cooking time for these fish is usually only a couple of minutes anyway, they are great candidates for deep-frying. Oysters are especially wonderful, since they remain succulent and tender encased in the crisp coating.

Other shellfish, especially shrimp, squid, and soft-shell crab, are also terrific when deep-fried. Fried squid has become something of a national craze, but is perhaps the most challenging fish to fry at home because of its tendency to spatter wildly. Shrimp is almost foolproof. You can deep-fry lobster, too, out of the shell. Use any coating you like; flour, bread crumbs, or a light batter are all quite fine.

STEAKS

Most steaks are too big to deep-fry, and you can get a similar crisp crust and moist interior by sautéing. If you want to, however, you can cut steaks into chunks and deep-fry them that way, coated with flour. Deep-fried steaks of smaller fish—whiting is my personal favorite—are fabulous.

FILLETS

Fillets of white-fleshed fish, even thick ones such as cod and tilefish, are delightful when fried; the crust seems to accentuate the tender, delicate nature of the fish. Cut large fillets into pieces three or four inches long, and use flour, cornmeal, or a light or even heavy batter. Oily fish—bluefish, mackerel, mahi-mahi, tuna, and so on—are already oily enough without deep-frying them.

Whole Fish

The only whole fish you can deep-fry easily are very small ones, such as sardines, anchovies, baby flounder, whitebait, and the like. You could also cut up somewhat larger fish, as long as they're no more than an inch thick, but not many people would bother to do this, since sautéing or roasting are much easier and eminently satisfying.

Cooking with Moist Heat: Braising, Steaming, Poaching, and Stewing Fish

These are among the simplest methods of cooking fish. As with all others, care must be taken not to overcook, but since each of these methods uses liquid as at least part of the cooking medium, there is a little bit more leeway. It's easier to dry a fish out by holding it over hot coals than it is by simmering it in liquid. Another advantage: Cooking with moist heat makes added fat superfluous; though some braised dishes and stews begin with browning in fat, the amounts used are minimal.

Almost any fish can be cooked with moist heat, and some are at their best when poached or steamed. A perfectly poached salmon, served cold, is incomparable, and some of the most wonderful scallops I ever had were simply steamed and drizzled with a few drops of good soy sauce. Large specimens of some fish often eaten whole, such as carp, tilefish, or red snapper, take on entirely new dimensions when they are braised. Braised squid (as prepared on page 300) is a revelation. Skate is rarely cooked without a preliminary poaching. And nothing compares to a good fish stew, to which I have devoted an entire entry.

Some definitions are in order here: By "brais-ing," I mean cooking, either in the oven or on top of the stove, in a covered vessel with a small amount of liquid. Some braised dishes begin with browning the fish, which enhances its color and flavor. Others allow the dish to derive its ultimate flavor from the exchange of essences between the fish and the liquid in which it steeps as it cooks. Braising is especially useful in cooking whole fish, or large cuts which are too big to sauté successfully. It's also a nice way to add extra flavor to a thick fillet or steak without much hassle. Some people call braising in the oven "baking," or "oven steaming." I reserve the term "baking" for pastries; I don't believe there is a right or wrong in this case, which is why I'm defining my terms.

Stewing, on the other hand, involves covering the fish with the same liquid in which you will serve it. Bouillabaisse and the like (pages 46–47) are all fish stews. You also cover the fish with liquid to poach it, but don't serve the poaching liquid with the fish; it is, however, occasionally reduced for sauce. In addition, poaching usually involves cooking at the gentlest of simmers, or even in liquid that has been boiled and removed from the heat. Don't let fish poach at a boil, which will cook it too quickly. This not only may lead to overcooking, but the vigorous action of the water may cause the fish to disintegrate before you know it.

Steaming, of course, is cooking over rather than in liquid. The liquid is usually water, and is usually not used in the finished dish, but there are exceptions.

A Note About Microwaving

Microwaving fish usually involves adding a tiny amount of liquid to a small amount of fish on a plate covered with plastic wrap or in a small, covered casserole. Because fish is mostly water, the net effect is similar to steaming, or to braising without the initial browning. There are no microwave recipes in this book, for a number of reasons. Chief among them is that I have experimented with the microwave for years and have found that microwaving is usually more trouble than it's worth. In addition, it's hard to use the microwave for more than one or at the most two servings at a time. Third, most microwave recipes give inconsistent results. I refer those readers who are interested in cooking fish in the microwave to Pat Tennison's excellent *Glorious Fish in the Microwave* (Contemporary Books, 1989), or to Barbara Kafka's authoritative *Microwave Gourmet* (William Morrow, 1987). You won't have much trouble applying the techniques in Kafka's book to my recipes, although I obviously believe you are better off with stovetop, grill, oven, or broiler.

General Guidelines for Cooking Fish with Moist Heat

SHELLFISH

There is no better way to prepare mussels and clams than by steaming, and hard-shell clams and mussels produce a fabulous liquor as they steam; with the addition of a few aromatics, you have a ready-made sauce. For this reason, there are quite a few steaming recipes for these bivalves.

These same fish are an integral part of many stews. You don't want to poach them, however, because their internal liquids, which are such an important part of their flavor, will be wasted in the process. And they cook too quickly to consider braising, although many of the steaming concoctions are so flavorful that they border on braising liquids.

Large scallops are fabulous simply steamed; they may also be poached with great success. Smaller scallops should not be steamed or poached for fear of overcooking. All scallops can be braised or used in stews.

Shrimp, lobster, and crab are often poached or steamed before being served cold. And steaming or poaching (boiling) is the essential way to cook not only lobster but crab, crayfish, and shrimp, usually with added spices. I like to poach squid, octopus, and other certain other shellfish—for seconds or hours—to tenderize them before using the meat in salads or, in the case of octopus and conch, before using in recipes. Braised squid and octopus are sensational. And all shellfish are frequent visitors to the stew pot.

STEAKS

I poach or steam steaks of various fish from time to time, but I must admit I'd rather sauté them unless I'm planning to serve them cold. One exception is halibut, which takes to poaching and steaming extremely well; see page 146. Before including steaks in a stew, you must cut them into chunks. Braised fish steaks—especially those of shark and other tough, meaty fish, for example, see Braised Mako Steaks with Lemon Pesto on page 171—can be quite good, but care must be taken not to overcook.

FILLETS

The one cut of fish that usually doesn't take well to moist cooking is the fillet; in most cases, it's simply too delicate. You can steam fillets—on a plate, to make serving easier—but you must be very careful not to overcook them. All but the thickest fillets will overcook quickly in poaching liquid, no matter how much care you take. And braising delicate fillets, or including them in a stew, will usually provide you with a flavorful thickening agent, but not much more; the fish dissolves into flakes almost instantly. There are exceptions to this, of course, and they are the tougher fillets of monkfish, grouper, blackfish, and so on, all of which make welcome additions to most stews when cut into chunks.

Cooking en papillote—in small, closed packages of paper or foil—is a form of steaming that is great for fillets. There are recipes for this technique scattered throughout the book, especially in the entry on red snapper.

WHOLE FISH

I love to steam whole fish, as long as they fit in the steamer. Sea bass, which has the meatiest texture and least complicated bone structure of the small fish, is perfect for this (see page 253), and red snapper runs a close second. If you want to spring for a classic fish poacher—a long, thin, covered pan that will span two burners on your stove and which you will use probably twice a year—you will have the ideal utensil for poaching or steaming larger fish. Big, whole poached salmon, served cold, is a classic. Personally, I like to poach smaller pieces of salmon, which taste just as good and are a whole lot easier. But then, I don't throw a lot of buffet parties for fifteen or twenty people; if I did, I might poach whole salmon.

Braising whole fish—probably the most complicated of all fish preparations, but still usually an hour or less in cooking time—gives you a special dish. Tilefish and carp are both terrific candidates for braising, as are grouper, red snapper, and sea bass. Stick with larger fish for braising, at least two pounds and preferably three or more; small fish cook too quickly. Cut off the head and tail if you have trouble fitting them in your skillet or casserole.

IMPROVISING A STEAMER

You can buy "steamers," but none of them is more effective than this: Take a large pot and cover the bottom with an inch or so of water (or whatever the steaming liquid is). Invert a custard cup, bowl, or a couple of coffee mugs in the pot, then place a round rack whose diameter is just smaller than that of the pot's interior on top. Steam on the rack or on a plate placed directly on the support structure. The pot, of course, must be covered.

BASICS AND STAPLES

Here is an assortment of recipes that don't readily fit elsewhere—toppings that can be used on a wide variety of fish; sauces, stocks and other basic preparations; and a couple of side dishes.

STOCKS

I never use canned stock (bear with me: I am not a snob). When I don't have stock, I use water, or water and wine, or water and a bit of vinegar and some herbs—whatever. I just can't stand the metallic, oversalted taste of canned stock.

You can make fish stock in fifteen or twenty minutes. Save scraps of fish, bones, and heads, along with carrot, onion, and other vegetable peelings; just keep a bucket or bag in the freezer, and empty it into a stockpot when it is full. Or, when you're buying fish, ask for a bunch of heads and skeletons, which will either be free or very, very cheap.

Avoid any dark-fleshed oily fish in stock-making, and don't use salmon unless you want its distinctive flavor. Shrimp shells and lobster and crab bodies are also excellent in stock.

Making chicken stock is not much more difficult; if you poach a whole chicken, along with some vegetables, for an hour or so, you not only have a light stock but a meal of chicken and vegetables. And light chicken stock can usually fill in nicely for fish stock.

Here are a variety of stocks, from quite light and quick to full-flavored and rich. They're interchangeable in virtually all recipes. All stock freezes well, for a long, long time. If you would rather refrigerate it, bring it to a boil and simmer for 3 minutes every 3 days to keep it from spoiling.

QUICKEST CHICKEN STOCK

Makes 3 quarts
Time: 40 to 70 minutes

1 whole chicken, 3 to 4 pounds
1 cup roughly chopped onion
1 cup roughly chopped carrot
½ cup roughly chopped celery
Pinch ground thyme
1 bay leaf
Several sprigs fresh parsley
1 tablespoon salt
3 ½ quarts water

Cut the chicken up if you like; it will speed cooking. Combine all the ingredients in a stockpot. Bring to a boil and simmer over medium heat just until the chicken is cooked through, 30 to 60 minutes. Strain and refrigerate or freeze; reserve the chicken for another use.

FULL-FLAVORED CHICKEN STOCK

Makes 3 quarts
Time: About 3 hours

Don't use meatless chicken bones by themselves or the stock will lack a meaty flavor. But a combination of bones and meat, or very meaty bones alone, is fine.

3 to 4 pounds chicken parts and/or bones
1 cup roughly chopped onion
1 cup roughly chopped carrot
½ cup roughly chopped celery
Pinch ground thyme
1 bay leaf
Several sprigs fresh parsley
1 tablespoon salt
4 quarts water

Combine all the ingredients in a stockpot. Bring to a boil and simmer over medium heat until the meat falls from the bones and the bones themselves no longer hold together, about 2 hours. Strain, skim, and simmer for about an hour longer. Refrigerate or freeze.

FAST FISH STOCK

Makes 1 quart
Time: 30 minutes

This is a light, all-purpose fish stock that you can make whenever you have just filleted a fish, or when a fishmonger is able to give you a couple of heads and some skeletons. It's not a luscious stock—I wouldn't use it as the sole basis for a soup—but it works well in reductions and other sauces. For more flavor, add some mushrooms (stems are fine), parsley, leeks, and a tablespoon or two of butter or olive oil.

1 quart water
1 onion, not peeled, quartered
1 carrot, cut into chunks
1 clove garlic, lightly crushed and peeled
10 black peppercorns
1 teaspoon salt
½ cup dry white wine (optional)
1 pound or more fish heads (gills removed) and/or skeletons, taken from white-fleshed fish

Bring all the ingredients to a boil over medium heat and cook at a slow simmer for 20 minutes; strain. Cool to room temperature and freeze or refrigerate.

FLAVORFUL FISH AND VEGETABLE STOCK

Makes about 4 quarts
Time: 1 hour, plus resting time

This is a fresh-tasting base for any fish soup;

reduced by 50 percent, it also makes a lovely consommé.

4 quarts water
4 to 5 pounds assorted fish heads (gills removed), skeletons, and scraps, taken from white-fleshed fish
1 pound tomatoes, cored and roughly chopped
½ pound carrots, cut into chunks
½ pound onions, left unpeeled and whole
½ pound celery, cut into chunks
3 cloves garlic, unpeeled
1 whole clove
10 black peppercorns
2 bay leaves
Several sprigs fresh thyme or 1 teaspoon dried
½ cup roughly chopped fresh parsley
2 tablespoons olive oil
1 cup dry white wine
Salt and freshly ground black pepper to taste

Combine all the ingredients except the salt and pepper in a stockpot. Bring to a boil, lower the heat to medium, and simmer for 45 minutes. Cool slightly and strain through a fine sieve or cheesecloth. Refrigerate, skim any fat and scum, and season with salt and pepper. Freeze or refrigerate until needed.

COURT BOUILLON

Makes about 3 quarts, enough to poach 4 to 6 fish steaks or 1 or 2 whole fish simultaneously
Time: 40 minutes
You don't have to make court bouillon too often, because it freezes well and improves with each use. When it becomes quite gelatinous—which it will after you've poached in it a few times—use it for stock or as the basis for a great fish stew or soup.

The following should be seen as guidelines; there is a lot of latitude in making court bouillon (and fish can, of course, be poached in water). Gar-

deners can experiment with exotic herbs here—lovage and lemon verbena, for example, are both wonderful when used sparingly.

3 quarts water
1 cup dry white wine
1 lemon, sliced
1 onion, left unpeeled and cut in half
2 carrots, cut into chunks
2 cloves garlic, crushed and peeled
10 to 20 black peppercorns
1 to 2 tablespoons minced fresh herbs as available: thyme, parsley, chervil, savory, marjoram, tarragon, or more exotic herbs, combined judiciously or used alone
2 bay leaves
1 tablespoon salt

Combine all the ingredients in a large kettle and bring to a boil over medium (not high) heat. Simmer gently over medium-low heat until the broth is fragrant and delicious. Poach fish immediately or strain and reserve.

SAUCES

There are dozens of sauces and variations scattered throughout this book, but here are some of the most frequently used basics.

PESTO

Makes about 1 cup
Time: 5 minutes
I don't add Parmesan to pesto that I'll be using on fish.

2 cups firmly packed fresh basil leaves
½ cup good olive oil
2 tablespoons pine nuts or walnuts
2 cloves garlic, crushed and peeled
Salt to taste

Combine all the ingredients in a blender or food processor and turn on the machine. Scrape down the sides of the container to ensure that everything is pulverized. Store in the refrigerator, covered with a thin layer of olive oil. Use within 1 week (or freeze) on any broiled, grilled, or poached fish.

SPICY PEPPER SAUCE
FOR FRIED FISH

Makes about 1 cup
Time: 10 minutes

1 tablespoon peanut or vegetable oil
1 tablespoon minced garlic
1 tablespoon peeled and minced fresh ginger
1 tablespoon good-quality soy sauce
1 teaspoon chili-garlic paste or to taste (available in Asian markets)
1 cup any chicken or fish stock (pages 40–41)
1 tablespoon cornstarch (optional)

Heat the oil in a small saucepan over medium heat for 2 minutes; add the garlic and cook, stirring, until it turns dark golden. Add the ginger and cook 1 minute more, then add the soy sauce and chili paste and stir. If you choose to use cornstarch, which will give the sauce some body (but do nothing for its flavor), mix it with 1 tablespoon of the stock. Add the stock to the sauce and bring just to a boil; then add the cornstarch mixture and cook, stirring, until just thickened. Use immediately.

ONION-TOMATO RELISH
FOR GRILLED FISH

Makes about 2 cups
Time: 5 minutes

2 cups chopped fresh, ripe tomatoes (canned are acceptable, but should be drained)
½ cup minced onion, preferably red
¼ cup olive oil
Balsamic, sherry, or other vinegar to taste
Salt and freshly ground black pepper to taste

Combine all the ingredients and check for seasoning. Pass at the table. This keeps for a day or two, but is best used immediately.

RED PEPPER SAUCE FOR
STEAMED OR GRILLED FISH

Makes about 1 cup
Time: 15 minutes

1 tablespoon butter
1 tablespoon minced shallot
1 medium red bell pepper, seeded and chopped
½ teaspoon minced fresh thyme or 1 pinch dried
Salt and freshly ground black pepper to taste
1 cup any fish or chicken stock (pages 40–41)

Melt the butter in a small saucepan over medium heat; add the shallot and cook, stirring, until soft, then add the bell pepper. Cook, stirring occasionally, until the pepper begins to soften, about 5 minutes. Add the thyme, salt, pepper, and stock and simmer gently about 5 minutes. Let cool, then puree in a blender. Reheat before using. You can store this, refrigerated and covered with plastic wrap, for 3 or 4 days.

AVOCADO SALSA FOR GRILLED OR BROILED FISH

Makes about 1 cup
Time: 10 minutes

1 ripe but not too mushy avocado, peeled, pitted, and diced
1 medium-size firm, ripe tomato, diced
Salt and freshly ground black pepper to taste
1 scallion, minced
1 tablespoon olive oil
2 tablespoons minced cilantro (fresh coriander)
1 tablespoon fresh lime juice

Combine all the ingredients and use immediately; this salsa does not keep well.

BASIC VINAIGRETTE

Makes 1 cup
Time: 5 minutes

Vinaigrette is among the most flavorful, useful, and versatile dressings. You can put it on any simply cooked fish, and you can make it with any vinegar you like, lemon, lime, or other citrus juice (or a combination), and nearly any combination of herbs and/or spices you can think of. Many of these variations appear elsewhere in this book; here is the basic recipe.

¼ cup good wine, sherry, balsamic, or other vinegar, or fresh lemon juice, more or less
¾ cup olive oil, more or less
Salt and freshly ground black pepper to taste
1 small shallot, minced
1 teaspoon Dijon mustard

Add most of the vinegar to the oil, along with the salt and pepper, shallot, and mustard. Stir and taste. Add more vinegar if necessary and adjust the seasoning. Stir, shake, or whisk until emulsified.

You can refrigerate this, covered, for 3 or 4 days with little deterioration in flavor.

BASIC MAYONNAISE

Makes 1 cup
Time: 10 minutes

Don't snub mayonnaise just because it's little more than an emulsion of egg and oil. You don't need much for flavor, and there's almost no limit to what you can do with it. This is another of those recipes for which variations are scattered about the book.

1 large egg
Dash cayenne pepper
½ teaspoon dry mustard
Salt and freshly ground black pepper to taste
1 tablespoon wine, balsamic, sherry, or other vinegar or fresh lemon juice
1 cup good olive or other flavorful oil, more or less

Place all the ingredients except the oil in a blender or food processor; turn on the machine and, with the machine running, add the oil in a thin, steady stream. After you've added about half of it, the mixture will thicken; you can then begin adding the oil a bit faster. Check the seasoning and serve or store in the refrigerator; mayonnaise keeps well for several days. It may be thinned with warm water or sweet or sour cream.

GARLIC MAYONNAISE (AÏOLI):

Make a basic mayonnaise, as above, with 1 to 4 whole, peeled cloves garlic added at the beginning. If you like, add a small boiled potato to the mixture for extra body. Thin as necessary with stock or water.

ROUILLE:

Rouille is frequently served with fish stews in the south of France. To the basic mayonnaise ingredients, add ½ cup roasted (page 55) and seeded or canned red bell pepper, Tabasco sauce to taste, and 2 peeled cloves garlic. As in aïoli, a small boiled potato may be added. Proceed as above, and thin as necessary with stock or water.

TARTAR SAUCE:

This is superior to any prepared tartar sauce. Combine 1 recipe mayonnaise with 10 to 15 finely chopped cornichons, the small, super-sour French pickles. Add a little prepared horseradish if you have any.

MUSTARD SAUCE

Makes 1 cup
Time: 10 minutes
Great for gravlax, smoked fish, or cold poached fish. If you add the egg, you will have a thick, mayonnaiselike sauce; without it, the sauce is thinner but equally tasty.

1 large egg (optional)
2 tablespoons Dijon mustard
2 tablespoons white wine vinegar
1 tablespoon sugar
Salt and freshly ground black pepper to taste
6 tablespoons extra virgin olive oil or other flavorful oil
1 tablespoon minced fresh dill

Combine the first five ingredients (four if you omit the egg) in a blender or bowl. Blend or whisk, adding the oil a little at a time, until the mixture thickens. Stir in the dill and serve.

COMPOUND BUTTERS

Makes 4 to 8 servings
Time: 10 minutes
If you have a variety of compound butters on hand

(they freeze perfectly), or the ability to make one (they take no time), you can jazz up just about any grilled or broiled fish with no work at all. To use compound butter, just put some—from a teaspoon to a tablespoon—on a hot fillet or steak. Here are a few suggestions. All of them can be made in a small food processor, but it's usually just as easy to cream the butter with a fork.

ANCHOVY BUTTER:

Canned anchovies are better than the salted variety for this purpose. Cream ¼ cup (½ stick) butter, then add 3 minced anchovy fillets and 1 teaspoon fresh lemon juice.

HERB BUTTER:

Some herbs, as you know, are stronger than others. Vary the amount based on the individual herb. Add about 2 tablespoons minced mixed or single herbs—parsley, chervil, tarragon, chives, garlic chives, dill, sage, rosemary, cilantro, etc.—to ¼ cup (½ stick) creamed butter. Season with salt and freshly ground black pepper to taste. Add fresh lemon juice with herbs such as parsley and dill.

MUSTARD BUTTER:

Use any kind of mustard you like; for a really hot butter, add dry mustard to taste. Add 1 tablespoon Dijon mustard to ¼ cup (½ stick) creamed butter, then season with salt and freshly ground black pepper to taste.

HORSERADISH OR WASABI BUTTER:

Add 1 tablespoon prepared horseradish, drained, or 1 teaspoon wasabe (Japanese dried horseradish, available in Asian food stores), or to taste, to ¼ cup (½ stick) creamed butter.

GARLIC BUTTER:

Essential. Make this once, and it will become a staple. Melt 1 tablespoon butter in a small saucepan over low heat. Add 1 tablespoon minced garlic and cook just until the garlic softens, 2 to 3 minutes. Let cool. Add the garlic to ¼ cup (½ stick) creamed butter, along with salt, freshly ground black pepper, and fresh lemon juice to taste.

GINGER BUTTER:

Follow the garlic butter directions, adding 1 teaspoon peeled and minced fresh ginger to the garlic just before it is done cooking and a few drops of soy sauce along with the lemon juice.

JALAPEÑO BUTTER:

Make this as hot as you like. Add 2 seeded and minced jalapeño peppers or other small chiles, the juice of ½ lemon, and salt and freshly ground black pepper to taste to ¼ cup (½ stick) creamed butter.

BALSAMIC BUTTER:

Add 1 tablespoon minced shallot, 1 tablespoon balsamic vinegar, and salt and freshly ground black pepper to taste to ¼ cup (½ stick) creamed butter.

LIME OR LEMON BUTTER:

You can also make this butter with orange or other citrus fruit. Add 1 teaspoon minced or grated lemon or lime zest, 1 tablespoon fresh lemon or lime juice, salt and freshly ground black pepper to taste to ¼ cup (½ stick) creamed butter.

TWO CLASSIC SIDE DISHES

SPICY COLE SLAW

Makes about 2 quarts
Time: 20 minutes

2 tablespoons Dijon mustard
2 tablespoons sherry or balsamic vinegar
½ cup olive, peanut, or vegetable oil
1 tablespoon sugar
6 cups shredded Napa, Savoy, green, and/or red cabbage
2 cups seeded and diced red bell pepper
1 cup diced scallion, both green and white parts
Salt and freshly ground black pepper to taste
¼ cup minced fresh parsley

Whisk together the mustard and vinegar; add the oil a little at a time, whisking all the while. Add the sugar and whisk to dissolve. Combine the cabbage,

bell pepper, and scallion, and toss with the dressing. Season with salt and pepper and refrigerate until ready to serve (it's best to let this rest for 1 hour or so before serving to allow the flavors to mellow). Just before serving, toss with the parsley.

HUSH PUPPIES

Makes 4 to 6 servings
Time: 30 minutes

In the North, fried fish is served with fried potatoes, and sometimes onion rings. In the South, this is the traditional—and wonderful—accompaniment. Fry the hush puppies before the fish; they will stay crisp in a low oven.

1 ½ cups cornmeal
½ cup all-purpose flour
1 tablespoon baking powder
1 teaspoon freshly ground black pepper or ½ teaspoon cayenne pepper or to taste (optional)
1 teaspoon salt
½ teaspoon ground sage or thyme (optional)
1 cup milk
3 scallions, minced
1 large egg, beaten
Vegetable oil for deep-frying

Mix the dry ingredients together in a bowl. Stir the milk and scallions into the egg and combine with the dry ingredients, stirring well to moisten but not beating. Refrigerate for 1 to 2 hours if desired.

Heat at least 2 inches of oil to 375°F. (If your fryer doesn't have a thermostat, or you don't have a frying thermometer, drop a small piece of bread or hush puppy batter in the oil; it should sink, then rise to the top and begin bubbling away.)

Drop the batter in by the tablespoonful; do not crowd. Fry until dark and crisp, about 1 minute on each side. Drain on paper towels and keep warm in a low oven until ready (they keep fairly well for 30 minutes or so).

MIXED SEAFOOD DISHES

Here are a few recipes for fish stews, and one for a mixed salad. The stews all have this in common: You build a base of seasonings and liquid and simmer a variety of fish therein. They differ little in technique, but widely in the type of fish and, especially, the seasonings used. Substitute wildly when making any fish stew; as long as you're in the ballpark, you'll be fine. And, whenever possible, use a wide variety of fish.

ZARZUELA

Makes 4 to 6 servings
Time: 40 minutes
This classic Catalonian mixed shellfish dish is not so much a stew as it is a plate of fish covered with broth.

Pinch saffron
2 ½ cups any fish or chicken stock (pages 40–41), heated
2 tablespoons olive oil
1 large onion, chopped
4 cloves garlic, minced
2 red bell peppers, roasted (page 55), seeded, and minced (canned pimentos may be substituted)
1 dried hot pepper, crushed
1 cup roughly chopped tomato
½ cup blanched almonds, roughly chopped
Salt and freshly ground black pepper to taste
1 cup dry white wine
1 whole lobster or ½ pound monkfish, cut into chunks
24 of the smallest hard-shell clams available, cleaned (page 79)
24 of the smallest mussels available, cleaned and debearded (page 183)

1 pound scallops, preferably large
½ pound shrimp, shelled and cut into bite-size pieces
2 dozen of the tiniest squid available, cleaned (page 293) and cut into rings
½ cup roughly chopped fresh parsley

Dissolve the saffron in ½ cup of the stock. Put the olive oil in a large, heavy skillet which may later be covered. Add the onion and garlic and cook, stirring, over medium-low heat until the onion softens. Add the roasted and crushed red peppers, tomato, almonds, salt, and pepper. Simmer slowly, uncovered, for about 5 minutes.

Add the stock, the saffron mixture, and the wine. Bring to a boil, reduce the heat to medium, and simmer gently, covered, for about 5 minutes. Add the lobster, clams, and mussels and cook, covered, until the first of the shellfish is starting to open, about 5 minutes. Add the scallops, shrimp, and squid and cook, covered, until the shrimp turns pink and the clams and mussels are all open, about 5 more minutes.

Remove the lobster and cut it up (page 152), then return it to the pot and add the parsley. Serve immediately.

BOUILLABAISSE

Makes 6 to 8 servings
Time: 60 minutes
If you needed convincing that intimidating-sounding French dishes can in fact be quite simple to prepare, this should do it. What is bouillabaisse? A mess of fish, cooked in a garlicky tomato-based broth. It can be a lot of work or a little, expensive or cheap. This one is easy, and no less delicious for the fact that it can be made in an hour. Serve this with Aïoli (page 43) and call it bourride, or with Rouille (page 43), another traditional accompaniment.

¼ cup fruity olive oil

1 large onion, chopped

3 tomatoes, chopped, with their liquid (canned are fine)

½ teaspoon fennel seeds

4 or 5 sprigs fresh thyme or 1 teaspoon dried

1 bay leaf

4 or 5 sprigs fresh parsley

4 or 5 pieces orange rind

4 cups any fish stock (pages 40–41) or water

Twelve 1-inch-thick slices crusty bread

1 clove garlic, cut in half

24 small clams or mussels, cleaned (page 79 or 183)

1 ½ pounds fish fillets or steaks, a combination of halibut, cod, red snapper, sea bass, grouper (almost anything but dark-fleshed fish such as tuna, salmon, or bluefish), cut into large chunks

1 ½ pounds shellfish, preferably a combination of scallops and shrimp; lobster, crab, or monkfish are good alternatives

1 tablespoon minced garlic

2 tablespoons minced fresh basil

1 tablespoon Pernod or other anise-flavored liqueur (optional)

Salt and freshly ground black pepper to taste

Heat 3 tablespoons of the oil in a large saucepan or casserole that can later be covered, then add the onion and cook over medium-low heat until it softens. Add the tomatoes, fennel seeds, thyme, bay leaf, parsley, and orange rind. Stir to blend.

Add the stock and raise the heat, bring to a boil, cover, and cook over medium-low heat for about 10 minutes. While the broth simmers, toast the rounds of bread in a preheated 350°F oven until dried, about 20 minutes, or under a broiler until lightly browned, 2 to 3 minutes per side. Rub the toast with the garlic halves and put a piece in as many soup bowls as there are diners.

Reserve the remainder to pass at the table.

Add the clams to the broth and continue to cook, covered, for about 5 minutes. Add the fish chunks to the broth and cook another 5 minutes. When the first of the clams begins to open, add the remaining shellfish to the broth, along with the minced garlic, basil, Pernod, salt, pepper, and the remaining tablespoon of olive oil. Cover and cook for 3 to 5 minutes. Spoon some fish and broth into each bowl over the toasted French bread and serve.

EVEN SIMPLER BOUILLABAISSE

Makes 4 servings

Time: 30 minutes

Yes, you need fish stock to make this New Orleans-style stew. But if you have it, nothing could be easier. This basic recipe contains just one fish, but you can make it with ten if you like (see *alternative fish for this recipe*). You can also serve it—using a slotted spoon so you have control over the amount of broth—on top of couscous.

2 tablespoons olive oil

2 cups chopped onions

1 tablespoon minced garlic

4 cups Fast Fish Stock (page 40) or Flavorful Fish and Vegetable Stock (page 40)

1 cup dry white wine

Juice of 1 lemon

2 cups chopped tomatoes, fresh or canned (not drained)

2 bay leaves

Several sprigs fresh thyme or ½ teaspoon dried

Salt and freshly ground black pepper to taste

Cayenne pepper to taste

One 1 ½-pound whole red snapper, gutted, scaled, fins and gills removed

Minced fresh parsley for garnish

Heat the olive oil in a casserole, then add the onions and cook, stirring, over medium-high heat until they begin to brown. Add the garlic and cook 30 seconds more. Add the fish stock and wine, bring to a boil, and simmer for 5 minutes. Add the lemon juice, tomatoes, herbs, salt, pepper, and cayenne. Simmer for about 5 more minutes.

Cut the fish into chunks, put it in the broth, and simmer for about 5 minutes. Remove a chunk and cut it in half. If it's opaque throughout, turn off the heat (if not, cook another 1 or 2 minutes). Serve immediately in bowls garnished with parsley with crusty bread.

ALTERNATIVE FISH FOR THIS RECIPE:

This is an "anything goes" dish, and you can combine freely. Try whole blackfish, grouper, rockfish, sea bass, tilefish, wolffish, or fillets or steaks of those same fish or catfish, dogfish, eel, monkfish, or Atlantic pollock. Shellfish are also good here.

WHOLE MEAL FISH SOUP

Makes 4 to 6 servings
Time: 45 minutes
This thick, creamy chowder makes a fabulous winter lunch.

¼ cup (½ stick) butter
1 cup chopped onion
1 teaspoon minced garlic
1 carrot, chopped
1 stalk celery, chopped
1 red bell pepper, seeded and chopped
6 cups any fish stock (pages 40–41)
1 fresh or canned tomato, chopped
1 bay leaf
2 tablespoons minced fresh basil
Salt and freshly ground black pepper to taste
4 medium-size potatoes (the "boiling," waxy kind work best), peeled or scrubbed and diced

2 to 3 pounds assorted firm boneless fish, such as catfish, dogfish, monkfish, grouper, etc., combined with scallops, shrimp, and/or other shellfish
1 cup heavy cream

Melt the butter over medium heat in a casserole or large saucepan that can later be covered. When the butter foam subsides, add the onion, garlic, carrot, celery, and red pepper and cook, stirring, until the onion softens. Add the stock, tomato, bay leaf, basil, salt, and pepper and bring to a slow boil over medium heat. Add the diced potatoes and simmer, covered, for about 10 minutes.

When the potatoes are nearly tender, add the fish, cover, and continue to simmer slowly until the fish is almost cooked through, 5 minutes or so. Remove the cover, turn the heat down as low as possible, and add the cream. Do not boil, but heat thoroughly. Adjust the seasoning and serve immediately with salad and bread.

WHOLE MEAL FISH SOUP PORTUGUESE STYLE:

Use olive oil in place of the butter. Sauté ½ pound chopped linguiça or chorizo with the vegetables. Substitute parsley for the basil, and finish the stew with ¼ cup red wine vinegar in place of the cream. Garnish with minced fresh parsley and top with lots of black pepper.

ASIAN SEAFOOD BROTH

Makes 4 servings
Time: 45 minutes
If you have a local Asian market and can find pea shoots, they make a wonderful substitute for bean sprouts.

5 cups any chicken or fish stock (pages 40–41)
1 red or green jalapeño pepper, cut in half and seeds removed
3 slices peeled fresh ginger

Juice of 1 lime
1 cup minced cilantro (fresh coriander) leaves
1 stalk lemon grass, cut into 1-inch pieces
(available in Asian markets)
1 tablespoon good-quality soy sauce
Salt and freshly ground black pepper to taste
24 small hard-shell clams, cleaned (page 79)
8 razor clams, cleaned (page 79)
12 mussels, cleaned and debearded (page 183)
8 medium to large shrimp
½ pound large scallops
2 cups bean sprouts
½ cup minced Chinese garlic chives or regular
chives
2 limes, quartered

Simmer together the stock, jalapeño, ginger, half the lime juice, half the cilantro, and the lemon grass for 15 minutes over medium heat. Strain into a steep-sided sauté pan, large saucepot, or casserole. Add the soy sauce, salt, and pepper, taste, and correct the seasoning. Heat the broth until it simmers, then add the clams and mussels, cover again, and cook until the mollusks open, about 10 minutes. Add the shrimp and scallops and cook over medium heat, stirring, until the shrimp turn pink, about 5 minutes.

Place the bean sprouts in the bottoms of four large bowls. Add half the garlic chives and half the remaining cilantro. Stir the remaining lime juice into the broth. Divide the shellfish among the bowls and ladle in a portion of the broth. Garnish with the remaining cilantro and garlic chives and serve with lime quarters.

SEAFOOD SALAD ADRIATIC STYLE

Makes 10 to 15 servings
Time: 2 hours, plus marinating time

I had a salad like this one in the not especially charming town of Rimini, on the Adriatic coast of Emilia-Romagna, a place where fish is treated as it should be: simply and respectfully. It's best as part of a feast; you can vary the ingredients as you like, including more raw vegetables, and a larger or smaller variety of fish, depending on what is available. The preparation of this dish takes some time, but there is nothing complicated about it.

8 cups Flavorful Fish and Vegetable Stock
(pages 40–41) or 8 cups water and salt and
freshly ground black pepper to taste, 1 onion,
cut in half but unpeeled, 3 cloves garlic, lightly crushed and peeled, 1 carrot, peeled and
cut into chunks, ½ bunch fresh parsley, 2 bay
leaves, 1 tablespoon vinegar, and ½ cup dry
white wine
1 octopus, about 3 pounds
3 pounds squid, cleaned (page 293)
3 pounds medium to large shrimp
40 small fresh sardines or anchovies, 1 to 2
pounds, cleaned (page 51) and marinated as
instructed on page 51
One 3-pound salmon fillet, poached as instructed on page 236
1 recipe white beans, cooked as instructed on
page 267
An assortment of vegetables: raw fennel, roasted red pepper (page 55), steamed carrots
and/or new potatoes, greens
Salt and freshly ground black pepper to taste
Fruity olive oil
Lemon wedges

Bring the stock to a boil or simmer together the water and stock ingredients for about 10 minutes. Add the octopus and simmer until tender (page

195), about 1 hour. Add the squid and shrimp and cook until the shrimp begin to turn pink, 2 to 3 minutes. Turn off the heat and let the seafood cool in the water for 10 minutes. Strain and reserve the stock for another use (you can use this stock to poach some vegetables for the salad if you like). Shell the shrimp and cut the octopus, squid, and shrimp (if necessary) into bite-size pieces.

Arrange the shellfish in small piles on a platter, along with the marinated sardines, poached salmon, beans, and vegetables. Sprinkle all with salt and pepper. You can cover and refrigerate at this point for a couple hours, but let the salad return to room temperature before serving. To serve, drizzle everything with olive oil and pass the platter, along with more olive oil and lemon wedges.

ANCHOVY

Latin name(s): *Engraulis* (from the Mediterranean and other European waters) and *Anchoa* (North American); many species of each.

Other common names: Sardine (there is much confusion between the two, and they are often sold interchangeably); very small anchovies may be sold as whitebait.

Common forms: Whole and beheaded fresh (unfortunately, not often enough); whole and beheaded salted; the familiar fillets, packed in oil in two-ounce cans.

General description: Small, shiny silver fish, often with red eyes. Small, virtually nonexistent scales; edible skin.

For other recipes see: Sardines, smelts, whitebait.

Buying tips: Fresh anchovies really stink when they start to go bad, so it's easy to tell when they're fresh. Don't count on finding unbruised specimens; these are soft-fleshed fish, and, unfortunately, are rarely handled with the care they deserve.

Almost every country, every region, has its "anchovy," although it is not always the same fish. A number of species are caught off our shores—mostly members of the Engraulidae family—and the catch is not small. But, unfortunately, fresh anchovies are something of a rarity, and will remain so until we develop a taste for them: Most are canned or exported, where they are salted, smoked, pounded into paste, or distilled to make the "fish sauces" of Southeast Asia, such as the Vietnamese *nuoc mam*. Anchovies were the main ingredient in garum, the ancient Greco-Roman dipping sauce.

In contemporary American kitchens, anchovies are most commonly used as an ingredient in Mediterranean cooking. You can buy salted anchovies, which are sold from large cans in Italian food stores. (To use them, rinse under cold running water, peel off one fillet, remove the bone and tail from the other fillet, and rinse again.) The familiar canned thin strips of anchovy fillets are also good, although you may not always need the oil in which they are packed. Neither of these preserved fish can be used in recipes for fresh anchovies, although they do have their uses.

Fresh anchovies, like sardines, are delicious, with a rich, fat, but quite muted flavor. (And, like sardines and all dark-fleshed fish, they must be well iced from the moment of catch until the moment they are cooked to ensure good quality.) But canned and salted anchovies are far more common, and the recipes that follow reflect that balance.

SPICY MARINATED FRESH ANCHOVIES

Makes 4 to 6 servings

Time: 30 minutes, plus 3 to 6 hours or more for marinating

This is a flavorful seviche-style recipe. Don't let the fish marinate too long or the flesh will become mushy; they'll be ready to serve within a couple of hours, and shouldn't be kept for more than a day or two.

1 pound fresh anchovies (20 to 30)
1 tablespoon olive oil
¼ cup fresh lemon juice
1 tablespoon minced garlic
¼ cup minced cilantro (fresh coriander)
1 fresh jalapeño, seeds and stems removed, cut into slivers
Salt to taste

To bone the anchovies, snap off the heads by grasping the body just behind the head and pulling down on the head. Most of the innards will come out with the head. Run your thumb along the belly flap, tearing the fish open all the way to the tail and removing any remaining innards. Then grab the backbone between your thumb and forefinger and pull it out, gently. Remove any spiny fin material and drop the fillet into a bowl of ice water. (See the illustrations in Sardine entry, page 240.)

Rinse the fish and dry them with paper towels. Place them in a shallow bowl. Mix together the olive oil, lemon juice, garlic, half the cilantro, the jalapeño, and salt; marinate the anchovies in this mixture until they turn white (you can keep them, refrigerated, for a day or two). Garnish with the remaining cilantro and serve.

ALTERNATIVE FISH FOR THIS RECIPE:

Sardines or small smelts; the larger the fish, the longer the marinating time.

VARIATION:

Increase the garlic to 2 tablespoons and reserve 1 teaspoon or so. Substitute fresh Italian parsley for the cilantro, and omit the jalapeño. When ready to serve, combine the remaining parsley and garlic with a bit of salt, and sprinkle this mixture over the fish.

CHRISTMAS EVE ANCHOVY "CRULLERS"

Makes 6 to 12 servings
Time: About 2 hours

This is a fun, traditional Italian-American dish, often served as a prelude to a larger all-fish dinner during the holiday season.

1 small potato
Pinch sugar
1 envelope yeast (not rapid rise)
One 2-ounce can anchovy fillets, drained and dried (reserve 1 tablespoon of the oil) or 6 to 10 salted anchovies, rinsed well, filleted, and dried
2 to 3 cups all-purpose or bread flour, or a bit more
Vegetable oil for deep-frying

Peel the potato and boil it in salted water until tender. Reserve 1 cup of the cooking water and mash the potato. When the water has cooled to lukewarm, mix it with the sugar and yeast; let sit for 10 minutes. Add the potato, the reserved oil from the anchovies (or 1 tablespoon of olive oil if you've used dried anchovies), and 1 cup of the flour. Stir well (you can use an electric mixer or food processor for this) and let sit for 10 minutes.

Gradually add enough flour to the mixture to make a soft but not sticky dough, mixing after each addition. Knead for a couple of minutes, then place in a greased bowl, turning the dough ball over in the grease to coat it all over. Cover with a clean kitchen towel, or use plastic wrap, and let rise in a warm place for 30 to 60 minutes. The dough will not double, but will swell slightly.

Pinch off small pieces of dough and roll into fingers about 4 or 5 inches long by thumb width. Flatten a section, place an anchovy fillet on top, then pinch the dough around the anchovy to enclose. Cover and allow to rise again, covered, for 15 to 30 minutes. Heat 3 to 4 inches of oil in a deep-fryer or deep kettle to 350° to 375°F (use a frying thermometer to measure temperature, or put a pinch of dough in the oil; when it sinks to the bottom and quickly rises to the top, the oil is ready). Fry the "doughnuts" in the hot oil, a few at a time; drain on paper towels and serve hot or warm.

ANCHOVY SAUCE FOR COLD FISH

Makes about ½ cup
Time: 30 minutes
A strong-flavored sauce that can be used hot or cold.

1 tablespoon minced garlic
One 2-ounce can anchovies, minced, oil reserved
½ cup good quality wine vinegar, red or white
1 tomato (canned is fine; drain it first), chopped
Salt and freshly ground black pepper to taste

Place the garlic and reserved anchovy oil in a cold, 10-inch skillet, and turn the heat to medium-low; simmer the garlic in the oil just until it begins to color. Add the anchovies and stir; cook for 1 minute over low heat. Add the vinegar, raise the heat to medium, and reduce the sauce slightly. Add the tomato and cook until the sauce separates, about 10 minutes. Season, place in a bowl, and whisk with a fork for a minute or so. Use over pasta such as spaghetti or linguine.

PASTA WITH ANCHOVY AND WALNUT SAUCE

Makes 4 servings
Time: 30 minutes

½ cup walnut pieces, roughly chopped
2 tablespoons olive oil
1 tablespoon minced garlic
Two 2-ounce cans anchovies, with their oil, minced
Salt
1 pound linguine
Minced fresh parsley for garnish

Place the walnuts on an ungreased baking sheet and toast in a preheated 350°F oven until fragrant, shaking occasionally, 10 to 15 minutes; set aside. Start a large pot of water for the pasta.

Meanwhile, heat the oil in a large skillet over medium heat, add the garlic, and cook, stirring, until lightly colored. Add the anchovies, along with their oil, cook for 1 minute, then turn off the heat.

Salt the water and cook the pasta until it is tender but retains some "bite"; dilute the anchovy sauce with ¼ to ½ cup of the pasta water. Toss together the pasta, sauce, and walnuts, garnish with the parsley, and serve.

BARRACUDA

Latin name(s): *Sphyraena barracuda* (Atlantic); *Sphyraena argentea* (Pacific).
Other common names: Great barracuda, sea pike (Atlantic); Pacific barracuda, scoots.
Common forms: Whole, steaks, fillets.
General description: Although its flesh is usually somewhat lighter and more firm, barracuda is not unlike the more popular bluefish, and generally can be treated as such. Whole fish range to ten pounds; most commonly sold are fish of five pounds or so, beheaded and dressed.
For recipes see: Bluefish, mackerel.
Buying tips: For reasons discussed below, barracuda should only be eaten on the West Coast; its flesh is generally somewhat firmer than that of bluefish. Barracuda spoils quickly; be sure it is well iced and sweet-smelling before you buy it.

All barracuda are warm-water fish; they are found in the Caribbean and off the coasts of Florida, Southern California, and Mexico. Great (Atlantic) barracuda can cause ciguatera poisoning (page 16); my recommendation is that home cooks living anywhere but on the West Coast should avoid barracuda entirely in order to avoid the possibility of buying Atlantic barracuda. Scoots—West Coast barracuda—are perfectly safe. Extra care must be taken to keep barracuda well iced at all times; it's fragile and spoils rather quickly.

BLACKFISH

Latin name(s): *Tautoga onitis*.
Other common names: Tautog, black porgy, oysterfish.
Common forms: Whole fish, fillets, and (occasionally) steaks.
General description: A delicious firm fish with mottled, off-white flesh, averaging three to five pounds in the market.
For other recipes see: Carp, cod, dogfish, grouper, haddock, mako shark, monkfish, ocean perch, pollock, rockfish, red snapper, striped bass, tilefish, wolffish.
Buying tips: Blackfish are usually quite inexpensive, but there is one caution: The skin, which is difficult to remove, is extremely tough and completely inedible. Therefore, if you want skinless fillets, make sure the fishmonger does the work for you.

All the fish that feed on shellfish are especially meaty, and blackfish is no exception. This is an extremely regional fish, one that rarely makes it out of New England waters or markets (the similar cunner is found farther south, also in a limited area). The commercial catch is not large, but blackfish are popular among sport fishermen—they're great fighters—and can be found in markets from time to time.

Mild-flavored and very firm, blackfish yield white fillets that grill beautifully. Fillets are also superb in soups and stews—in fact, blackfish is known as chowderfish in some coastal areas, because it's cheap and doesn't fall apart in the cooking.

GRILLED BLACKFISH WITH CUMIN-SCENTED RED PEPPER RELISH

Makes 4 servings
Time: 45 minutes

Blackfish fillets look like those of Atlantic pollock, but there is a major difference: Blackfish is oilier and far more sturdy. Still, it's wise to use a grill basket (page 26), since the fish will start to flake when it is done.

4 medium-size red bell peppers
2 tablespoons olive oil
1 teaspoon balsamic vinegar
½ teaspoon ground cumin
Salt and freshly ground black pepper to taste
4 blackfish fillets, 1 to 1 ½ pounds total

Roast the peppers on a grill, over a flame, in a very hot oven, or under the broiler, until the skins are blistered and blackened. As soon as they are cool enough to handle, peel the skins off and remove the seeds. Chop the flesh coarsely and mix with 1 tablespoon of the olive oil, the balsamic vinegar, and cumin and season with the salt and pepper. This can be done a day or even two in advance; refrigerate the relish.

If the relish has been refrigerated, bring it to room temperature. Preheat a covered grill or broiler. Rub the fillets with the remaining tablespoon of oil and some salt and place them in a grilling basket (use a rack in a broiling pan if you are using the broiler). Grill, turning once, until the thinnest part of the fish shows signs of flaking (don't turn the fish if you are broiling), 8 to 10 minutes. To check for doneness, make a cut in the thickest part of the fish; the knife will meet little resistance and the flesh will be tender and opaque when fully cooked. Serve immediately, topped with the relish.

ALTERNATIVE FISH FOR THIS RECIPE:

On the grill, I'd limit the selection to grouper, Atlantic pollock, rockfish, red snapper, or wolffish. If you're broiling the fillets, they're much less likely to fall apart, so you could add more tender fillets such as catfish, cod, dogfish, haddock, Pacific pollock, and tilefish to the list.

BLACKFISH FILLETS
EN PAPILLOTE WITH CITRUS

Makes 4 servings
Time: 30 minutes
Don't let the name scare you; few preparations are as easy—or as much fun—as cooking in little packages. See Red Snapper Fillets en Papillote, page 288, for more ideas.

4 blackfish fillets, 1 to 1 ½ pounds total
1 navel orange, peeled and sectioned
1 grapefruit, peeled and sectioned
1 lemon, sectioned as you would a grapefruit
¼ cup olive oil
Salt and freshly ground black pepper to taste

Preheat the oven to 450°F. Tear off a 1-foot-square piece of aluminum foil (the more traditional parchment paper is, of course, acceptable). Place a fillet of fish on it, then top with a quarter of each of the citrus fruits, sprinkle with 1 tablespoon of olive oil, and salt and pepper. Seal the package and repeat the process with the remaining fillets.

Place all the packages in a large baking dish and bake until the fish is opaque and flaky, about 20 minutes. Serve the closed packages, allowing each diner to open his or her own at the table.

ALTERNATIVE FISH FOR THIS RECIPE:

Fillets of catfish, cod, dogfish, flatfish, grouper, haddock, perch, Atlantic and Pacific pollock, rockfish, red snapper, tilefish, weakfish, or wolffish.

Steaks of similar fish are also good; increase the cooking time accordingly (generally, by about 50 percent).

BLACKFISH PROVENÇAL STYLE

Makes 4 servings
Time: 30 minutes
Blackfish will stand up to braising as long as it isn't overcooked.

2 tablespoons olive oil
2 medium-size onions, chopped
1 teaspoon minced garlic
2 cups chopped tomatoes, fresh or canned (not drained)
½ cup dry white wine
1 cup tiny Niçoise olives
½ cup chopped fresh basil
1 sprig fresh rosemary or ½ teaspoon dried
1 sprig fresh thyme or ½ teaspoon dried
Salt and freshly ground black pepper to taste
1 ½ to 2 pounds blackfish fillet, cut into serving pieces

Heat the olive oil in a large, steep-sided skillet or casserole over medium heat; add the onions and cook, stirring, until softened. Add the garlic and tomatoes, raise the heat slightly, and cook, stirring occasionally, until some of the tomato juice bubbles away. Add the wine and cook, stirring occasionally, another 5 minutes.

Add the olives, half the basil, the remaining herbs, and some salt (remember that the olives are salty) and pepper. Cook 1 minute; submerge the fish in the sauce and cook over medium heat until the fillets are tender and white, about 8 minutes. Garnish with the remaining basil. Serve immediately, with crusty bread.

ALTERNATIVE FISH FOR THIS RECIPE:

Grouper, monkfish Atlantic pollock, rockfish, red snapper, or wolffish.

BLUEFISH

Latin name(s): *Pomatomus saltatrix*.
Other common names: Snapper (especially young fish), chopper, tailor.
Common forms: Whole fish, fillets, steaks (with less frequency as the average size of bluefish declines due to overfishing).
General description: A silvery, dark-fleshed fish, full-flavored and oily, with edible skin. Bluefish run from tiny snappers (best treated like butterfish) to ten-pounders and more; market size is generally three to five pounds. Mild-flavored when fresh, stronger a day or two out of water.
For other recipes see: Striped bass, mackerel, mahi-mahi, Atlantic pollock.
Buying tips: Bluefish must smell and look "clean"; fillets should glisten, whole fish look alive. Make sure it is iced when you buy it, keep it iced, and cook it quickly.

Although bluefish has its fans, many of them are people who fish for recreation and are more interested in fighting this fierce, voracious fish than in eating it (three quarters of the 100-million-pound annual catch of blues is taken by recreational fishermen). There's no denying that bluefishing is fun: As these piranhalike predators cruise the seas, devouring menhaden (bunker), croaker, mackerel, and other fish with an unduplicated frenzy, they will strike viciously at almost anything that moves (they have been known to attack fishermen), sometimes just tearing it to bits and not stopping to eat. Needless to say, they are tough: Many eight-pound blues have more fight than the average welterweight. The first time I caught a blue, I thought someone had sneaked underwater and tied a refrigerator to the line.

Bluefish has had trouble shedding its "poor man's" reputation, which began during the Depression, when trolley cars, subways, and railroads ran "Fisherman's Specials" to the shoreline. After a day of surfcasting, people returned lugging burlap bags filled with mature bluefish or young "snappers," so called because their sharp little teeth chatter.

To add to the challenges to its popularity, bluefish is reputed to be "fishy"; it takes courage for the uninitiated to sample it. Like mackerel and tuna, bluefish travel in schools in most of the world's warmer waters (but not the Pacific) and—like those fish—they are oily and rich, with a big, fat texture that calls for strong flavors; bluefish is best cooked with acidic ingredients.

When people say that bluefish is "too fishy," they're responding to poor quality fish. Like all fish, and especially dark-fleshed fish, bluefish must be iced immediately after the catch. The oil in bluefish—and there is lots of it—begins to turn rancid quickly after death if the internal temperature of the fish is not brought down immediately.

Nor does bluefish freeze or travel well; your best bet is to buy it (or catch it) when it is in season locally. High-quality bluefish looks and smells good; if the fish looks beat up, it probably is—look elsewhere. Although bluefish is coarser in texture and not as fine-tasting as tuna, it is quite delicious and, when not overcooked, exceptionally moist.

If you are sampling bluefish for the first time, buy fillets, and begin with my more-or-less standard recipe for grilled bluefish fillets (page 58).

Note, however, that whole bluefish, soaked in garlic- and cumin-scented soy sauce before grilling (below), wins more converts than anything else.

Note: Bluefish, especially larger ones, have been associated with high levels of PCBs. To be safe (see the discussion of contaminants in fish on page 16), stick with smaller fish (four to six pounds, or under two feet long). If you're especially concerned, don't eat the skin, and—using the "V" cut illustrated here—cut out the dark strip of meat that runs through the fillet. Taking these steps will minimize ingestion of PCBs. Most experts, however, would remark that occasional consumption of bluefish poses no threat to your health.

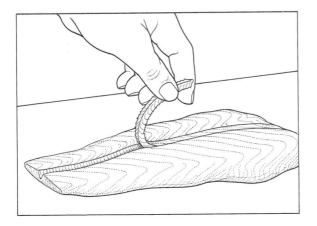

To remove the dark line of meat that runs through bluefish fillets, make a V-shaped cut on either side of it and pull it out. This technique works well for removing pinbones from bluefish, salmon, and other large fillets.

GRILLED BLUEFISH FILLETS

Makes 4 servings
Time: 60 minutes, including marinating time
Rosemary and lemon juice work together here to cut through the rich taste of the bluefish. The result is a striking combination of moist flesh and pleasantly acidic flavor.

2 bluefish fillets, skin on and scaled, about 2 pounds total
1 small onion, minced
Juice of 1 lemon
½ cup olive oil
Salt and freshly ground black pepper to taste
1 tablespoon minced fresh rosemary or 1 teaspoon crumbled dried, plus extra for the fire and garnish

Cut the fillets in half; combine all the remaining ingredients except for the extra rosemary. Pour this mixture over the fillets and marinate for 30 minutes, turning occasionally.

Preheat a gas grill or start a charcoal fire; the heat should be medium-high. Place the fillets in a fish basket (alternatively, brush both sides of the fish with additional olive oil). Toss a branch of fresh or a small handful of dried rosemary directly onto the coals and grill the fish, skin side up, for 4 to 5 minutes (if you're not using a fish basket, slide a spatula under the fish every minute or two to prevent sticking). Baste with the remaining marinade and turn, then grill until the skin is nicely browned, another 4 or 5 minutes. Bluefish becomes white when it is done; use a thin-bladed knife to peek at the interior of the fillet at its thickest part.

ALTERNATIVE FISH FOR THIS RECIPE:

This is a basic preparation for well-flavored fish; try fillets of bonito, jack, mackerel, mahi-mahi, or striped bass, or steaks of swordfish or tuna.

GRILLED WHOLE BLUEFISH

Makes 4 to 6 servings
Time: 30 minutes, plus marinating time
Everyone I know likes this dish—even those who claim to hate bluefish. Make sure the skin is well scaled, because you'll probably want to eat every

bit of it. Like many bluefish dishes, this goes well with boiled or scalloped new potatoes.

One 4- to 6-pound bluefish, cleaned and scaled, preferably with head on
1 cup high-quality soy sauce
½ cup dry red wine
Dash red wine or balsamic vinegar
One 1-inch piece fresh ginger, peeled and minced
2 tablespoons ground cumin
4 cloves garlic, peeled and crushed

Cut shallow (¼-inch) gashes, running from top to bottom, every inch or two along the length of the fish; place it in a large bowl or baking dish. Mix together all the other ingredients and pour over the fish. Marinate the fish, in the refrigerator, for at least 1 hour, or as many as 24. (If you have problems fitting the fish in a pan, place it in a double garbage bag and pour in the marinade. Squeeze the air from the bag and seal.)

When you're ready to cook, preheat a gas grill or start a charcoal fire; the heat should be medium. Brush both sides of the fish with olive oil, or use a fish basket if you have a large one. Grill the fish slowly about 6 inches from the heat. Slide a spatula under the fish from time to time to keep it from sticking. Turn the fish only once—using two spatulas to keep it intact—after about 10 minutes, and grill the other side until the fish is done (use a thin-bladed knife to peek into the thickest part of the fish, and make sure the meat near the bone is opaque). Remove the fish carefully and serve by scooping the fish off the central bones along the gashes made previously. Don't forget to eat the cheeks, which many consider the best part.

ALTERNATIVE FISH FOR THIS RECIPE:

Any full-flavored whole fish, especially jack, mackerel, pompano, or small tuna. Adjust cooking times accordingly.

STIR-FRIED BLUEFISH WITH SCALLOPS

Makes 2 servings
Time: 15 minutes

Bluefish meat remains moist and firm as long as it isn't overcooked, so it can be stir-fried. The addition of scallops and crunchy snow peas varies the texture, flavor, and color here.

One ½- to ¾-pound bluefish fillet, skinned and cut into 1-inch chunks
Cornmeal for dredging
¼ pound calico ("bay") scallops (page 244)
¼ cup peanut oil
1 cup snow peas or snap peas, trimmed
2 tablespoons high-quality soy sauce
Salt to taste
2 tablespoons dry sherry
1 tablespoon rice or white wine vinegar
1 teaspoon sesame oil

Preheat a wok or 12-inch nonstick skillet over medium heat. Dredge the bluefish chunks in the cornmeal, then shake them in a colander to remove any excess. Repeat the process with the scallops, keeping the fish separate. Add the oil to the wok, then raise the heat to high. When it smokes, stir-fry the peas for 30 seconds, then remove them with a slotted spoon.

Put the bluefish in the wok and cook, stirring, for 3 to 4 minutes; add the scallops and stir quickly. Add the soy sauce, salt, sherry, and vinegar and stir; return the snow peas to the wok, stir, and remove from the heat. Sprinkle with the sesame oil and serve.

ALTERNATIVE FISH FOR THIS RECIPE:

Chunks of blackfish, bonito, dogfish, grouper, mahi-mahi, mako shark, monkfish, striped bass, swordfish, tilefish, or wolffish.

BLUEFISH SEVICHE

Makes 6 to 8 appetizer servings
Time: 4 to 6 hours, including marinating time
Because bluefish is so strong-flavored, you can use it to make a highly spiced, Caribbean-style seviche. Great on crackers.

1 pound perfectly fresh bluefish fillets, skinned and cut into pieces no larger than ½ inch on any side
1 medium-size onion, chopped
Hot pepper sauce to taste
½ cup fresh lime juice, about 4 to 8 limes
1 small clove garlic, minced
¼ cup seeded and chopped red bell pepper
Salt and freshly ground black pepper to taste
1 teaspoon minced fresh thyme or ½ teaspoon dried
1 medium to large fresh, ripe tomato, peeled, seeded, and chopped
2 tablespoons minced cilantro (fresh coriander)

Combine all the ingredients except the tomato and cilantro. Mix well, cover, and place in the refrigerator. The fish will turn white gradually; when "cooked" through, it is ready to serve. Toss with the tomato and garnish with cilantro.

ALTERNATIVE FISH FOR THIS RECIPE:

This is too strong a marinade for most fish; I'd reserve it for mackerel and striped bass; it will also work for conch, although the meat will remain quite tough.

BROILED BLUEFISH WITH LIME MUSTARD

Makes 4 servings
Time: 20 minutes
Like mackerel, bluefish is great with acidic sauces that cut its richness. This one is supremely simple.

½ cup Dijon or coarse-grained mustard
Juice and grated zest of 1 lime
Salt and freshly ground black pepper to taste
1 tablespoon olive or peanut oil
1 ½ pounds bluefish, in 1 or 2 fillets (skin on or off; scaled if skin is left on)
1 medium to large ripe fresh tomato, seeded and coarsely chopped
Lime wedges

Mix together the mustard, lime juice and zest, salt, and pepper. Preheat the broiler. Brush a cookie sheet or broiler pan with the oil, and lay the bluefish on it. Brush it with the mustard-lime mixture.

Broil about 6 inches from the heat source for 6 to 10 minutes, depending on the thickness of the fish (bluefish is white throughout when done; peek between the layers of flesh with a thin-bladed knife). Sprinkle with the tomato and return to the broiler for 1 minute. Serve immediately, with lime wedges.

ALTERNATIVE FISH FOR THIS RECIPE:

Any rich-tasting fish will be nicely complemented by this treatment: try fillets or steaks of bonito, mackerel, mahi-mahi, mako shark, or striped bass. Adjust cooking times accordingly.

ROASTED BLUEFISH FILLETS WITH EGGPLANT CAPONATA

Makes 6 servings
Time: 60 minutes
This caponata is the creation of Lynne Aronson, the talented chef of Lola, a restaurant in New York City's Flatiron neighborhood.

2 pounds eggplant
1 medium-size red bell pepper
1 cup olive oil
2 ribs celery, diced
1 large red onion, sliced

1 medium-size zucchini, diced
⅓ pound calamata olives
5 tablespoons capers
2 large fresh tomatoes, seeded and chopped
1 tablespoon tomato paste dissolved in ¼ cup warm water
2 pounds bluefish fillets (skin on or off; scaled if skin is left on)
Salt and freshly ground black pepper to taste
¼ cup good quality red wine vinegar
1 tablespoon sugar

Slice the eggplants into rounds, salt liberally, and set in a colander; let drain for 30 minutes. Roast the red pepper on a grill, over a flame, or under a broiler until the skin is blistered and blackened; cool, peel, seed, and julienne.

Pat the eggplant dry and cut into ½-inch dice. Heat ½ cup of the oil in a large skillet over medium heat and cook the eggplant, stirring occasionally, until very tender, 15 minutes or so. Remove from the pan, add another ¼ cup of the olive oil, let it heat up, and cook the celery and onion, stirring, until limp; add the zucchini, red pepper, olives, capers, tomatoes, and dissolved tomato paste, stir to combine, cover, and cook over low heat for 10 minutes.

Meanwhile, preheat the oven to 500°F. Brush the bluefish fillets top and bottom with the remaining olive oil. Place them on a baking sheet and season with salt and pepper. Roast, shaking the pan occasionally, until opaque throughout, about 10 minutes.

When the caponata is done, remove it from the heat and season with the salt, pepper, vinegar, and sugar. Taste for seasoning, spread it atop the bluefish, and serve.

ALTERNATIVE FISH FOR THIS RECIPE:

Fillets or steaks of bonito, mackerel, mahi-mahi, mako shark, or striped bass. Adjust cooking times accordingly.

SIMMERED BLUEFISH WITH LEMON GRASS

Makes 4 servings
Time: 20 minutes

The clean, fragrant flavor of lemon grass, spiked with cayenne, offsets the oiliness of bluefish beautifully.

One 1 ½- to 2-pound bluefish fillet, skinned
2 tablespoons peanut oil
1 tablespoon minced garlic
1 stalk lemon grass, roughly chopped, or 2 tablespoons chopped dried lemon grass (available in Asian and specialty markets)
¼ teaspoon cayenne pepper or to taste
2 tablespoons high-quality soy sauce
1 teaspoon sugar
½ cup water

Heat a large nonstick skillet over medium-high heat for 3 to 4 minutes. Cut the bluefish in two (or four) pieces if necessary. Add the oil to the skillet, wait a minute, and add the garlic. Stir once or twice and add the fillets. Raise the heat to high and sear about 1 minute on each side. Add the remaining ingredients and stir. Turn the fish once or twice in the liquid, reduce the heat to low, cover, and simmer until done (the bluefish will be opaque throughout; use a thin-bladed knife to check), about 10 minutes. Remove the bluefish to a bowl and strain the broth over it. Serve immediately, with white rice.

ALTERNATIVE FISH FOR THIS RECIPE:

Fillets or steaks of bonito, mackerel, mahi-mahi, mako shark, or striped bass. Adjust cooking times accordingly.

ROASTED BLUEFISH FILLETS
WITH TOMATOES

Makes 4 servings
Time: 30 minutes

When bluefish oils combine with other ingredients during baking, the result is a wonderful sauce. There are many possibilities; see the variations below for additional ideas.

4 medium-size fresh, ripe tomatoes, sliced ¼ inch thick
½ cup minced scallions, green and white parts
¼ cup olive oil
1 teaspoon minced fresh rosemary or basil
¼ cup minced fresh parsley
Salt and freshly ground black pepper to taste
1 ½ pounds bluefish, in 1 or 2 fillets, skin off

Preheat the oven to 450°F. Layer about two thirds of the tomatoes on the bottom of a nonstick or lightly oiled baking dish, and sprinkle with half the scallions, most of the olive oil, half the herbs, and some salt and pepper. Top with the bluefish and the remaining ingredients except the remaining parsley.

Roast, uncovered, until the bluefish is done (it will be white throughout; use a thin-bladed knife to peek) and the tomatoes have liquefied, about 15 minutes. Serve immediately, with the sauce spooned over the fish and sprinkled with the remaining parsley.

ALTERNATIVE FISH FOR THIS RECIPE:

Fillets or steaks of bonito, mackerel, mahi-mahi, mako shark, or striped bass. Adjust cooking times accordingly.

BLUEFISH ROASTED ON GREENS:

Roast the fish on a bed of well-seasoned cooked greens, such as those on page 136 for Grouper Sandwich with Spinach or page 228 for Crispy Skin Salmon with Gingery Greens.

BLUEFISH WITH PARSLEYED BREAD CRUMBS:

Combine ½ cup plain bread crumbs in a food processor with a couple of garlic cloves and a handful of parsley, and process until well mixed and chopped. Cover the top layer of tomatoes with this mixture. Brown very briefly under the broiler after roasting.

BLUEFISH WITH CILANTRO AND LIME:

Substitute cilantro (fresh coriander) for the herbs; add a seeded, slivered jalapeño or other hot pepper to the bottom layer (optional); squeeze the juice of a lime over the bottom layer of tomatoes. Garnish with minced cilantro, minced scallion, and a little more lime juice.

BLUEFISH WITH CRISP POTATOES:

This takes longer but is worth it. Cover the bottom of the dish with about 2 pounds peeled, thinly sliced potatoes. Toss these with ½ cup olive oil, 1 tablespoon minced garlic, a handful of minced parsley or basil, and salt and pepper to taste. Roast the potatoes, gently mixing them up occasionally, until they are nicely browned and almost cooked through, 20 to 40 minutes. Top with the bluefish, a little more olive oil, and salt and pepper. Roast until the bluefish is cooked through. (You can add tomatoes and/or other herbs to this dish, also, on top of the bluefish.)

BLUEFISH FILLETS
IN SOUR CREAM

Makes 2 servings
Time: 20 minutes

An old-fashioned recipe, but a very pleasant one. Serve it over white rice, and keep the portions small—this is very rich.

3 tablespoons butter
1 tablespoon light vegetable or olive oil
1 small onion, chopped
1 tablespoon fresh paprika

Pinch dried thyme
1 bay leaf
Salt and freshly ground black pepper to taste
½ cup dry white wine
1 pound bluefish fillets, skinned
1 cup sour cream
Minced fresh parsley for garnish

Melt the butter and oil in a heavy skillet over medium-low heat. Add the onion and cook, stirring, until soft. Add the paprika, thyme, bay leaf, salt, and pepper and stir. Add the wine, stir, and raise the heat, letting the liquid boil away for 1 minute or so.

Add the fillets. Cook gently over medium heat until the fish is white throughout (use a thin-bladed knife to check the fillets' interior), about 8 minutes. Turn the heat to low and add the sour cream. Heat through but do not boil. Garnish with the parsley and serve over white rice.

ALTERNATIVE FISH FOR THIS RECIPE:
Mackerel, which should be very fresh.

PICKLED BLUEFISH SALAD

Makes 6 to 8 servings
Time: 30 minutes

A fine recipe for leftover bluefish.

3 tablespoons olive oil
2 medium-size onions, thinly sliced
4 medium-size carrots, chopped
2 medium-size red bell peppers, seeded and thinly sliced
1 tablespoon minced garlic
¼ cup dry white wine or vermouth
¼ cup white wine vinegar
1 bay leaf, crumbled
Salt and freshly ground black pepper to taste
1 to 1 ½ pounds skinless bluefish fillets, cooked, cooled, and flaked
4 to 6 cups mixed greens, washed and dried
About 20 cherry tomatoes

Heat the olive oil in a large skillet over medium heat, and cook the onions, carrots, peppers, and garlic, stirring, until the carrot is softened. Remove from the heat and add the wine, vinegar, bay leaf, salt, and pepper. Let cool. Combine the bluefish with the vegetable mixture in a glass bowl. Serve over the greens with the cherry tomatoes.

ALTERNATIVE FISH FOR THIS RECIPE:
Leftover fillets or steaks of bonito, mackerel, mahi-mahi, mako shark, or striped bass.

BONITO

Latin name(s): *Sarda sarda* (Atlantic), *Sarda chiliensis* (Pacific).
Other common names: Striped bonito, skipjack, short-finned tuna.
Common forms: Whole fish to ten pounds or so; steaks; dried flakes for use in the Japanese soup base called dashi.
General description: Often sold as tuna, bonito most definitely is not. In fact, it is more like bluefish, and should be priced accordingly. Bought right—fresh and inexpensively—it is a fine fish. Found worldwide, but never in great quantities.
For recipes see: Bluefish, mackerel.
Buying tips: The chances are good that any bonito you buy will have been caught locally, because the fish is not that popular and doesn't travel well. This increases your chances of buying a nice piece of fish; whole fish should be well iced, look alive, and smell of seawater. Steaks should glisten and have no browning.

BUTTERFISH

Latin name(s): *Peprilus triacanthus* and others.
Other common names: Pacific pompano, dollarfish, starfish.
Common forms: Whole.
General description: Small fish weighing in at a few ounces each; figure at least two per person. Fairly flat, round, shiny silver (hence the name dollarfish), fatty (hence the name butterfish), and flavorful. High-quality, dark-fleshed panfish, similar to the European pomfret. Underappreciated and usually inexpensive.
For other recipes see: Pompano (especially), spot, and almost any sauté recipe; whole butterfish cook as quickly as most fillets.
Buying tips: Skin should be silvery and bright; fish should be unbruised, with no strong odor. Many butterfish are gutted before sale, which is fine; if not, ask the fishmonger to gut them and remove the fins. Scales are not a problem.

Many of us ignore butterfish, thinking the tiny things to be more trouble than they're worth. The Japanese, however, import them in huge quantities, and I don't know anyone who has tried these babies and not liked them. The price is low, the cleaning and cooking time short (the scales can be rinsed off, and, by the time the skin browns, the fish is cooked through), and, unlike some whole fish, they're easy to eat. Far from a nuisance, the butterfish is pure pleasure.

PAN-FRIED BUTTERFISH WITH SPICY TOMATO PUREE

Makes 2 servings
Time: 30 minutes
Butterfish are so sweet that they cry for an assertive sauce. This crosscultural tomato puree works nicely, and is delicious over rice or other grains, but also with crisp bread.

4 to 6 whole butterfish, gutted, with heads on (about 1 ½ pounds)
½ cup plus 2 tablespoons peanut oil
2 cloves garlic, peeled and crushed
2 dried hot red peppers
1 tablespoon cumin (seeds or ground)
1 cup canned, drained or fresh, peeled plum tomatoes
2 tablespoons high-quality soy sauce
2 teaspoons sugar or to taste
Salt and freshly ground black pepper to taste
½ cup dry white wine, more or less
Flour for dredging
Minced scallions, green and white parts, for garnish

Rinse the fish well and dry them between paper towels. Heat the 2 tablespoons of oil in a medium-size saucepan over medium heat; add the garlic and red peppers and cook, stirring, until the garlic is golden. Add the cumin and stir. Add the tomatoes, crushing them with a fork or spoon. Bring to a boil, turn the heat to low, and add the soy sauce. Simmer gently for 10 minutes, then taste and add sugar as necessary; season with salt and pepper. Thin with a little wine, cool slightly, fish out the red peppers, and puree the sauce in a blender. Thin with more of the wine if necessary. Place in a serving bowl and keep warm.

Preheat a 12-inch nonstick skillet over medium-high heat. Add the ½ cup of oil and heat until a pinch of flour sizzles when added. Dredge the butterfish in the flour, place them in the pan, and raise the heat to high. Cook until lightly browned, about 3 minutes per side. Remove from the pan and drain quickly on brown paper bags or paper towels. Serve immediately, napped with 1 to 2 tablespoons of the puree and garnished with the scallions. Pass the remaining puree at the table.

ALTERNATIVE FISH FOR THIS RECIPE:

This is a wonderful recipe for any panfish: croaker, small mackerel, mullet, pompano, porgy, sardines, smelts, or spot. Adjust cooking times accordingly.

CRISPY SAUTÉED BUTTERFISH

Makes 2 servings
Time: 30 minutes
This is a basic recipe for pan-fried panfish.

4 to 6 whole butterfish, gutted, with heads on, about 1 ½ pounds
2 cups milk, more or less
1 cup unbleached all-purpose flour
1 cup cornmeal
Salt and freshly ground black pepper to taste
Olive, peanut, or vegetable oil
Lemon wedges

Rinse the fish well and let them soak in milk to cover while you preheat a 12-inch nonstick skillet

over medium-high heat. Mix together the flour and cornmeal and season liberally with salt and pepper. Add enough oil to the pan to cover the bottom to a depth of ⅛ to ¼ inch. Dredge the fish in the flour-cornmeal mixture and, when the oil is hot—a pinch of flour will sizzle—sauté them over high heat until lightly browned, about 3 to 4 minutes per side. Serve immediately, with lemon or Spicy Pepper Sauce for Fried Fish (page 42).

ALTERNATIVE FISH FOR THIS RECIPE:

Croaker, small mackerel, mullet, pompano, porgy, sardines, smelts, or spot. Adjust cooking times accordingly.

SESAME BUTTERFISH:

Mix 1 cup sesame seeds with the flour-cornmeal mixture for extra crunch. Serve with Sesame Dipping Sauce for Deep-fried Calamari (page 295).

MARINATED BUTTERFISH:

Drain the fish well after cooking. Heat 1 tablespoon olive oil in a large skillet over medium heat. Add 1 medium-size onion, sliced, 1 medium-size carrot, peeled and chopped, and 2 cloves garlic, peeled and smashed, and cook, stirring, until the onion is clear. Add 1 teaspoon sugar, ½ cup red wine vinegar, ½ cup red wine or water, 1 bay leaf, 1 teaspoon fresh or dried rosemary, 1 teaspoon black peppercorns, and 1 teaspoon salt and let boil for 1 minute; pour over the fish. Let marinate, refrigerated, for 6 hours or more before serving. Garnish with minced fresh parsley.

ROASTED BUTTERFISH WITH HERBS

Makes 4 servings
Time: 40 minutes

8 to 12 butterfish, gutted, with heads on, about 3 pounds
2 tablespoons olive oil

Salt and freshly ground black pepper to taste

½ cup dry white wine

½ cup any fish or chicken stock (pages 40–41), more white wine, or water

A handful chopped fresh herbs: rosemary, tarragon, sage, basil, parsley, thyme, alone or in combination

1 tablespoon butter

Preheat the oven to 400°F. Rinse the fish well and dry them between paper towels. Put the olive oil in a skillet or baking dish that can later be heated on top of the stove. Place the fish in the oil, season with salt and pepper, turn the fish over, and season again.

Roast the fish for about 8 minutes, shaking the pan occasionally to prevent sticking. When the fish are done (there will be no trace of blood in the body cavity), remove them from the pan to a platter; put the platter in a low oven. Add the wine and stock to the pan juices and reduce slightly over high heat. Add the herbs, stir, and add the butter; lower the heat to a minimum, and stir gently just until the butter melts. Taste for seasoning, pour the sauce over the fish, and serve.

ALTERNATIVE FISH FOR THIS RECIPE:

Croaker, small mackerel, mullet, pompano, porgy, or spot. Adjust cooking times accordingly.

CARP

Latin name(s): *Cyprinus carpio*.
Other common names: German carp, Chinese carp.
Common forms: Mostly whole fish, although fillets and steaks can be cut.
General description: Freshwater fish, frequently farmed, best in winter months. Carp are rarely harvested at under three pounds, but can grow to fifty pounds; most are sold in the five- to eight-pound range. Although most carp meat is white, fillets have a stripe of dark flesh that is usually trimmed before cooking. Carp skin is edible but not especially delicious.
For other recipes see: Striped bass, blackfish, catfish, cod, dogfish, grouper, haddock, halibut, monkfish, pollock, red snapper, rockfish, tilefish, turbot.
Buying tips: Carp is often kept alive in tanks, to be killed just before cleaning. Just because the fish is alive, however, doesn't necessarily mean it is fresh; the tanks should not be overly crowded, and the fish within should be active rather than sluggish. Carp is difficult to scale at home; leave this task to the fishmonger.

The Chinese began cultivating carp before the birth of Christ. It's an extremely hardy fish, and easy to raise—all it takes is a hole filled with fresh water and temperatures above freezing. In fact, the disadvantage of carp is that other fish simply cannot compete with it; there was a time in the late nineteenth century when carp were eradicated as pests.

Like catfish and tilapia, farm-raised carp can have a muddy flavor. But, for the most part, these are good-flavored fish sold at reasonable prices. Make sure you get the fish scaled; it's not an easy job (some people just remove the skin, but it is edible). In addition, trim the dark meat from fillets; it is tough and not especially appetizing. When eating whole fish, trim the dark meat as you eat.

BRAISED CARP

Makes 6 servings
Total time: 60 minutes
A Chinese-style recipe, slightly Americanized.

One 4-pound carp, cleaned, gutted, and scaled, preferably with head on
Salt
Flour for dredging
½ cup peanut oil
20 pearl onions, peeled
1 pound white mushrooms, halved
¼ pound oyster mushrooms
½ pound lotus root, peeled and sliced ¼ inch thick (available in Asian markets; optional)
5 pieces star anise (available in Asian markets or any store with a good selection of spices)
1 tablespoon minced garlic
1 tablespoon high-quality soy sauce
4 cups rich chicken stock
¼ cup sherry wine vinegar
Freshly ground black pepper to taste
½ cup minced fresh chives or garlic chives for garnish

Preheat the oven to 400° F. Rinse and dry the fish; cut three or four vertical slashes on each side of the fish, 1 or 2 inches apart. Heat a baking dish or similar pan long enough to fit the fish (cut off the fish's head if necessary) over medium-high heat for a few minutes. Salt the fish inside and out and dredge lightly in flour; shake to remove any excess. Add the peanut oil to the pan and raise the heat to high. When the oil is hot—a pinch of flour will sizzle—add the fish and sear on both sides; remove from the pan.

Add the onions and mushrooms to the pan and cook, stirring, over medium-high heat until lightly browned. Add the lotus root, anise, garlic, soy sauce, stock, and vinegar, season with salt and pepper, and stir. Return the fish to the pan, cover (aluminum foil is fine), and put it in the oven. Bake until the fish's flesh comes off the bone with ease, about 30 minutes.

Remove the fish to a platter and keep warm. Over high heat, reduce the liquid in the pan by half. Take out the star anise and check the sauce for seasoning. Serve by spooning portions of the fish off the bone, topping with the sauce, and garnishing with the chives.

ALTERNATIVE FISH FOR THIS RECIPE:
Whole grouper, red snapper, or tilefish.

HELEN ART'S GEFILTE FISH

Makes 10 or more servings, at least a dozen pieces depending on their size
Time: About 2 hours
This is my grandmother's recipe although, of course, she never used a food processor. I always do.

2 to 3 pounds fish scraps—bones, heads (gills removed), skin—from carp and other white-fleshed fish
3 cups sliced onions
3 pounds carp fillets or a mixture of carp and other freshwater fish such as pike and white-fish, skinned and trimmed of dark meat

3 large eggs, lightly beaten
2 tablespoons matzo or cracker meal
1 cup water, more or less
Salt and plenty of pepper (white pepper is traditional)
5 medium-size carrots, peeled and cut into chunks
Prepared red and white horseradish

Put the fish scraps in a large pot with about a third of the onion. Cover with plenty of water (top the scraps by 3 or 4 inches), bring to a boil, then reduce to a simmer.

In a food processor fitted with the steel blade, pulse the remaining onions and the fish fillets until coarsely chopped (overprocessing is a danger here, so be careful). Add the eggs, one at a time, pulsing after each addition. Add the matzo meal and about ½ cup water and process for a few seconds; the mixture should be light, smooth, and almost fluffy. Add a little more water if it seems too dry. Season with salt and pepper and taste; the mixture should be well seasoned and delicious.

Drop the carrots into the simmering stock. With wet hands, shape the fish mixture into small ovals, about the size of eggs. Lower each one of them into the simmering stock; don't worry about crowding. Simmer for 1 ½ hours, covered. Turn off the heat and allow the fish to cool in the liquid.

With a slotted spoon, remove the fish balls and the carrots to a platter. Reduce the stock, if necessary, to about 4 cups. Strain it over the fish balls, cover the platter, and refrigerate. Serve the fish cold, with a bit of the jelly, a few carrot pieces, and plenty of horseradish.

ALTERNATIVE FISH FOR THIS RECIPE:
Any white freshwater fish, plus any fairly light, gelatinous white-fleshed fish, such as dogfish, john dory, rockfish, red snapper, turbot, or wolffish.

FILLET OF CARP WITH
SMOTHERED ONIONS

Makes 4 servings
Time: 60 minutes

I associate carp with onions and other sweet vegetables, and so I cook these onions in butter; you can use olive oil if you like.

¼ cup (½ stick) butter
3 or 4 large Spanish onions, thinly sliced
Salt and freshly ground black pepper to taste
½ teaspoon minced fresh thyme or 1 pinch dried
1 tablespoon tomato paste or 1 medium-size fresh tomato, peeled, minced, or pureed
½ cup white wine
1 or 2 carp fillets, skinned and trimmed of dark meat, about 1 ½ pounds
Minced fresh parsley for garnish

Melt the butter over medium heat in a large skillet. When the foam subsides, add the onions and cook them, stirring occasionally, until they are very soft and dark; do not let them burn. Season with salt and pepper, then stir in the thyme and tomato paste. Add the wine, raise the heat to high, and let the liquid bubble away for 1 minute or so. Place the carp in among the onions, spooning some of the onions over the fish. Simmer over low heat until the fish is opaque throughout, about 10 minutes (use a thin-bladed knife to peek within). Garnish with the parsley and serve.

ALTERNATIVE FISH FOR THIS RECIPE:
This is best with very firm fillets: blackfish, grouper, monkfish, or Atlantic pollock.

CARP QUENELLES WITH DILL

Makes 6 appetizer servings
Time: About 1 hour

The most essential difference between quenelles and gefilte fish can be summed up in one word: cream. This addition not only makes quenelles lighter, it allows them to cook more quickly. Traditionally, quenelles were made with pike, but carp is both more widely available and more flavorful.

2 pounds fish scraps—bones, heads (gills removed), skin—from carp and other white-fleshed fish or about 1 quart Flavorful Fish and Vegetable Stock (pages 40–41)
1 bunch fresh dill, the stalks separated from the leaves
1 quart water
1 teaspoon salt
1 pound carp fillets, skinned, trimmed of dark meat, and cut into chunks
2 large egg whites
1 teaspoon fresh lemon juice
1 ½ cups heavy cream
Freshly ground black pepper to taste
6 tablespoons (¾ stick) butter, cut into bits

Begin by making the stock: Combine the scraps and dill stalks with the water and salt and simmer over medium heat for about 20 minutes. Turn off the heat and let the stock cool while you prepare the quenelles. Strain it into a large pot.

To make the quenelles, place ½ cup of the dill leaves and the carp fillets in a food processor. Pulse until they're chopped and blended, then add the egg whites one at a time, processing for about 10 seconds after each addition. Add the lemon juice, and 1 cup of the cream, season with salt and pepper, and process until smooth. Work quickly so the mixture remains cool.

Bring the stock to a gentle simmer; its surface should be shimmering. Make 12 egg-shaped quenelles, shaping them with two tablespoons or your wet hands. Gently lower them into the poaching liquid and simmer for about 10 minutes, turning once.

Remove the quenelles with a slotted spoon, drain them on paper towels, and keep them warm by covering them with an inverted bowl. Boil the stock until it is reduced to about 1 cup. Mince the remaining dill. Stir the butter into the stock, a piece at a time, until the sauce thickens. With the sauce simmering, add the remaining cream and most of the remaining dill. Taste for seasoning. Serve the quenelles with the sauce; garnish with a bit of dill.

ALTERNATIVE FISH FOR THIS RECIPE:

Any white freshwater fish, plus any fairly light, gelatinous white-fleshed fish, such as dogfish, john dory, rockfish, red snapper, turbot, or wolffish.

STEAMED CARP

Makes 4 servings
Time: About 20 minutes
A simple and basic Chinese preparation.

1 whole carp, gutted and scaled, with head on, about 3 pounds
1 tablespoon white wine vinegar
1 tablespoon high-quality soy sauce
1 teaspoon sesame oil
Salt and freshly ground black pepper to taste
½ cup whole scallions, cut into 1- to 2-inch lengths
1 cup snow peas, trimmed
One 1-inch piece fresh ginger, peeled, thinly sliced, and slivered
1 clove garlic, thinly sliced and slivered
Cooked white rice
Minced cilantro (fresh coriander) for garnish

Make three or four slashes, from top to bottom, on each side of the fish. Mix together the vinegar, soy sauce, and sesame oil and rub all over the fish. Sprinkle it with salt and pepper, then place it on a plate. Scatter the scallions and snow peas over and

around it. Press about half of the ginger and garlic into the slashes and sprinkle the rest over it.

Remove the carp's head if necessary, then steam, on the plate, in a bamboo or improvised steamer (page 38), for about 15 minutes, then check for doneness (the flesh of the fish will be opaque clear down to the bone). For each serving, scoop some of the flesh off the bone and place it on a portion of white rice, with some vegetables and accumulated juices. Garnish with a bit of minced cilantro.

ALTERNATIVE FISH FOR THIS RECIPE:

This technique can be used with almost any whole fish, but it's best with those that combine flavor and texture, such as grouper, porgy, sea bass, red snapper, or tilefish.

POACHED CARP

Makes 4 servings
Time: 40 minutes
Lake fish such as carp are staples in landlocked Burgundy, where cooks tend to prepare them as if they were meat. Most places that sell carp will be happy to cut you a few steaks from a whole fish. The variations here are more Eastern European in style and spirit.

1 tablespoon olive oil
4 to 6 slices good bacon (about ¼ pound), minced
Four 1- to 1 ½-inch-thick slices of carp
Flour for dredging
8 to 10 cloves garlic, roughly chopped
2 cups chopped onion
1 bay leaf
Several sprigs fresh thyme or ½ teaspoon dried
1 ½ cups red wine
Minced fresh parsley for garnish

Heat the olive oil over medium heat in a 12-inch skillet for 1 or 2 minutes. Add the bacon and cook, stirring, until browned; remove the bacon with a slotted spoon.

Dredge the carp slices in the flour and brown, in the same skillet, for about 2 minutes per side over medium-high heat. Remove to a plate and keep warm. Reduce the heat to medium and add the garlic and onion to the pan; cook, stirring, until the onion softens, about 5 minutes. Add the bay leaf, thyme, and wine. Let the wine bubble away for 1 minute or so. Return the carp to the pan, cover, and simmer until tender, about 10 minutes (a thin-bladed knife will pierce the carp easily when it's done). Remove the cover and put the carp on a platter. Reduce the liquid if necessary. Garnish the carp with the bacon and parsley and spoon a bit of the sauce over all. Serve immediately, with crusty bread.

ALTERNATIVE FISH FOR THIS RECIPE:

Any steaks of firm, white-fleshed fish: blackfish, grouper, Atlantic pollock, rockfish, red snapper, sablefish, or sturgeon.

CARP POACHED WITH ROOT VEGETABLES:

Combine 2 cups chopped onion, 2 cups chopped peeled potatoes (or beets, turnips, carrots, or parsnips, or a combination), 2 cups water, a handful of minced fresh dill, and some salt and freshly ground black pepper. Simmer until the root vegetables begin to soften, about 10 minutes, then add 4 slices of carp. Simmer until the carp is cooked through, another 15 to 20 minutes. Serve hot or chilled, garnished with minced fresh parsley.

CARP WITH SOUR CREAM AND DILL:

Simmer the carp, covered, in about 1 inch of court bouillon (page 41) or a mixture of 8 parts water or fish stock to 1 part vinegar. When the fish is cooked through, remove it to a platter and keep it warm. Reduce the liquid to a cup or so, then stir in ½ cup sour cream, ¼ cup minced fresh dill or parsley, some salt and freshly ground black pepper, and prepared horseradish to taste (at least 1 tablespoon). Spoon the sauce over the fish, garnish with minced parsley or dill, and serve.

CATFISH

Latin name(s): *Ictalurus punctatus*.

Other common names: Bullhead, channel cat. For ocean catfish, see wolffish.

Common forms: Whole, fillets. Wild fish range to five pounds; more common farmed fish average about a pound each. There is an increasing quantity of good quality frozen fillets available.

General description: Widely farmed medium-firm white-fleshed fish. Cultured fish have fairly insipid flavor, wild fish can be muddy, although not unpleasantly so. Fish have no scales, but are always skinned before eating.

For other recipes see: Blackfish, carp, cod, dogfish, flatfish, grouper, haddock, ocean perch, pollock, rockfish, red snapper, sablefish, scrod, sea bass, tilefish, weakfish, whiting, wolffish.

Buying tips: Catfish fillets are sold all over the country, but raised mostly in the South, so be sure that they appear fresh before buying: The flesh should be white rather than grayish or brown, and the flavor should be sweet and fresh, not at all muddy or moldy.

I caught catfish in the lakes of upstate New York when I was young, but since no one told me I could eat them, I didn't. My first, then, was from the Mississippi River, at one of Illinois's many fried fish restaurants along the banks. I was lucky: This was one of the restaurants that treated the fish with the respect it deserved, and it was delicious—crunchy, sweet, and slightly muddy, tasting just the way the river smelled.

Just twenty years ago, almost all catfish came straight from the great rivers; some were found in lakes and estuaries. They were dipped in cornmeal and deep-fried (I'm not sure anyone thought about doing much else with them). The annual catch was about five thousand tons. Now, catfish farming is Mississippi's biggest industry—it surpassed cotton a few years ago—with annual production surpassing 150,000 tons.

Farm-raised catfish—which is what you'll find in supermarkets and most fish stores—has little of the character that distinguishes river cats. In some ways, that's been its selling point; there's nothing to dislike. So if you're looking for a plain-jane white fillet, look no further. They're even being bred small, so portion sizes are convenient (gone are the two-hundred-pound catfish such as the one Huck Finn pulled out of the Mississippi).

PEPPER-FRIED CATFISH

Makes 2 to 4 servings
Time: 30 minutes

See the general guidelines for deep-frying fish, pages 34–36, before making this dish.

1 cup milk
1 pound catfish fillets
Vegetable oil for deep-frying
1 ½ cups cornmeal
2 tablespoons freshly ground black pepper
½ teaspoon cayenne pepper
Salt to taste
Lemon wedges
Spicy Pepper Sauce for Fried Fish (page 42)

Pour the milk into a bowl and let the catfish soak in it while you heat 3 to 4 inches of oil to about 375°F. Mix the cornmeal in a plastic bag with the peppers and salt. Drain the fillets, then shake them in the cornmeal in the bag; shake off any excess coating and fry them until golden on both sides, about 5 minutes. Drain on brown paper bags or paper towels and serve immediately, with lemon wedges or the pepper sauce.

ALTERNATIVE FISH FOR THIS RECIPE:

Blackfish, cod, dogfish, grouper, haddock, orange roughy, pollock, rockfish, red snapper, tilefish, weakfish, whiting, or wolffish. Adjust cooking times accordingly.

SPICY FRIED CATFISH:

You can season the cornmeal with thyme, sage, curry powder, cinnamon, chili powder, cumin, or five-spice powder (available in Asian markets). Use at least 1 tablespoon of most spices per cup of cornmeal.

CURRY-SAUTÉED CATFISH

Makes 4 servings
Time: 20 minutes

1 to 1 ½ pounds catfish fillets
Juice of ½ lemon
Salt to taste
½ teaspoon freshly ground black pepper
1 tablespoon curry powder
¼ cup peanut or vegetable oil
Flour for dredging
Lime wedges
Salsa Fresca (page 209)

Rub the fillets all over with the lemon juice. Heat a 12-inch nonstick skillet over medium-high heat for 3 to 4 minutes. Mix together the salt, black pepper, and curry powder. Pat this mixture onto the fish. Add the oil to the pan and, when it is hot (a pinch

of flour will sizzle), begin dredging the fillets in the flour. Place them in the oil and cook them. Do not crowd; turn the fillets when they are brown, about 3 minutes. Cook until browned on the other side. Keep the fillets warm in a low oven until the cooking is all done. Serve immediately with the lime wedges and/or salsa.

ALTERNATIVE FISH FOR THIS RECIPE:

Blackfish, cod, dogfish, grouper, haddock, orange roughy, pollock, rockfish, red snapper, tilefish, weakfish, whiting, or wolffish. Adjust the cooking times accordingly.

CATFISH SANDWICHES WITH ARUGULA AND SPICY MAYONNAISE

Makes 4 servings
Time: 20 minutes

¼ cup sour cream
¼ teaspoon cayenne pepper or to taste
¾ cup mayonnaise, homemade (page 43) or storebought
¼ cup peanut or olive oil
4 catfish fillets, 3 to 4 ounces each
Cornmeal for dredging
2 cups arugula, washed and dried
4 good rolls or sections of French or Italian bread
Salt and freshly ground black pepper to taste

Heat a 12-inch nonstick skillet over medium-high heat for 3 to 4 minutes. Mix the sour cream and cayenne into the mayonnaise.

Add the oil to the skillet and, when it's hot (a pinch of cornmeal will sizzle), dredge the fish in the cornmeal. Place the fillets in the oil—do not crowd them—and cook until golden, about 3 minutes per side; do not overcook. Drain briefly on paper towels. Make sandwiches with the catfish, arugula, and mayonnaise. Season with salt and pepper.

ALTERNATIVE FISH FOR THIS RECIPE:
Blackfish, cod, dogfish, grouper, haddock, orange roughy, pollock, rockfish, red snapper, tilefish, weakfish, whiting, or wolffish. Adjust the cooking times accordingly.

STIR-FRIED CATFISH WITH NAPA CABBAGE AND RED PEPPERS

Makes 2 servings
Time: 30 minutes
The fillets of very few white fish—catfish, dogfish, grouper, and rockfish—are perfect for stir-frying. The pieces are done in a couple of minutes and, as long as they are removed from the pan before they overcook, they will not fall apart.

½ to ¾ pound catfish fillets, cut into chunks for stir-frying
1 tablespoon rice or distilled vinegar
¼ cup peanut or vegetable oil
1 teaspoon minced garlic
1 teaspoon minced peeled ginger
2 scallions, green and white parts, minced
1 medium-size red bell pepper, seeded and cut into strips
2 cups shredded Napa cabbage
Salt and freshly ground black pepper to taste
½ cup any fish or chicken stock (pages 40–41) or water
1 tablespoon high-quality soy sauce

Preheat a wok over high heat. Toss the catfish chunks with the vinegar and set aside. Add the oil to the wok and immediately add the garlic, ginger, and scallions. Stir-fry for 30 seconds, then add the pepper strips. Cook 1 minute, stirring, and add the cabbage. Season with salt and pepper; if you feel that the cabbage is cooking too slowly, cover the wok. If not, toss and cook for about 5 minutes. Add the stock, soy sauce, and fish and cook, stir-

ring, until the fish is cooked through, about 3 minutes. Serve immediately, with rice.
ALTERNATIVE FISH FOR THIS RECIPE:
Blackfish, dogfish, grouper, Atlantic pollock, rockfish, red snapper, or wolffish. Adjust the cooking times accordingly.

"OVEN-FRIED" CATFISH

Makes 4 servings
Time: 15 minutes
This fifties-style recipe works. If you want to get really authentic, use cornflake crumbs.

1 ½ pounds catfish fillets
1 ½ cups milk
Plain bread crumbs for dredging
Salt and freshly ground black pepper to taste
3 tablespoons butter, melted
Lemon wedges

Soak the catfish in the milk while you preheat the oven to its highest temperature, short of broiling. Season the bread crumbs with salt and pepper; dredge the still-wet fish in the bread crumbs, patting them to make sure they adhere. Drizzle a little of the butter over the bottom of a baking pan, then put the fillets in. Drizzle with the remaining butter. Bake near the top of the oven for about 8 minutes; the catfish will be tender and opaque when done. Serve immediately, with lemon wedges.
ALTERNATIVE FISH FOR THIS RECIPE:
Any white fillet you like: Blackfish, carp, cod, dogfish, flatfish, grouper, haddock, orange roughy, ocean perch, pollock, rockfish, red snapper, sablefish, scrod, sea bass, tilefish, weakfish, whiting, or wolffish. Adjust the cooking times accordingly.

ROASTED CATFISH FILLETS WITH CREAMY PESTO

Makes 4 servings
Time: 30 minutes

This mayonnaiselike pesto is a bit of an indulgence. You can, if you prefer, substitute the more standard pesto recipe on page 41.

1 to 1 ½ pounds catfish fillets
¾ cup olive oil, plus extra for brushing
Salt and freshly ground black pepper to taste
1 clove garlic, peeled
1 teaspoon Dijon mustard
1 large egg
1 tablespoon balsamic vinegar or fresh lemon juice
30 fresh basil leaves, rinsed and dried

Preheat the oven to 500°F. Brush both sides of the catfish with olive oil, season with salt and pepper, and place on a baking dish. Roast for about 6 to 8 minutes, shaking the pan occasionally; the fish is done when it is opaque throughout.

Meanwhile, combine the garlic, mustard, egg, vinegar, salt, and pepper in a blender or food processor. Blend for 30 seconds. Add the basil leaves and blend again. Add the oil, a bit at a time, until the mixture achieves a thin, mayonnaiselike consistency. Top the fish with the creamy pesto and serve.

ALTERNATIVE FISH FOR THIS RECIPE:

Blackfish, cod, dogfish, flatfish, grouper, haddock, perch, Atlantic pollock, rockfish, red snapper, tilefish, weakfish (sea trout), or wolffish. Adjust the cooking times as necessary.

CHAR

Latin name(s): *Salvelinus alpinus*.
Other common names: Arctic char, alpine trout, salmon trout.
Common forms: Whole fish, fillets.
General description: To the nonprofessional, virtually indistinguishable from salmon; almost always farm-raised, and almost always in the three- to four-pound range. As with salmon, the skin is edible and delicious.
For other recipes see: Salmon, trout.
Buying tips: As a farm-raised fish, char is usually in splendid shape; the only question is how long has it been sitting at the retailer's? Look for bright, silvery skin and clear, unmarred, orange-pink flesh. The smell should be fresh and clean.

There are several types of char (the entire salmon-trout family is a mass of confusion to the uninitiated) and some of them are caught wild. These fish vary widely in size, geographical distribution (some are caught in lakes, most are circumpolar), color (white to pink to orange), and texture.

None of this matters much, however, since the only char most of us see is the farm-raised product from the North Atlantic. This fish, which is usually of excellent quality, is much like salmon in every way except size (it is smaller) and price (it is more expensive). Treat it exactly as you would salmon.

PAN-GRILLED CHAR

Makes 2 or 3 servings
Time: 15 minutes

Char is delicate, more like trout than salmon in flavor, so it must be treated with respect. This is the simplest preparation possible.

1 char fillet, about 1 pound, skin on (it need not be scaled)
¼ cup coarse salt
Salt and freshly ground black pepper to taste
2 teaspoons butter, melted

Heat a 12-inch nonstick skillet over high heat for 5 minutes; the pan should be really hot. Sprinkle it with the coarse salt. Place the fillet in the pan and cook, undisturbed, over high heat, for 8 to 10 minutes. The skin will burn, but the fish will cook through quite nicely. The top may appear underdone, but by the time you get it to the table it will be ready; if, however, this makes you uncomfortable, flip the fillet and cook the other side for 30 seconds, *no more*. Sprinkle with salt and pepper, drizzle it with the melted butter, and serve.

ALTERNATIVE FISH FOR THIS RECIPE:
Salmon; adjust the cooking time according to the thickness of the fillet.

CLAMS

Latin name(s): *Mercenaria mercenaria* (hard-shell clam); *Mya arenaria* (soft-shell clam); and others.
Other common names: Hard-shell clams: quahog, chowder clam, littleneck, top neck, count neck, cherrystone, hard clam, Manila clam, butter clam, cockle, pismo clam, baby clam; soft-shell clams: steamer, squirt clam, gaper, nannynose, belly clam, horse clam, mud clam, geoduck, razor clam, long clam.
Common forms: Whole (live), shelled (rarely), chopped (canned, fresh, or frozen).
General description: One of the most widespread and popular of all bivalve mollusks; species vary from region to region but are easily divided into two types (see below).
For other recipes see: Conch, mussels, oysters.
Buying tips: Whole clams *must* be alive when sold (page 8). Minced clams may be fresh or frozen; if fresh, the package should be dated.

Clams have not always been popular; although Native Americans ate them, and turned their shells into wampum, some Pilgrims fed them to their pigs. Now, however, we like them enough to make them scarce. One result is that prices of smaller clams, those best for eating on the half shell and steaming, have skyrocketed in the past decade. Another is that giant sea clams—which may weigh hundreds of pounds, obviously too large and tough for eating on the half shell—are often processed for canning and freezing, to be used in chowders and sauces.

Still, live clams are widely available. Although the selection can be confusing—especially when you travel from one region to another—all clams are either hard-shell or soft-shell (razor clams, which look like straight razors and can have sharp edges, can be considered soft-shells). Within each category, the smaller clams are more tender, the larger ones tougher. The smallest hard-shells, such as littlenecks—less than two inches across, and sometimes half that—are highly prized, while the largest, roughly three to six inches wide and usually called quahogs or chowder clams, are best minced and used in chowders, fritters, hash, and the like.

A similar division can be made in the soft-shell category; the small clams—steamers—are best after a brief steaming, with little adornment. The largest, such as the enormous geoduck (pronounced "gooey-duck"), whose neck may protrude several feet from its shell, require special preparations: Only their necks are used and, following a brief parboiling, these are skinned. They are then usually minced or ground before being included in recipes, although they can be sliced and treated like squid.

Most clams grow in tidal flats; the hard-shells in sandier bays and along beaches, the soft-shells in muddier areas. Both hard- and soft-shell clams can be found on the East and West coasts, though most of the commercial production is from the East Coast. Hard-shells come in a wide range of colors—from white to slate gray to brown—and are, of course, quite hard. Soft-shells, which gape, are usually stark white and quite brittle.

Clams may be dug at any time of year, but since it is easier to dig in the summer months, they may be more plentiful and less expensive at that time.

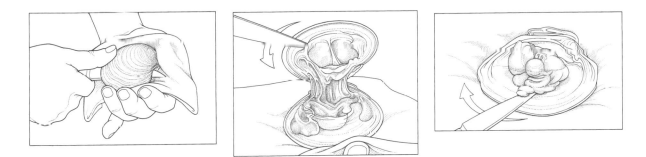

(Left): Using a towel to protect your hand, hold the clam with its "hinge" facing you. Wiggle a strong paring or clam knife between the two shells. Once you get it in there, slide it around to separate the shells. *(Center):* Open the clam and, with the point of the knife, scrape the meat attached to the top shell into the bottom shell, taking care to keep as much of the clam liquid as possible in the shell. *(Right):* Detach the meat from the bottom shell and remove or serve on the half-shell.

You can, of course, dig your own, once you check with the local regulators (or a good sporting goods shop, which can also sell you the appropriate rake or other tool) to see whether the beds are unpolluted and whether a license is required. Commercially harvested clams are subject to a fairly strict inspection and, by law, all clams should be shipped with a certification tag. You can ask to see this when you buy clams if you are wary of the dealer. Eating raw clams may be risky; see the general discussion on safety in seafood, pages 14–17.

Buying clams is easy, since those in the shell must be alive. When hard-shells die, you can move their shell apart; otherwise, they're shut up pretty tight, and you cannot even slide their shells from side to side. Live soft-shells react visibly to your touch, retracting their necks and closing slightly (they are never closed all the way—hence the name "gapers"). Dead clams smell pretty bad, so it's unlikely you'll be fooled.

Never store clams in sealed plastic (needless to say, never buy them in sealed plastic, either) or under water; they'll die. Just keep them in a bowl in the refrigerator, where they will remain alive for several days. The sooner you eat them, though, the better.

Soft-shells, which are never eaten raw, usually contain large quantities of sand, and it's worth trying to purge them of some of this before you cook them. Rinse them in water a few times, then soak them for a few hours in salted or seawater to which a couple handsful of cornmeal have been added. Then rinse them again. Shucking soft-shells is easy; see the recipe for Fried Clams (page 87) for directions. Figure two to three dozen steamers per person. If you're lucky enough to find fresh razor clams, treat them like soft-shells; they're very easy to shuck. Once completely purged of their sand, they are also wonderful in Sautéed Clams with Pasta, page 80.

Hard-shells require little more than a cleaning of their shells. I use a stiff brush to scrub them under running water. To shuck them, see the illustrated steps above. A traditional serving of littlenecks on the half-shell is six or twelve, although I like to eat nine; sauces are completely superfluous, although a squeeze of fresh lemon is nice if the clams are on the bland side. Small hard-shells—under two inches across—are also nice lightly steamed, like mussels.

SAUTÉED CLAMS WITH PASTA

Makes 2 servings
Time: 30 minutes

Some call a watery mess made with canned chopped clams "spaghetti with clam sauce." This is the real thing, a quickly made, intensely flavored sauce that leaves you with a few delicious (and not overcooked) clams to eat before you get down to the business of the pasta. Wonderful and authentic.

1 dozen littlenecks or other hard-shell clams, more or less, as small as you can find
⅓ cup olive oil
2 cloves garlic, peeled and crushed
1 dried hot red pepper
½ cup dry white wine
½ cup minced fresh parsley
1 teaspoon minced garlic
Salt and freshly ground black pepper to taste
⅔ pound linguine or other long pasta

Bring a large pot of water to a boil.

Wash and scrub the clams well, then dry them. Heat the olive oil in a 10-inch skillet over medium-high heat. Add the crushed garlic and hot pepper and cook, stirring occasionally, until the garlic is lightly browned. Add the clams, one or two at a time, stir briefly, and cover. Put the pasta in the boiling water and cook according to the package instructions.

Check the clams every minute or two; when the first one pops open (it will take just a few minutes), remove the cover and add the wine. Continue to cook over medium-high heat, shaking the pan occasionally. When most of the clams are open, add the parsley, minced garlic, and salt and pepper. Drain the pasta when it is done, put it in a warm bowl, and top with the clams and sauce. Serve the clams on the side of each plate. If any remain closed, open them with a knife.

ALTERNATIVE FISH FOR THIS RECIPE:
Mussels, cleaned according to the directions on page 183.

CLAMS WITH PESTO AND PASTA:
Prepare the clams as instructed above; when the clams begin to open, uncover and stir in ¼ cup dry white wine and 1 cup pesto (page 41). This is excellent without pasta, but you will need more clams.

CLAMS WITH PARSLEY PESTO:
Mix 1 cup chopped clams (from steamed or canned clams) with Parsley Pesto (page 208). Toss with 1 pound cooked pasta, adding additional olive oil if needed.

GRILLED FRESH CLAM PIZZA

Makes 4 to 8 servings
Time: 2 hours or less, including making the dough

I live in New Haven, where almost all the good restaurant food is Italian. The pizza here has a well-deserved reputation, and none is better than the fresh clam pizza at Pepe's. This is my adaptation of their recipe. You can make it in the oven or on any covered grill.

1 ¼ cups lukewarm water
1 teaspoon dry yeast
3 to 4 cups unbleached all-purpose flour (bread flour is best)
2 teaspoons salt
¼ cup olive oil or a bit more
2 dozen littlenecks or other hard-shell clams
2 cloves garlic, slivered
Coarse salt to taste
Chopped fresh parsley to taste

Combine the water and yeast in a bowl (you can use an electric mixer or a food processor, if you prefer; I do). Add about 2 cups of the flour and stir or mix until well blended. Add the salt, and 1 tablespoon of the olive oil, then continue to add flour ½ cup at a time, until you have a soft, slightly sticky, but manageable dough. Knead for a few minutes (30 seconds if you are using a food processor), then place in a covered bowl with another tablespoon of the olive oil, turning the dough to coat it with the oil. Let rest an hour or so (you can refrigerate or freeze the dough if you prefer to prepare it in advance); the dough will swell but not necessarily double. (You can let the dough rise in a cool place for as long as you like, punching it down once or twice when it doubles in bulk; this way, you can make the dough in the morning and the pizza in the evening; you can even refrigerate the dough to further retard its rising.)

Preheat a covered grill, or turn the oven on 30 minutes before you are ready to bake as high as it will go, short of broiling. If you have pizza stones, so much the better.

Flatten the pizza dough into a thick disk and let it relax, covered, while you prepare the clams. Rinse and scrub them well, then shuck them (page 79). You don't have to be too careful about keeping the meat whole or preserving the liquor (although it is nice to have around); what you want is some pieces of clams to scatter over the dough.

Roll the dough out on a well-floured board or pizza peel until it is about ¼ inch thick. (If you're grilling it, brush the top with olive oil and slide the dough onto the grill; cook, uncovered, until that side is firm and lightly browned, about 5 minutes, then flip the dough over and proceed according to the directions in the next paragraph.)

Brush the dough with olive oil (working quickly if you're using a grill), then sprinkle it with the clam pieces, garlic, and salt. Slide it into the oven, or cover the grill, and bake or grill until the crust is crisp and the clams and garlic sizzling in the oil, about 10 minutes. Sprinkle with parsley and serve immediately.

ALTERNATIVE FISH FOR THIS RECIPE:

Of course you can put almost anything on top of pizza dough, but I especially like chopped tenderized conch, shucked mussels, scallops, sea snails (removed from the shell), or peeled shrimp.

STIR-FRIED LITTLENECKS IN HOT SAUCE

Makes 4 servings
Time: 20 minutes

Use the smallest clams you can find for this dish. Since the recipe makes abundant sauce, you can increase the amount of clams by a pound or two and still have plenty of liquid for the rice.

3 pounds or more littlenecks or other hard-shell clams
2 tablespoons peanut or vegetable oil
1 tablespoon minced garlic
1 teaspoon peeled and minced fresh ginger
½ cup any chicken or fish stock (pages 40–41), white wine, or water
1 tablespoon dry sherry
1 tablespoon high-quality soy sauce
1 teaspoon chili-garlic paste (available in Asian markets) or to taste
Freshly ground black pepper to taste
Minced cilantro (fresh coriander) for garnish

Rinse the clams in several changes of water, until the water runs clear; drain. Make rice—it will take longer than cooking the clams (I recommend about 2 cups of raw short-grain rice for this dish).

In a wok or large, deep pot, heat the oil over medium-high heat. When it shimmers, add the garlic and ginger and stir for 30 seconds or so. Add the clams, raise the heat to high, and stir. Add the stock and cook, stirring occasionally, until the clams begin to open, 3 to 5 minutes. Add the sherry, soy sauce, chili-garlic paste, and black pepper, lower the heat to medium, and continue to cook and stir until almost all the clams are open, a few minutes more. (Those clams that do not pop open can be easily opened at the table with a knife.) Garnish with cilantro and serve immediately over rice.

ALTERNATIVE FISH FOR THIS RECIPE: Mussels, shrimp, or sea snails.

GRILLED MIXED MOLLUSKS

Makes 4 appetizer servings
Time: 30 minutes

Use any mixture of clams, mussels, and oysters you can put together. On vacation by the sea, for example, you might easily get all three; on sale at the supermarket you might only use one. No matter; for most people, the novelty of grilled molluscan shellfish—and their wonderful flavor—comes as a completely enjoyable surprise. This dish can be made in the oven, too.

30 to 40 hard-shell clams, mussels, and/or oysters
¼ cup (½ stick) butter
Hot pepper sauce or chili-garlic paste (available in Asian markets) to taste (I use ¼ teaspoon, just enough to add some zing)
Fresh lemon juice to taste

Preheat a gas grill or start a charcoal fire (to make this dish in the oven, preheat to 500°F). Meanwhile, debeard and wash the mussels according to the directions on page 183, rinse the clams, and scrub the oysters (page 201). Gather them all together and, when the fire is hot, dump them unceremoniously onto the grill. (If you are using the oven, place the mollusks in a baking pan and slide it into the oven.) Melt the butter, add the hot sauce and the lemon juice, and let the mixture sizzle for a couple of minutes over low heat.

As the mollusks open—some will take 1 or 2 minutes, others several—remove them to a platter and move the more stubborn members to hotter parts of the fire. Try to keep the liquor in the shells of those that open, but don't be a fanatic about it; you're bound to lose some. When they're all cooked, drizzle the butter over them and bring to the table for a messy snack, warning your fellow diners that the hot shells can be damaging to careless lips.

MIXED MOLLUSKS BARCELONA STYLE: Cook the clams, mussels, and/or oysters on a very hot griddle (it should preheat over high heat for at least 10 minutes), with nothing else. Do only a few at a time so that the heat does not dissipate. Serve with ground black pepper and lemon wedges.

STEAMED LITTLENECKS WITH BUTTER AND HERBS

Makes 2 appetizer servings
Time: 20 minutes

I think nine is the perfect number of littlenecks for an appetizer; six is too few when they're so delicious, and twelve can be a bit much. Be sure not to salt the broth until you taste it; clams can be quite salty.

18 littleneck or other hard-shell clams, the smaller the better
½ cup dry white wine
3 shallots, chopped
Several sprigs fresh parsley
Several sprigs fresh mint
1 tablespoon chopped fresh chervil, if available
¼ cup (½ stick) unsalted butter, softened

Wash and scrub the clams well. Place them in a kettle with the wine, shallots, parsley, mint, and chervil. Cover the pot and cook over high heat, shaking occasionally, until the clams are open, 5 to 10 minutes. Remove the clams to two bowls and reduce the sauce over high heat by about half (if any of the clams did not open, leave them in the sauce while you reduce it—they will "pop" eventually). Lower the heat to medium and stir in the butter, 1 tablespoon at a time, until melted. Pour the sauce over the clams and serve.

ALTERNATIVE FISH FOR THIS RECIPE:
Well-scrubbed mussels (double the quantity) or oysters.

CURRY-SPICED CLAMS WITH GREENS

Makes 4 servings
Time: 30 minutes
Vary this recipe by substituting cornmeal for the flour, and other spices—lots of black pepper, sage, or chili powder, for example—for the curry.

6 tablespoons olive oil
2 tablespoons balsamic vinegar
2 teaspoons Dijon mustard
3 tablespoons peanut, olive, or vegetable oil
½ cup all-purpose flour
2 tablespoons curry powder
Salt and freshly ground black pepper to taste
30 to 35 fresh littleneck or other hard-shell clams, shucked
6 cups mixed greens, your choice, washed and dried

Mix together the olive oil, vinegar, and mustard. Set aside.

Heat a 12-inch nonstick skillet over medium-high heat for about 5 minutes. Add the peanut oil. Season the flour with the curry powder, salt, and pepper. When the oil is hot (a pinch of flour will sizzle), dredge the clams in the flour and add them, a couple at a time, to the skillet. Raise the heat to high and cook until golden, turning once, about 2 minutes total.

Drain the clams on paper towels and toss the greens with the dressing. Divide the greens among four plates and top each with a portion of clams. Serve immediately.

ALTERNATIVE FISH FOR THIS RECIPE:
Oysters.

CLAMS IN BROTH WITH ROASTED GARLIC

Makes 4 servings
Time: 1 ½ hours
A wonderfully hearty soup, and a great alternative to clam chowder.

1 whole head garlic, separated but not peeled
2 tablespoons olive oil
1 large onion, minced
4 cups any chicken or fish stock (pages 40–41)
24 littleneck or other hard-shell clams, well-scrubbed
Zest of 1 orange
Juice of 2 limes
Salt and freshly ground black pepper to taste
1 lime, cut into small wedges
1 small chile pepper (such as jalapeño), seeded and minced (optional)

Preheat the oven to 350°F. Place the garlic cloves in a small ovenproof bowl with 1 tablespoon of the oil. Cover with aluminum foil and roast, covered, until tender, about 1 hour. Cool.

Squeeze the garlic meat from its husks and reserve. In a large saucepan, heat the remaining oil over medium-high heat, add the onion, and cook until soft. Add the stock and bring to a simmer. Add the clams, cover, and cook until they open, 5 to 10 minutes. Add the garlic, orange zest, lime juice, salt, and pepper. Stir and taste for seasoning. Serve immediately, passing the lime wedges and jalapeño at the table.

ALTERNATIVE FISH FOR THIS RECIPE:
You can mix shellfish (shrimp and scallops are

especially good), pieces of whole fish (red snapper or rockfish, for example), and any fillets. Be careful not to overcook.

RICE AND CLAMS

Makes 4 servings
Time: 45 minutes
Risotto with Shrimp and Greens (page 268) is the more-or-less classic rice and shellfish dish, but this South American specialty is no less interesting. Use a number of shellfish—scallops, shrimp, mussels, oysters—for variety.

2 tablespoons olive oil
1 small onion, minced
1 ½ cups long-grain rice
1 tablespoon ground cumin
Salt and freshly ground black pepper to taste
2 ½ cups any chicken or fish stock (pages 40–41)
24 littleneck or other hard-shell clams, the smaller the better, shucked, liquor reserved
Minced cilantro (fresh coriander) for garnish

Heat the oil over medium heat in a saucepan or skillet; add the onion and cook until it wilts. Add the rice and stir to coat with oil; add the cumin, salt, and pepper and cook another minute, stirring. Add the stock, bring to a boil, lower the heat to medium, cover, and cook for 15 minutes, until almost all the liquid is absorbed. Stir in the clams, cover, and cook an additional 2 minutes. Garnish with cilantro and serve immediately.

ALTERNATIVE FISH FOR THIS RECIPE:

As mentioned above, any shellfish will work here, but pieces of other sturdy fish can be used: blackfish, dogfish, grouper, monkfish, Atlantic pollock, rockfish, red snapper, or wolffish.

RICE WITH CLAMS NORTH AMERICAN STYLE:
Sauté the onion in 2 tablespoons butter. Add 1 teaspoon minced garlic and the rice. Add 1 cup dry white wine and let most of it bubble away. Add the stock and proceed as directed above.

NEW ENGLAND CLAM CHOWDER

Makes 4 servings
Time: 30 minutes
Basic and essential. Add corn for variety; use tomatoes and their juice in place of the milk and cream to make Manhattan clam chowder.

4 to 6 slices good bacon (about ¼ pound), minced
1 cup minced onion
2 cups peeled and chopped potatoes
2 tablespoons flour
2 cups any chicken or fish stock (pages 40–41), augmented by as much liquor as you can salvage from the clams
Salt and freshly ground black pepper to taste
1 cup milk
1 cup heavy cream, half-and-half, or more milk
24 hard-shell clams, shucked, cut in half or quarters if very large
1 tablespoon butter
Minced fresh parsley for garnish

In a casserole, fry the bacon until crisp. Remove it with a slotted spoon and set aside. Over medium heat, cook the onions and potatoes in the bacon fat until the onions soften. Sprinkle with the flour and stir. Add the stock and cook until the potatoes are almost cooked through, about 10 minutes.

Season with salt and pepper and add the milk and cream; bring to a simmer and add the clams. Float the butter on top of the chowder; by the time it melts, the clams will be ready. Garnish with parsley and reserved bacon and serve.

RHODE ISLAND CLAM CHOWDER:
Omit the bacon and potatoes. Sauté the onion

and 1 cup chopped celery in a little butter or oil. Omit the flour; use 4 cups stock, a portion of which should be clam liquor. Add the clams, salt, pepper, and nothing else.

CHICKEN WITH CLAMS

Makes 4 to 6 servings
Time: About 1 hour
The garlic-ginger-scallion trinity gives this a vaguely Chinese feel.

1 dozen littlenecks or other hard-shell clams, the smaller the better
1 chicken, about 3 pounds, cut up
2 tablespoons olive or vegetable oil
Flour for dredging
3 medium-size carrots, peeled and diced
3 cloves garlic, peeled and crushed
2 tablespoons butter
½ cup dry white wine
1 tablespoon peeled and grated fresh ginger or a sprinkling of ground
Salt and freshly ground black pepper to taste
1 scallion, including about half the green part, minced

Wash and scrub the clams; wash and dry the chicken. Heat a 12-inch nonstick skillet over medium-high heat for 3 to 4 minutes. Add the oil. When it's hot (a pinch of flour will sizzle), dredge the chicken in the flour, then brown it on both sides. Remove the chicken to a plate as it browns.

Meanwhile, cook the carrots and garlic in the butter in a pot or casserole over medium-low heat. When the carrots are a bit softened, add the wine. Let it bubble away a bit, then add the chicken, ginger, salt, and pepper. Cover and simmer slowly until the chicken is almost done, about 30 minutes, stirring occasionally. Lay the clams on top of the chicken, cover, and cook over medium heat until the clams open, about 10 minutes. Garnish with the scallion and serve on rice, or with fried potatoes or good bread.

CLAMS WITH GREENS AND LINGUIÇA

Makes 4 servings
Time: 30 minutes
Clams and linguiça are a popular combination among New England's Portuguese fishermen.

½ pound dry garlicky sausage, such as linguiça, kielbasa, or chorizo, cut into bite-size pieces
1 pound kale or chard or any other pot green
1 big starchy potato, thinly sliced
4 cups Quickest Chicken Stock (page 40) or Fast Fish Stock (page 40)
Salt and freshly ground black pepper to taste
1 medium-size onion, peeled and minced
1 dozen littlenecks or other hard-shell clams, washed well

Cook the sausage in a dry skillet until nicely browned, stirring occasionally.

Wash the greens in several changes of water. Chop them coarsely, then combine them, the potato, sausage, and stock in a 3- or 4-quart saucepan. Simmer over medium heat until the greens are tender, 10 to 20 minutes. Season with salt and pepper, add the onion and clams, cover, and simmer until the clams are open, about 10 minutes. Serve immediately.

ALTERNATIVE FISH FOR THIS RECIPE:

This is a very versatile preparation, and can be made with mussels, scallops, shrimp, or chunks of blackfish, cod, dogfish, grouper, orange roughy, pollock, rockfish, red snapper, scrod, tilefish, or wolffish. Remember that all fish cooks quickly, especially in liquid, and be careful not to overcook.

CLAM FRITTERS

Makes 5 or 6 appetizer servings
Time: 30 minutes

Clam fritters are a Rhode Island staple, especially in the area around Point Judith. Sad to say, however, those served in restaurants are usually fairly bland, and tend to be made with pieces from the largest, toughest clams imaginable. These are much more interesting, and, if you use good clams, impossible to stop eating. See the general guidelines for deep-frying fish, pages 34–36.

1 ½ cups unbleached all-purpose flour
2 teaspoons salt
1 teaspoon sugar
½ teaspoon freshly ground black pepper
½ teaspoon ground ginger
⅛ teaspoon cayenne pepper
12 ounces beer
Juice of 1 lemon
1 cup minced hard-shell clams
Vegetable oil for deep-frying
Lemon wedges

Mix together the flour, salt, sugar, pepper, ginger, and cayenne in a large bowl. Add the beer and lemon juice and stir to blend. Mix in the clams.

Heat at least 2 inches of oil in a deep-fryer or large saucepan. When oil is about 375°F (a piece of bread will bounce in lively fashion and brown in a few seconds) drop the batter, 1 tablespoon at a time, into the oil. Cook 6 or 8 fritters at a time, without crowding. Drain on paper towels and serve immediately with lemon wedges.

ALTERNATIVE FISH FOR THIS RECIPE:
Cooked conch, cooked octopus, oysters, or squid.

CLAM HASH

Makes 4 servings
Time: 60 minutes

Buttery and crunchy, this is a sure hit with any fan of corned beef hash.

5 tablespoons butter
About 2 cups minced or ground clams
About 2 cups finely chopped peeled potatoes
½ cup minced scallions, green and white parts,
  or onion
1 teaspoon minced garlic
Salt and freshly ground black pepper to taste
4 poached or soft-boiled eggs (optional)

Melt 2 tablespoons of the butter in a 12-inch non-stick skillet over medium heat. Mix together the clams, potatoes, scallions, and garlic; when the butter foam subsides, spread the mixture in the pan and flatten with a spatula. Lower the heat, season with salt and pepper, and cook slowly until browned on the bottom, about 20 minutes (check by lifting a corner with a spatula).

Slide the cake onto a plate, top with another plate, and invert. Melt another 2 tablespoons butter in the pan and, when it melts, return the cake to the pan. Cook until browned. Spread with the remaining tablespoon of butter and serve, with or without poached eggs.

ALTERNATIVE FISH FOR THIS RECIPE:
Tenderized conch or minced shucked oysters.

BAKED STUFFED CLAMS

Makes 4 to 6 appetizer servings
Time: 30 minutes

Like pasta with clam sauce, this is a legitimate dish that was done wrong by restaurants and lazy cooks. Try them; they're not much work, and are a wonderful starter.

12 hard-shell clams, each under 2 inches in diameter
1 tablespoon olive oil
1 tablespoon minced garlic
1 cup unseasoned bread crumbs, preferably fresh
2 tablespoons minced parsley
Dash cayenne pepper
Salt and freshly ground black pepper to taste
Fresh lemon juice as needed
Lemon wedges
Tabasco sauce to taste

Preheat the oven to 450°F. Shuck the clams, reserving half the shells and as much of the liquid as possible. Mince the clams (you can do this in a small food processor if you are careful; don't over-process).

Heat the olive oil over medium heat in an 8- or 10-inch skillet. Add the garlic and cook, stirring, just until it begins to color. Add the bread crumbs and cook, stirring, until the mixture browns. Add the parsley, cayenne, salt, and pepper, stir, and taste for seasoning. Add the reserved liquor and, if the mixture seems dry (or simply if you want a moister, more acidic mixture), some lemon juice. Add the minced clam meat.

Stuff the shells with this mixture, place them on a cookie sheet or baking pan, and bake until lightly browned, 10 to 15 minutes. Serve hot or warm, with lemon wedges and Tabasco.

BASIC STEAMED CLAMS ("STEAMERS")

Makes 4 servings
Time: Several hours soaking, 15 minutes preparation
I've had Maine steamers so sweet and good I've ignored the lobster they were served with. When they're like that, forget the melted butter.

4 to 6 pounds soft-shell clams ("steamers")
Melted butter

Clean and purge the clams of their sand: Rinse them in water a few times, then soak them for a few hours in salted (or sea-) water to which a couple handsful of cornmeal have been added. Then rinse them again.

In a covered pot over medium-high heat, steam the clams in an inch or so of boiling water, shaking the pot until the clams open, 5 to 10 minutes. Place the steamed clams in one bowl and strain the broth into another. Serve immediately, with melted butter. Eat by removing each clam from its shell, then taking the black membrane off of its "neck" or "foot," dipping it in the broth to clean it of any remaining sand, then into the butter.

ALTERNATIVE FISH FOR THIS RECIPE:
Small hard-shell clams (littlenecks), mussels.

FRIED CLAMS

Makes 4 appetizer servings
Time: 24 hours soaking, 30 minutes preparation
Fried clams are usually made with steamers because they are so easy to shuck. But if you have a hankering for a mess of fried clams, I would say get thee to a clam shack, because shucking even two dozen soft-shell clams takes the average nonprofessional a good 15 minutes, and eating two dozen fried clams is the work of an instant. Furthermore, they spatter as they fry.

So, if you want to fry clams, I suggest you limit the production to a few; see the general guidelines for deep-frying, pages 34–36. Serve them with pesto (page 41), any light tomato sauce (page 209), or one of the dipping sauces for squid (page 299), and keep it light and elegant.

24 to 30 steamers, purged according to the directions on page 87
Vegetable oil for deep-frying
3 cups unbleached all-purpose flour, more or less
Salt and freshly ground black pepper to taste
1 tablespoon baking soda (optional)

Shuck the clams by inserting a paring knife on either side of the hinge (you'll soon see why some New Englanders call these "piss clams") and running it between the shells, scraping along the top shell to loosen the clam. Open the shell and cut the clam from the bottom shell. Use the paring knife to slit and remove the black membrane covering the "foot"; that's where most of the sand hides. Drop the clams into cold water.

Rinse the clams in two or three changes of water; shake off excess water in a strainer or, even better, a salad spinner. Lay a clean kitchen towel flat on a table, and spread the clams evenly on it. Cover with another clean towel and roll the towels up together with the clams inside. Let sit for a few minutes while the oil is heating. (You may clean the clams early in the day and refrigerate them, wrapped in the towels.) The clams must be bone-dry before frying, or you and your kitchen will be attacked by spattering oil (if you have a covered fryer, such as that made by DeLonghi, use it).

Preheat 2 or 3 inches of the oil to 350°F. Place the flour in a bowl and season it liberally with salt and pepper; add the baking soda, which helps the flour brown. When the oil is ready (if your fryer doesn't have a thermostat, or you don't have a frying thermometer, drop a small piece of bread in the oil; it should sink, then rise to the top and begin bubbling away), remove about half of the clams from the towels—more if your fryer is a big one, less if it is small; a quart of oil can handle all of these clams at once—and toss them into the flour. Move them around until they are well coated with flour and shake off the excess. Place the clams in the frying basket and carefully lower it into the hot oil. Unless the fryer has a cover, stand back.

The clams are done when they are lightly browned, 2 minutes or so; do not overcook. Drain quickly in the frying basket, then on paper towels. Serve immediately with one of the sauces suggested above.

ALTERNATIVE FISH FOR THIS RECIPE: Littleneck clams or mussels.

COBIA

Latin name(s): *Rachycentron canadum*.

Other common names: Sargentfish (it has stripes on its side), bonito (it is not), ling (a name also misapplied to some cod), crabeater.

Common forms: Steaks, fillets.

General description: An attractive, fast-swimming, East and Gulf Coast fish ranging from twenty pounds (typical market size) to a hundred pounds (rare). Like most fish that feed on crustaceans, cobia has meaty, good-tasting flesh. Grill it as you would swordfish.

For recipes see: Mako shark, swordfish.

Buying tips: This is a good eating fish that is not fished commercially. If you see some, and the fish is firm, pearly white, and sweet-smelling, grab it. Make sure the tough skin is removed for you.

COD

Latin name(s): *Gadus morhua* (Atlantic); *Gadus macrocephalus* (Pacific).

Other common names: Scrod (a market name for small cod or haddock, also spelled schrod), Arctic cod, Greenland cod, true cod (Pacific), Alaska cod, etc.

Common forms: Whole (to ten pounds and larger), steaks, skinless fillets (most common), salt cod.

General description: Arguably the most important fish in the history of the world; lean, medium-firm, snow white meat with a big flake and mild flavor. The paradigm of white-fleshed fish.

For other recipes see: Blackfish, carp, catfish, dogfish, flatfish, grouper, haddock, halibut, monkfish, ocean perch, pollock, rockfish, red snapper, sablefish, sea bass, tilefish, turbot, weakfish, whiting, wolf-fish.

Buying tips: The thicker part of the fillet (the "loin," or "captain's cut") is generally preferred, because it is of more uniform thickness; I wouldn't make a fuss about it. Cod should be snow white, without a hint of dryness, browning, or off odors; when it's really fresh, you'll know it—the fillet is just gorgeous.

"At one time," wrote the late A. J. McClane, the dean of American fish writers, cod "filled the belly of the world." You might think of cod as the pig of the sea. Almost every part of it is eaten somewhere (cheeks, tongues, and sounds—air bladders—are all good), and you can do almost anything to it: salt it, smoke it, pickle it, and cook it by any method you can imagine, although grilling is difficult at best.

Yet somehow cod developed a reputation as common, as if its popularity detracted from its quality. This is absurd: If cod were rare, it would be a luxury item, treasured for its snow white, delicate flesh and subtle but far from characterless flavor. Cod is no longer dirt cheap, but it remains available in good quantity, and is less expensive than snapper, swordfish, tuna, and salmon.

Americans eat more cod than any other finfish, and almost always have. Though many Pilgrims starved to death or succumbed to disease within months of their arrival on the shores of the New World—about half failed to survive their first New

England winter—this was due to timing and stupidity rather than a paucity of natural resources. The Pilgrims' stubbornness, a trait which preceded the word "Yankee," kept them here. But it also caused them to ignore the bounty of the sea while they awaited supplies from England.

This changed, of course: By 1640 the new fishermen were producing hundreds of thousands of dried salted cod annually. And 150 years later, on the eve of the American Revolution, fishing was the cornerstone of the New England economy, and fishing meant cod. In the middle of the eighteenth century a crude wooden codfish was hung in the chambers of the Massachusetts legislature "as a memorial to the importance of Cod-Fishery to the welfare of this Commonwealth." An effigy of the "sacred cod" still hangs in the State House in Boston.

Salt cod fueled the New England coastal economy. Massachusetts produced so much of it that even after its citizens consumed enormous quantities of the stuff there remained so much that the

British, who were world-trade leaders at the time, couldn't dispose of it all. They didn't even have enough ships to carry it, and were forced, for the first time, to allow the colonies to engage in trade of their own.

Thus cod was sent directly from the colonies to the Mediterranean. (It was also sent to the Caribbean, where it directly involved the Yankees in the slave trade—future slaves were fed dried cod.) The "codfish aristocracy" had been born.

In March 1775 King George, angry over a number of inappropriate and insubordinate acts, decided to hit the codfish industry where it hurt. He issued the New England Restraining Act, which would have prevented the colonists from fishing the Great Bank, essentially denying them their most reliable industry. But the Boston Cod Party failed to become part of history when the Redcoats met the Minutemen at Concord while George's Restraining Act papers were in transit.

Today, salt cod has become a novelty item, and most of the cod trade is in fresh fillets. Buy the thickest section you can (sometimes called "captain's cut" or loin), but don't fret if only thinner cuts are available. Notice that most fillets have a thin, shiny section of fat where the skin has been removed; this dulls as the fish deteriorates, and is therefore a good indicator of freshness. Fillets of cod (and of many other fish) usually contain some bones, which can be removed with needlenose pliers before cooking if you like (see illustration, page 229); alternatively, make the V-cut used to remove the dark section from bluefish (page 58). My feeling is that most diners are perfectly capable of removing the few bones that remain in fillets at the table.

A word or two about really fresh cod—that is, cod you caught yourself or bought fresh from a dayboat fisherman: Many people, especially Scandinavians, who have been eating cod for eons, believe that the best preparation for fresh cod is the simplest: Boil it in lightly salted water and serve it with boiled potatoes and butter.

You can also make a fresh version of salt cod: Cover steaks or fillets with salt and let sit, refrigerated, for 24 hours, then pour off the brine. The cod will keep for a week or so. To prepare it, soak the fillet for a few hours, changing the water occasionally. Then cook as you like; the result will be firmer than fresh cod. To prepare store bought salt cod, see the recipe for Salt Cod Cakes, page 98.

BROILED COD FILLETS

Makes 2 to 3 servings
Time: 15 minutes
This is a basic recipe with almost infinite variations, a few of which I give here.

1 cod fillet, about 1 pound
2 tablespoons olive oil or butter
Salt and freshly ground black pepper to taste
½ lemon, quartered

Preheat the broiler while you prepare the cod. Brush a baking pan with a little oil or rub it with some butter, then brush the rest of the oil on the fish or dot it with butter and sprinkle with salt and pepper. Place the fillet about 4 inches from the source of the heat. Change the pan's position every 2 minutes or so in order to brown the cod evenly, and baste once or twice with the melted fat from the bottom of the pan. Generally, when the top of the fish is nicely browned, the fish is cooked through (figure about 8 to 10 minutes per inch of thickness, measured at the thickest point). If the fish is browning too quickly, turn off the broiler and finish the cooking with the oven set at 500°F. Cod begins to "gape"—its sections separate—when it is done, is opaque throughout, and will offer no resistance to a thin-bladed knife; avoid overcooking. Serve with lemon quarters.

ALTERNATIVE FISH FOR THIS RECIPE:

Fillets of almost any white-fleshed fish: Blackfish, carp, catfish, dogfish, flatfish, grouper, haddock, ocean perch, pollock, rockfish, sablefish, sea bass, red snapper, tilefish, turbot, weakfish, whiting, or wolffish. Adjust the cooking times accordingly.

COD BROILED WITH BREAD CRUMBS:

Sauté ½ cup unseasoned bread crumbs briefly in 2 tablespoons butter or oil over medium-low heat, with or without a minced clove of garlic. Spread the bread crumbs on top of the fish about 2 minutes before it finishes cooking.

COD BROILED WITH WHITE WINE AND HERBS:

Douse the fish with ¼ cup dry white wine and a sprinkling of chopped fresh herbs—tarragon, rosemary, parsley, chives, etc.—about halfway through the cooking. A teaspoon or so of minced garlic may be added at the same time. Serve with the liquid and good crusty bread.

BROILED COD PROVENÇAL STYLE:

Halfway through cooking, top the fish with a mixture of ½ cup chopped fresh tomato, ¼ cup chopped pitted calamata olives, 1 tablespoon chopped fresh parsley or basil, 1 teaspoon minced garlic, salt, and freshly ground black pepper, 1 tablespoon olive oil, and 1 teaspoon balsamic vinegar.

BROILED COD WITH PESTO:

Spread a few tablespoons pesto (page 41) atop the fish about 2 minutes before it finishes cooking.

COD À LA VASCA

Makes 4 to 6 servings
Time: 20 minutes
This recipe comes from my friend Ignacio Blanco, owner of Meson Galicia in Norwalk, Connecticut.

2 cod fillets, about 1 pound each
Flour for dredging
¼ cup olive oil

Salt and freshly ground black pepper to taste
3 cloves garlic, peeled and crushed
½ cup dry white wine
¼ cup minced fresh parsley
3 scallions or shallots, chopped, about ¼ cup

Preheat the oven to its highest temperature short of broiling, 500°F or more. Heat a 10-inch non-stick skillet with an ovenproof handle over medium-high heat for a minute or two. Dredge the top side of the cod in flour. Add the olive oil to the pan and heat it until a pinch of flour sizzles when dropped into the pan.

Cook the cod, floured side down, until it is browned, 3 to 4 minutes. Turn it and season with salt and pepper. Add the garlic, wine, parsley, and scallions. Immediately put the pan in the oven, and bake until the cod is done (cod begins to "gape"—its sections separate—when it is done, is opaque throughout, and will offer no resistance to a thin-bladed knife; avoid overcooking), 5 to 7 minutes. Serve immediately, with rice or fried potatoes.

ALTERNATIVE FISH FOR THIS RECIPE:

Fillets of almost any white-fleshed fish: Blackfish, carp, catfish, dogfish, flatfish, grouper, haddock, ocean perch, pollock, rockfish, sea bass, red snapper, tilefish, turbot, weakfish, whiting, or wolffish. Adjust the cooking times accordingly.

COD WITH SAGE BUTTER

Makes 4 servings
Time: 30 minutes
If you have good fish stock on hand, you might roast the cod fillet (8 to 10 minutes at 450°F should do it) and make the sauce separately, starting with the reduction. This method, however, gives delicious results.

2 cups water or 1 cup water and 1 cup dry white wine

Salt and freshly ground black pepper to taste
1 bay leaf
30 fresh sage leaves or 1 tablespoon dried
1 ½ pounds cod fillet, cut in two if necessary
¼ cup (½ stick) butter

Preheat the oven to 300°F. Place the water, salt, pepper, bay leaf, and 10 of the sage leaves in a deep skillet with a cover. Bring the water to a boil, simmer over medium heat about 5 minutes, then gently lower the piece(s) of cod into the liquid. Cover and simmer gently over low heat for 5 minutes. Remove the cod carefully (it will not be fully cooked), place it on a platter, cover the platter loosely with aluminum foil, and put it in the oven.

Over high heat, reduce the cooking liquid to about ½ cup (this will take about 10 minutes). Scoop out the bay leaf and stir in the butter, 1 tablespoon at a time. Add the remaining sage and cook over low heat, stirring, about 1 minute more. Taste for seasoning. The fish will have finished cooking in the oven (cod begins to "gape"—its sections separate—when it is done, is opaque throughout, and will offer no resistance to a thin-bladed knife). Serve the cod topped with the sauce.

ALTERNATIVE FISH FOR THIS RECIPE:

Fillets of almost any white-fleshed fish: Blackfish, carp, catfish, dogfish, flatfish, grouper, haddock, ocean perch, pollock, rockfish, sablefish, sea bass, red snapper, tilefish, turbot, weakfish, whiting, or wolffish. Adjust the cooking times accordingly.

PAN-FRIED COD FILLET WITH GINGERED SNOW PEAS

Makes 2 to 3 servings
Time: 30 minutes

I had been making this dish with snow peas for some time when my next door neighbor had a bumper crop of both "regular" peas and the edible-podded kind. The combination is pleasing to the eye and the palate, but any combination of peas (including frozen) and edible pods will work nicely here.

1 cod fillet, about 1 pound, cut into 2 or 3 pieces
¼ cup all-purpose flour
3 tablespoons high-quality soy sauce
1 teaspoon minced garlic
1 teaspoon peeled and minced fresh ginger
2 tablespoons peanut or vegetable oil
2 cups snow peas, edible-podded peas, pea pods, or any combination
¼ cup any fish or chicken stock (pages 40–41), sherry, or dry white wine
1 teaspoon sesame oil

Wash and dry the fillets. Preheat the oven to 200°F and begin warming a 12-inch nonstick skillet over medium heat. Make a thin batter by mixing the flour with 2 tablespoons of the soy sauce and water as needed (about ½ cup). Add half the garlic and ginger to the batter. Put 1 tablespoon of the oil in the skillet and heat for 2 to 3 minutes. Raise the heat to high, dip each of the fillets in the batter, and place them in the skillet.

Cook over medium-high heat, adjusting the heat so the oil is not smoking, until brown, about 3 to 4 minutes. Turn and brown the other side. When the cod is almost opaque all the way through, turn off the heat, remove it to a platter, and place the platter in the oven.

Turn the heat back to high, add the remaining tablespoon of oil along with the remaining garlic and ginger, and cook the peas over high heat, stirring or tossing occasionally, until they are lightly brown and their green color is vivid, about 2 minutes. Add the remaining tablespoon of soy sauce and the stock, and cook for 30 seconds. Add the sesame oil, stir, and turn off the heat. Use a slotted spoon to scatter the peas around the fish, then pour the sauce over all. Serve immediately over rice.

ALTERNATIVE FISH FOR THIS RECIPE:

Fillets of almost any white-fleshed fish: Blackfish, carp, catfish, dogfish, flatfish, grouper, haddock, ocean perch, pollock, rockfish, sea bass, red snapper, tilefish, turbot, weakfish, whiting, or wolffish. Adjust the cooking times accordingly.

EMMA'S COD
(Cod Roasted with Potatoes)

Makes 4 servings
Time: 60 minutes

There are many fish-and-potato recipes (such as that for Bluefish with Crisp Potatoes on page 62), but this, despite its simplicity—or because of it— is the ultimate. Like seviche, steamed mussels, grilled swordfish, or clams on the half shell, it showcases the fish perfectly. To vary this dish, use a layer of onions, scent the potatoes and fish with garlic and/or herbs, cook the potatoes in olive oil, and drizzle a few drops of balsamic vinegar over the fish when it's done, or see the variation below.

This dish is a guaranteed kid-pleaser, hence its alternative name; Emma is among my more discerning tasters.

6 tablespoons (¾ stick) butter
2 to 3 pounds waxy potatoes
Salt to taste
1 or 2 cod fillets, about 1 ½ to 2 pounds

Preheat the oven to 425°F; place 4 tablespoons of the butter in a baking dish—the shape doesn't matter, but it should be large enough to comfortably fit the fish—and melt it while the oven preheats. Peel the potatoes and slice them about ⅛ to ¼ inch thick (I use a mandoline). Remove the pan from the oven when the butter is melted. When the oven

is hot, stir the potatoes into the butter and salt liberally. Return the dish to the oven and set a timer for 10 minutes.

Every 10 minutes, turn the potatoes gently with a spatula. When they are nicely browned all over— 30 to 40 minutes—place the cod on top of them, dotting the fish with the remaining butter and some salt. Roast the cod for 8 to 12 minutes depending upon the thickness of the fillets (cod begins to "gape"—its sections separate—when it is done, is opaque throughout, and will offer no resistance to a thin-bladed knife; avoid overcooking). Serve immediately.

ALTERNATIVE FISH FOR THIS RECIPE:

Fillets of almost any white-fleshed fish: Blackfish, carp, catfish, dogfish, flatfish, grouper, haddock, ocean perch, pollock, rockfish, sablefish, sea bass, red snapper, tilefish, turbot, weakfish, whiting, or wolffish. Adjust the cooking times accordingly.

COD ROASTED WITH VEGETABLES:

Use any young or small vegetables with or in place of the potatoes: carrots, broccoli, onions, leeks, individually or in combination. Cook as above, baking until the vegetables are nearly done before adding the cod.

BAKED COD WITH SMOKED RATATOUILLE

Makes 4 servings
Time: 90 minutes

This is a time-consuming dish (although you can make it more quickly by sautéing or directly grilling rather than smoking the vegetables), but one that makes good use of late summer vegetables. Vary the ingredients according to what's available when you make the dish.

2 medium-size red bell peppers
6 to 8 tiny eggplant or 2 large

2 medium-size zucchini
3 large tomatoes
2 medium-size onions, peeled
8 cloves garlic, peeled and skewered together
Salt and freshly ground black pepper to taste
3 tablespoons olive oil, plus a little for drizzling
¼ cup minced fresh basil
1 or 2 cod fillets, about 2 pounds total
Minced fresh parsley for garnish

Build a charcoal fire or preheat a gas grill. Bank the fire to one side (if you're using a gas grill, turn off one of the burners) and toss a couple handfuls of soaked wood chips onto the hot part of the fire. Place the red peppers directly over the coals, the eggplant and zucchini next to them, in a slightly cooler spot, and the tomatoes, onions, and garlic over the cool part of the grill; cover the grill. Add charcoal and more wood chips to the fire if necessary, and turn the vegetables every 15 minutes, removing them as they begin to "collapse"; everything will be done within an hour, and some will be done earlier. Skin and core the tomatoes, remove the skin from the eggplants if it's thick, skin the peppers, and chop the onions. Mix everything together, keeping the garlic aside. Add the salt, pepper, olive oil, and basil.

Preheat the oven to 350°F. Line the bottom of a baking dish just large enough to hold the cod fillets with the ratatouille. Top with the fish, cutting it into pieces if necessary to cover most of the surface without overlapping. Stud the surface of the fish with the smoked garlic, then place the pan in the oven. Bake until the cod is done, about 30 minutes (the cod will become opaque and a thin-bladed knife will go right through the fish without encountering resistance). Garnish with the parsley and serve immediately.

ALTERNATIVE FISH FOR THIS RECIPE:

Fillets of almost any white-fleshed fish: Blackfish, carp, catfish, dogfish, flatfish, grouper, haddock, ocean perch, pollock, rockfish, sablefish, sea bass, red snapper, tilefish, turbot, weakfish, whiting, or wolffish. Adjust the cooking times accordingly.

COD IN GREEN SAUCE

Makes 4 servings
Time: 15 minutes
I make this dish, a Basque staple, with cod steaks, but fillets can be used as well, and substituting is easy; just reduce the cooking time.

½ cup olive oil
2 tablespoons minced garlic
4 cod steaks, about 1 ½ pounds total
Salt and freshly ground black pepper to taste
1 cup roughly chopped Italian (flat-leaf) parsley

Heat the olive oil and garlic in a 10- or 12-inch nonstick skillet over low heat. When the garlic floats and begins to color, add the cod steaks to the pan. Season them with salt and pepper and cook slowly, moving the fish in the oil from time to time. After about 5 minutes, turn the fish and add the parsley to the pan. Cook until the cod is done, 5 to 7 minutes more (it will easily pull away from the bone). Serve immediately, with white rice or crusty bread.

ALTERNATIVE FISH FOR THIS RECIPE:

Steaks of almost any white-fleshed fish: Blackfish, grouper, pollock, red snapper, tilefish, turbot, or whiting. Adjust the cooking times accordingly.

POACHED COD STEAKS WITH CORIANDER-MINT VINAIGRETTE

Makes 4 servings
Time: 45 minutes, plus time to chill
This dish begins with an assertive court bouillon and finishes with a sparkling vinaigrette. Pile left-

overs into pita bread and dress with vinaigrette for a terrific sandwich.

1 recipe Court Bouillon (page 41)
4 good-size cod steaks, about ½ pound each
½ cup extra virgin olive oil
Juice of ½ lime or lemon
Salt and freshly ground black pepper to taste
1 tablespoon minced shallot
1 tablespoon minced fresh mint
1 teaspoon minced cilantro (fresh coriander)
1 teaspoon minced fresh parsley

Over medium heat in a steep-sided skillet or broad casserole, bring the court bouillon to a boil. Lower the heat to a simmer and gently place the steaks in the liquid. Cook about 8 to 10 minutes, depending on thickness (about 8 minutes per inch of thickness). Remove the fish before it is fully cooked; it will retain enough heat to finish cooking. Cool, then chill.

Mix together the remaining ingredients. Taste and adjust seasoning. Spoon over the chilled cod steaks.

ALTERNATIVE FISH FOR THIS RECIPE:
Steaks of grouper, pollock, rockfish, red snapper, sturgeon, tilefish, or turbot.

COD AND VEGETABLE SOUP

Makes 4 to 6 servings
Time: 45 minutes
You can make this soup with water; the flavor, of course, will be less intense.

2 tablespoons olive oil
2 medium-size potatoes, peeled and diced
2 medium-size carrots, diced
2 medium-size onions, diced
2 cloves garlic, minced
8 to 10 cups any fish or chicken stock (pages 40–41), water, or a combination

Salt and freshly ground black pepper to taste
½ cup uncooked rice
1 to 1 ½ pounds cod fillet
½ cup minced fresh parsley

In a large saucepan, heat the oil over medium-high heat. Add the potatoes and carrots and cook, stirring, until the potatoes begin to brown. Add the onions and garlic and continue to cook, stirring, until the onion softens. Add the stock 2 cups at a time, stirring. Simmer over medium-low heat for 10 minutes, taste for seasoning, and add the rice. Cook until the rice and vegetables are tender, another 20 minutes or so. Cut the cod into four to six pieces (depending on how many you are serving) and add it to the soup; cook just until a thin-bladed knife passes easily through one of the cod pieces, about 6 to 8 minutes. Serve immediately, sprinkled with the parsley.

ALTERNATIVE FISH FOR THIS RECIPE:
Fillets of almost any white-fleshed fish: Blackfish, carp, catfish, dogfish, flatfish, grouper, haddock, ocean perch, pollock, rockfish, sea bass, red snapper, tilefish, turbot, weakfish, whiting, or wolffish. Adjust the cooking times accordingly.

ASIAN NOODLES WITH FISH HEAD SAUCE

Makes 4 appetizer or 2 main course servings
Time: About 45 minutes
The best stock is made from fish heads, and there's always plenty of meat left when you're done. Here's a recipe that gives you a quart of rich stock and uses less than half that much, leaving you some to freeze.

3 cod heads, about 1 ½ pounds, gills removed
4 cups water
1 medium-size onion, cut in half
1 tablespoon Thai or Vietnamese fish sauce (available in Asian markets)
1 tablespoon high-quality soy sauce

1 teaspoon sesame oil

½ teaspoon chili-garlic paste (available in Asian markets)

¾ pound wheat vermicelli (available in Asian markets; thin Italian pasta is a fine substitute)

2 scallions, minced

1 tablespoon minced cilantro (fresh coriander)

1 lime, cut into wedges

Put the cod heads, water, and onion in a pot, bring to a boil, and simmer gently over low heat for about 15 minutes. Let cool a little, then strain the stock. Measure out 1 ½ cups and save the rest for another use. Pick the meat off the fish heads and shred it with your fingers, removing any bones (most of the bones in the head are quite large, so this is not especially arduous). You will have a cup or more of meat.

Bring a large pot of water to a boil. Mix together the fish stock, fish sauce, soy sauce, sesame oil, and chili-garlic paste. Cook the pasta until it is not quite done, but retains a starchy interior. Drain it. Add the fish stock mixture to the pot, bring it to a boil, and add the cooked pasta and the meat from the fish heads. Continue to cook, stirring frequently, until the pasta is done. Divide into two or four bowls, and serve with scallions, cilantro, and pieces of lime for squeezing.

ALTERNATIVE FISH FOR THIS RECIPE:

It's not so much a question of which heads you can use, but which you will find. Likely candidates are grouper, red snapper, and tilefish.

NO-HOLDS-BARRED COD CHOWDER

Makes 4 servings

Time: 40 minutes

The trend in cooking is to try to make less be more; but nothing beats a real fish chowder. If you have accumulated some chunks of assorted white fish in your freezer, this is the place to use them.

⅛ pound good bacon, diced

1 large onion, chopped

3 medium-size potatoes (about 1 pound), peeled and cut into ½-inch cubes

4 cups Fast Fish Stock (page 40) or Quickest Chicken Stock (page 40)

1 to 2 pounds boneless cod, cut into 1-inch chunks

2 cups corn kernels (frozen are fine)

1 cup heavy cream

Salt and freshly ground black pepper to taste

In a 3- or 4-quart kettle, sauté the bacon over medium heat until nice and crisp. Remove the bacon with a slotted spoon and reserve. Still over medium heat, cook the onion and potatoes in the remaining bacon fat, stirring occasionally, until the onion is soft and the potato lightly browned, about 10 minutes. Meanwhile, heat the stock separately.

When the stock is warm, add it to the potatoes and onions and simmer over medium-low heat until the potatoes are just tender, about 10 minutes. Add the fish chunks and corn and cook until the fish is tender but not quite flaky, 8 minutes or so. Over low heat, add the cream, then taste for salt (it shouldn't need much) and pepper (this chowder is good with lots). When heated through, garnish with the reserved bacon and serve.

ALTERNATIVE FISH FOR THIS RECIPE:

Fillets of almost any white-fleshed fish: Blackfish, carp, catfish, dogfish, flatfish, grouper, haddock, ocean perch, pollock, rockfish, sea bass, red snapper, tilefish, turbot, weakfish, whiting, or wolffish. Adjust the cooking times accordingly.

SALT COD CAKES

Makes 4 servings
Time: 30 minutes, using cooked salt cod

No longer a staple, salt cod has become expensive and uncommon. The fish—called *morue* (French), *baccalà* (Italian), *bacalao* (Spanish), and *bacalhau* (Portuguese)—usually comes in wooden boxes or in large slabs of half a fish. Though the desalting process takes some time, it is easy, and the results are worth it: fish cakes made with salt cod are, quite simply, the best.

To prepare salt cod, remove its center bone (some salt cod is boneless) and cut the meat into large pieces. Soak them overnight, or up to 24 hours, changing the water at least four times. The fish must be cooked before using it in fish cakes: just poach it for 15 minutes or so (page 38), adding a clove of crushed garlic to the water if you like.

1 ½ cups flaked cooked salt cod
1 ½ cups cooked mashed potatoes
½ cup grated onion
2 large eggs
Salt and freshly ground black pepper to taste
Bacon fat or a mixture of butter and oil for sautéing
Flour or unseasoned bread crumbs for dredging

Mix together the fish, potatoes, onion, eggs, salt, and pepper. Cover the bottom of a 12-inch skillet with fat to a depth of at least ⅛ inch. Heat over high heat until the oil shimmers. Shape the salt cod mixture into cakes or small balls; dredge them in the flour, then fry until lightly browned all over, 3 to 4 minutes per side. Drain briefly on paper towels, then serve with lemon wedges, Spicy Pepper Sauce for Fried Fish (page 42), or Light Tomato Sauce (page 209).

ALTERNATIVE FISH FOR THIS RECIPE: Any leftover white-fleshed fish.

BRANDADE DE MORUE
(Creamed Salt Cod Mousse)

Makes 6 servings
Time: 45 minutes, using soaked salt cod

One of the great Provençal specialties, this rich, filling dish is a perfect example of the whole being greater than the sum of its parts: While you're assembling it, you will wonder why you're bothering. While you're eating it, you will wonder how you ever lived without it. Truly special, and easily made in a food processor, although you can use a mortar and pestle if you want to be traditional.

1 pound boneless salt cod, soaked overnight in several changes of cold water
2 cloves garlic, peeled
⅔ cup delicious olive oil
⅔ cup heavy cream or milk
Freshly ground black pepper to taste
Juice of 1 lemon
⅛ teaspoon grated nutmeg

Pick over the salt cod to remove any remaining bones or pieces of skin. Place it a skillet or saucepan with water to cover; bring the water to a boil, turn off the heat, and let cool for 15 to 20 minutes.

Place the cod in a food processor or blender along with the garlic and 2 tablespoons of the olive oil. Start processing and, through the feed tube, add small amounts of olive oil alternating with small amounts of cream. Continue until the mixture becomes smooth, creamy, and light. Add black pepper, some of the lemon juice, and the nutmeg. Blend and taste; the mixture may need a bit of salt and more lemon juice.

To serve, reheat the brandade in a double boiler or a covered baking dish in the oven (or even the microwave). Serve with crusty bread or, even better, make croutons by taking slices of bread, brushing them with olive oil, and baking them at 300°F until crisp, turning once. Make sure there are plenty of them.

FRIED SALT COD WITH GARLIC BATTER

Makes 4 servings
Time: 30 minutes, using soaked salt cod

1 pound salt cod, soaked overnight in several changes of water
1 cup unbleached all-purpose flour
1 teaspoon salt
1 teaspoon baking powder
1 large egg
1 cup milk
1 tablespoon olive oil
1 tablespoon garlic, minced with some salt as finely as possible
Freshly ground black pepper to taste
Vegetable oil for deep-frying
Lemon wedges

Pick over the salt cod to remove any remaining bones or pieces of skin. Cut the fish into strips about 2 inches long and 1 inch wide. In a bowl, mix together the flour, salt, and baking powder. In another bowl or measuring cup, beat the egg and mix it with the milk and olive oil. Add the wet ingredients to the dry ones, stirring just to blend; don't worry about leaving a few specks of flour (this is exactly like making pancake batter). Stir in the minced garlic and some pepper.

Heat at least 1 inch of oil in a deep skillet or fryer to about 375°F (if you don't have a thermostat or a frying thermometer, drop a small piece of bread in the oil; it should sink, then rise to the top and begin bubbling away). Dip the cod strips into the batter and fry, a few at a time—do not crowd—until golden and crisp, 3 to 4 minutes. Serve immediately, with lemon wedges.

MARINATED SALT COD SALAD

Makes 4 servings
Time: About 2 days, including soaking time

1 pound salt cod soaked over overnight in several changes of water
½ cup delicious olive oil
Freshly ground black pepper to taste
Fresh lemon juice to taste
1 cup minced fresh chives or garlic chives
4 to 6 cups assorted, well-washed greens (lettuces, arugula, mustard, mizuna, chicory, radicchio, etc.)

Pick over the salt cod to remove any remaining bones or pieces of skin. Cut it into small pieces and mix with the olive oil, pepper, lemon juice (at least 2 tablespoons), and about ½ cup of the chives. Marinate, refrigerated and covered, for about a day, stirring occasionally. Taste for seasoning and serve over the greens, garnished with the remaining chives.

GARLICKY SALT COD SALAD:

Cover the soaked cod with water and simmer for about 15 minutes. While it's still hot, cut it up and combine it with 1 teaspoon minced garlic, 3 tablespoons olive oil, and a handful of minced fresh parsley. Let cool, then serve atop greens, sprinkled with lemon juice and freshly ground black pepper.

SALT COD WITH GARLIC MAYONNAISE:

This is a basic aïoli: Cook the cod as in the first variation, then serve it warm, along with an assortment of poached vegetables—potatoes, carrots, cauliflower, or whatever you like—and the garlic mayonnaise on page 43.

ACCRAS DE MORUE

Makes 6 to 8 appetizer servings
Time: About 40 minutes, using soaked salt cod

These wonderful fritters are the staple appetizer of Guadeloupe and Martinique. They are addictive, and can be seasoned in a variety of ways; thyme and allspice (called pimiento in the islands) are standard.

1 pound salt cod, soaked overnight in several changes of water
1 small jalapeño or habanero pepper, seeded, deveined, and minced, or cayenne pepper to taste (optional)
1 teaspoon minced fresh thyme or ½ teaspoon dried
¼ teaspoon ground allspice
2 scallions, minced
1 tablespoon minced fresh parsley
1 cup unbleached all-purpose flour
1 teaspoon baking powder
1 large egg
⅔ cup milk, more or less
Vegetable oil for deep-frying
Lime wedges

Pick over the salt cod to remove any remaining bones or pieces of skin. Place it in a skillet or saucepan with water to cover; bring the water to a boil, turn off the heat, and let cool for 15 to 20 minutes. Remove it from the water, chop it finely, and mix it with the pepper, thyme, allspice, scallions, and parsley.

In a large bowl, mix together the flour and baking powder. Lightly beat the egg with ½ cup of the milk and pour them into the flour; stir together until well blended. The batter should be fairly stiff, but if it seems too dry, add the remaining milk. Stir in the salt cod mixture.

Heat 2 to 3 inches of oil to about 375°F. (If you don't have a thermostat or a frying thermometer, drop a small piece of bread in the oil; it should sink, then rise to the top and begin bubbling away.) Fry the batter by the tablespoonful, a few fritters at a time, turning once, until golden brown all over. Drain on paper towels and serve immediately or keep warm in a low oven until ready to serve. Serve with lime wedges.

ALTERNATIVE FISH FOR THIS RECIPE:

Clams (minced, raw or cooked), conch (minced, cooked), crab or lobster meat (minced, raw or cooked), or shrimp (minced, raw or cooked).

CURRIED ACCRAS:

Add curry powder and/or minced garlic to the batter; add about ½ cup seeded and minced red bell pepper to the batter.

CONCH

Latin name(s): Various species of Strombidae and Buccinidae (whelk).
Other common names: Whelk, scungilli, sea snail.
Common forms: Whole, out of shell (usually precooked); in shell (rare); cooked and frozen.
General description: The familiar large, whorled shell of the Atlantic and Caribbean; the texture and flavor of the meat are much like that of clams, and indeed minced conch may be substituted freely for minced clams.
For other recipes see: Clams, octopus, snails, squid.
Buying tips: Check whether the conch meat you buy has been precooked (this will usually be the case); if not, be aware that it is extremely perishable and that it will require extensive simmering—up to a couple of hours—before it becomes tender.

Conch (pronounced "konk") and whelk are different animals, but for culinary purposes they can be treated the same; essentially, they are both large sea snails. You might occasionally be offered live conch in the shell, but the chances are much greater that you will see a rather large (up to one-quarter pound) hunk of tan conch meat. This has been precooked, probably not to the point of tenderness, but enough so that cooking time is minimized. The only preparation necessary before cooking is cutting off the operculum, the hard, shell-like covering that protects the meat. After that you can chop or mince the meat and cook it until it softens, which usually takes fifteen to thirty minutes; if you by raw conch, plan on precooking for a couple of hours.

Conch is one of the least expensive mollusks. It still sells for under three dollars a pound for meat only, which, compared to the meat of related species, is a steal. It's available year-round, and can be used in almost any clam-meat recipe. Raw or cooked, conch meat is quite fragile; keep it as cold as possible, preferably on ice (see page 10 for tips on storing seafood).

CONCH FRITTERS

Makes 8 to 10 appetizer servings
Time: 60 minutes or a little more

1 cup unbleached all-purpose flour
1 teaspoon baking soda
1 teaspoon salt
½ teaspoon cayenne pepper or to taste
Freshly ground black pepper to taste
1 teaspoon fresh thyme leaves, chopped, or
   ½ teaspoon dried
1 cup water
2 large eggs, separated
Vegetable oil for deep-frying
Meat of 3 or 4 conchs, about 1 pound or a little
   less
1 medium-size onion, quartered
Lime wedges

Combine the flour, baking soda, salt, cayenne, black pepper, and thyme in a medium-size bowl. Add the water and beat with a whisk or electric mixer until well blended; add the egg yolks and beat again to combine. Let stand for 30 to 60 minutes.

When you're ready to cook, begin heating 3 or 4 inches of the oil to about 350°F. (If you don't have a thermostat or a frying thermometer, drop a small piece of bread in the oil; it should sink, then rise to the top and begin bubbling away.) Cut the operculum from the conch and cut the meat into chunks. Place the conch and onion in a food processor and pulse until both are minced. Beat the egg whites with an electric mixer until stiff peaks form; stir the batter once or twice, then stir half the egg whites into it. Gently fold in the other half. Fold in the conch-onion mixture.

Make fritters by dropping tablespoonsful of the mixture into the oil. Start with one, and taste it for seasoning. Then make a few at a time, without crowding; they only need about 1 minute per side. Scoop out the inevitable stray pieces of batter in between batches. Drain the fritters on paper towels and serve immediately with lime wedges. These can also be held for a few minutes in a warm oven.

ALTERNATIVE FISH FOR THIS RECIPE:
Clams or squid.

CONCH PANCAKES

Makes 12 appetizer servings
Time: 45 minutes
If you are a fan of sweetbreads, try this; the similarity is remarkable.

2 cups minced conch meat
1 medium-size onion, minced
½ teaspoon dried thyme or 1 teaspoon fresh leaves
¼ teaspoon cayenne pepper or to taste
1 teaspoon minced garlic
1 teaspoon peeled and minced fresh ginger
Salt and freshly ground black pepper to taste
2 or 3 large eggs

4 to 6 tablespoons unseasoned bread crumbs
Juice of 1 lime, if needed
Peanut or vegetable oil for sautéing
Lime or lemon wedges

In a large bowl, mix together the first seven ingredients. Beat the eggs and mix them in. Mix in enough bread crumbs to absorb any loose liquid and give the mixture a little body; it will not be a batter, but more like corned beef hash. Thin it with a little lime juice if necessary. Refrigerate, covered, until ready to cook.

Heat 2 tablespoons of peanut oil in a 12-inch nonstick skillet over medium-high heat. When the oil shimmers, shape the conch into small patties and place three or four in the pan. Don't crowd; you will have to cook in batches. Taste one and correct the seasoning if necessary. Cook until nicely browned on one side, about 3 minutes, adjusting the heat if necessary. Turn gently and brown the other side. Cook the remaining pancakes, adding oil as needed. Serve immediately, with lime or lemon wedges.

ALTERNATIVE FISH FOR THIS RECIPE:
Clams or squid.

CONCH SALAD, VERSION I

Makes 4 servings
Time: 1 hour, plus chilling time
You need not make this salad exclusively with conch, but can mix it with other shellfish such as shrimp, squid, octopus, or scallops. I do like the singular flavor of conch, however.

3 to 4 cups any chicken or fish stock (pages 40–41) or water
2 stalks celery, cut into big chunks
2 medium-size carrots, cut into big chunks

1 onion, peeled and quartered

1 tablespoon whole peppercorns

2 bay leaves

½ cup minced cilantro (fresh coriander)

1 pound conch meat, operculums removed, cut into ¼-inch dice

Salt and freshly ground black pepper to taste

¼ cup fresh lime juice

½ cup good olive oil

¼ cup minced scallions, green and white parts

Bring 3 cups of the stock to a boil, lower the heat, and add the celery, carrots, onion, peppercorns, bay leaves, half the cilantro, and the conch. After 30 minutes, check the conch for tenderness. Continue to cook, checking from time to time and adding more stock if necessary, until the conch is tender. When it is, remove the conch with a slotted spoon; reduce the remaining liquid to a glaze; strain, discarding the aromatics. Mix the liquid with the conch, salt, pepper, lime juice, olive oil, scallions, and remaining cilantro. Chill until ready to serve. Serve on a bed of mixed greens.

ALTERNATIVE FISH FOR THIS RECIPE:

You can use almost any shellfish for this—such as squid, octopus, clams, oysters, or shrimp—but only octopus would require such long cooking; the rest will cook in two or three minutes, so be sure to start with a flavorful stock, since the fish will be adding little to it.

CONCH SALAD, VERSION II

Makes 12 or more servings

Time: 1 to 4 hours

This is minimalist conch salad, to be eaten on crackers, preferably on a sailboat in the Caribbean.

1 pound conch meat, operculums removed, ground or finely minced

About ½ cup fresh lime juice

1 tablespoon Tabasco or other hot pepper sauce

Salt and freshly ground black pepper to taste

Combine all the ingredients and marinate, refrigerated, for 1 hour or more; the conch will be chewy but delicious.

CONCH WITH GARLIC AND LIMES

Makes 3 to 4 servings

Time: About 1 hour

I like this dish over white rice, but it's also good with bread.

1 pound conch meat, operculums removed, cut into ¼-inch dice

3 limes

5 cloves garlic

1 bay leaf

1 tablespoon sherry wine vinegar or other good vinegar

Salt and freshly ground black pepper to taste

1 large onion, cut in half

2 tablespoons olive oil

1 jalapeño or other hot pepper, deveined, seeded, and minced

2 tablespoons minced cilantro (fresh coriander) or to taste

Simmer the conch meat in water to cover with 1 of the limes, cut in half, 2 cloves of the garlic (unpeeled), the bay leaf, vinegar, salt, pepper, and half the onion. When it is tender, after about 30 minutes, turn off the heat and let the conch cool in its liquid.

Mince the remaining onion and garlic. Heat the olive oil over medium heat in a large skillet. Add the onion and jalapeño and cook until the onion softens. Add the garlic, along with the tenderized conch meat, to the skillet and cook for 5 minutes, stirring occasionally. Juice the remaining limes and add their juice to the skillet; taste for seasoning, garnish with the cilantro, and serve.

ALTERNATIVE FISH FOR THIS RECIPE:
Clams, octopus (precooked), or squid.

CONCH WITH TOMATOES:
Marinate the conch in about half the lime juice for 1 hour. Heat the oil and cook about 1 tablespoon minced garlic, stirring, until lightly colored. Add the bay leaf, vinegar, the minced half onion, and jalapeño and cook until the onion softens. Add the conch, scallions, and 2 ripe fresh tomatoes, roughly chopped. Simmer until the tomatoes liquefy, about 10 minutes. Garnish with minced scallions.

PASTA E SCUNGILLI

Makes 4 servings
Time: 45 minutes

½ cup olive oil
2 cloves garlic, slivered

4 or 5 dried hot red peppers or to taste
3 cups chopped tomatoes (canned are okay; drain first)
Salt and freshly ground black pepper to taste
½ pound conch meat, operculums removed, ground or finely minced
1 pound long pasta, such as linguine
½ cup minced fresh parsley

Set a large pot of water to boil for the pasta.

Heat the olive oil over medium heat in a large skillet. When it begins to shimmer, add the garlic and peppers. Cook, stirring, until the garlic browns; turn off the heat and wait a minute before adding the tomatoes. Cook over medium heat until the tomatoes begin to liquefy, about 5 minutes, then add the salt, pepper, and conch. Simmer, stirring occasionally, until the conch is fairly tender, about 30 minutes.

Salt the pasta water well, then cook the pasta according to package instructions. Drain and toss with the sauce; toss with half the parsley, sprinkle with the remaining parsley, and serve.

ALTERNATIVE FISH FOR THIS RECIPE:
Clams or squid.

CRAB

Latin name(s): *Callinectes sapidus* (blue crab); *Cancer magister* (Dungeness crab); *Paralithodes camtschaticus* (king crab); *Cancer irroratus, C. borealis* (rock or jonah crab); *Chionoecetes tanneri* (snow crab); *Menippe mercenaria* (stone crab); and others.

Other common names: Calico, green, tanner, lady, land, spider, etc. crab.

Common forms: Whole, live (especially blue and rock); whole, cooked (especially Dungeness); cooked (and often frozen) claws and sections (snow, king, stone).

General description: Dozens of species of these familiar crustaceans dot our coasts; their meat is valuable and widely appreciated. Like lobster, they should be sold live, or cooked and refrigerated or frozen.

For other recipes see: Lobster.

Buying tips: Crabs must be either alive, cooked, or frozen when they are sold. Live crabs should be lively and active; if they don't move, don't buy them. Cooked crabs will keep for several days as long as they're chilled, but they will lose flavor with each passing day. Most picked and packed crabmeat is pasteurized; this process robs some flavor, but few of us have the patience to pick our own crabmeat (although it's easy enough, if you start with king, Dungeness, or snow crabs).

Crabs of all types are among the most delicious and treasured crustaceans. There are dozens of species we don't eat, some because they don't taste great, some because they're hard to catch, but most—I think—because they are "icky-looking." It can't be because they're a hassle to eat, because the best-selling crab in the country—the blue crab—is a nuisance to take apart, especially for the novice. If you stumble across a bushel or two in crab country, find yourself trapped at a crab boil, or just want a leisurely, messy lunch, you'll learn how to get the meat out quickly enough. But for most purposes, I suggest you go with blue crab in one of its other, far more accessible forms—soft-shell or picked meat—or find another species.

All crabs have some things in common: They must be sold live, or cooked and frozen or refrigerated; they have sweet, white delicious meat; they can be cooked by simple boiling (even if they have been frozen); and they taste as good cold as hot.

You can take frozen king crab legs, defrost them (slowly, in the refrigerator), serve them with any mayonnaise (page 43) or a thin mustard sauce (page 44), and have an eating experience you couldn't duplicate if you worked for two hours. That's essentially how stone crab claws are served in many of South Florida's seafood restaurants.

Crabs do have differences, mostly in size and form.

Blue crab: The familiar four- to six-inch blue crustacean, often with red claw tips. Its Latin name means "savory blue swimmer," and it is all of those. Often sold live and nipping, to be boiled or used in sauces, it's also picked from the shell from Maryland on south, and all around the Gulf Coast, to be sold throughout the country, refrigerated or frozen. When sold as picked meat, "lump" means large pieces from the body, "flake" means smaller pieces, and "claw" . . . you can guess. Fresh blue crabmeat is expensive, but incredibly convenient so long as all bits of shell and cartilage have been removed, and wonderfully flavorful; frozen, canned, or pasteurized "fresh" crabmeat are all decidedly inferior.

Soft-shells are a stage of blue crabs; see below.

Dungeness crab: This great-tasting Pacific crab, which runs from three to four pounds, is better compared to Maine lobster than to the blue crab; it's that good and that meaty. Almost always cooked and refrigerated (for local sales) or frozen (for shipping) immediately after the catch, Dungeness is sold whole and easy to eat. The rock crab is similar in appearance and flavor, but smaller, about the size of the blue crab.

King crab: The largest crab, which may weigh twenty-five pounds and measure six feet from tip to tip. This northwestern (mostly Alaskan) delicacy is not available fresh elsewhere in the country. The crabs are simply too big to ship live, and the meat deteriorates too quickly once they're dead. So the crabs are cooked, dismembered, and frozen. Sometimes the legs are split, which is nice, because it makes eating them so easy. But they're not difficult in any case—certainly the easiest-eating crab (except for soft-shells, of course), and actually less trouble than lobsters. Two or three legs can make a good serving.

Snow crab: A three-pound Pacific crab; most sales are of frozen legs, which contain good meat.

Soft-shell crab: Mid-May brings one of the best treats of all to fish counters: the live soft-shell crab. This strange delight—I doubt whether one in a hundred devotees wasn't at least a little bit squeamish when first biting into a whole crab—is nothing more than a plain old blue crab, caught just after it has molted—shed—its hard outer shell. But since the crab only stays soft for a couple of hours, an entire industry has grown up around removing them from the water the instant they shed.

Once out of the water the crabs will not form new shells. But they only live a couple of days, and are therefore either shipped immediately, by air, or

cleaned and frozen. When you get a live soft-shell crab home, you have three choices: Clean it and eat it, clean it and refrigerate it (which will give you a couple of days to think about it), or clean it and freeze it. Though soft-shells freeze fairly well, this last option is a bit wasteful, since frozen soft-shell crabs are available year-round. (You can sometimes buy dressed soft-shell crabs, which can be stored at 33°F and kept for a few days before cooking.) Figure two soft-shells per serving for average appetites, although eating a half dozen is not that difficult, and one can be enough if there is other food around.

To clean a live soft-shell, use a scissors to snip off the eyes and mouth, then the gills found under both sides of the shell. Then, if you like, turn the crab over and pull off the "apron"—that little flap that looks like a "T" on the male and a bell on the female. You don't have to do this, but the apron is a bit on the chewy side.

Stone crab: The recyclable crab of Florida; claws are broken off by fishermen, and the crab returned to the water, where it generates another limb (it's illegal to be in possession of whole crabs). It has a very hard shell, usually cracked with a small wooden mallet.

Note: "Seafood salads" made to resemble crab are made from surimi, a heavily processed fish product that contains a variety of other, mostly unsavory, ingredients. Unless the label says crabmeat—and unless it's expensive—it probably isn't.

BOILED BLUE OR ROCK CRAB

Makes 1 serving
Time: 10 minutes

Note the yield on this recipe, which follows Bittman's first law of crab cooking: You will eat all the crabmeat that you pick. Do not think you can pick enough to make one of the other recipes below; buy already picked crabmeat for those. This is for a lazy summer afternoon when you feel like making a pig of yourself. If someone else wants to join you, fine; just make sure they're willing to work for their lunch or dinner. Incidentally, fresh blue or rock crabs need no salt, lemon, or butter to be delicious. But, since some people like them spicy, I offer an alternative to packaged crab boil mixes.

6 to 12 live blue or rock crabs

Bring abundant water to a boil. Plunge the crabs in, one by one (use tongs—when crabs don't try to pinch you they're probably dead). Cook about 5 minutes. Remove to a colander and eat (it's also nice to ice them down and eat them cold, an hour later).

To eat: Twist off the claws and break them open to pick and suck out the meat. Break off the apron, then pull off the top shell. Rub off the feather gills and break the body in two; then break it in two again. Go to work, picking and sucking that meat out of there and forgetting your manners entirely.

SPICY CRAB BOIL:

To 1 gallon of well-salted water, add 2 onions, roughly chopped, 2 stalks celery, roughly chopped, the juice of 2 limes (or ¼ cup vinegar), 1 tablespoon fresh thyme or 1 teaspoon dried, 1 teaspoon ground allspice, 2 dried or fresh hot peppers or 1 teaspoon cayenne pepper, 1 tablespoon paprika, and 1 teaspoon ground black pepper. Simmer for 15 minutes before adding the crabs.

BASIC METHODS FOR KING CRAB

Time: 20 minutes

King crab legs are delicious, and expensive enough so that you probably don't want to mess about with them too much. Although the meat has a tendency to dry out, I like to grill them; the slightly burned shell has an aroma I find irresistible. Steam-ing is another alternative, and a good one. In either case, serve the legs with drawn butter (page 154) or lemon wedges.

Allow 1 or 2 legs per person. To grill, keep the fire on the cool side, and grill just until hot; if the shells have been split, keep the meat side up so the juices remain in the shells.

To steam, throw the legs in a covered pot with an inch or so of water, bring to a boil, and steam until hot, about 5 minutes. Serve immediately.

WHOLE COLD DUNGENESS CRAB SALAD

Makes 2 servings
Time: 1 hour, using cooked defrosted Dungeness

2 Dungeness crabs, cooked and defrosted if frozen
Mirin-soy Vinaigrette (page 250) or the simple vinaigrette from Sautéed Soft-shell Crabs, Version II (page 111)
4 cups mixed greens

Crack all the Dungeness claw shells and break the body in half. Drizzle them with the vinaigrette and refrigerate an hour or so before eating, stirring occasionally. Serve over mixed greens, which will catch not only the excess vinaigrette but the delicious juices from the crab.

CRAB SALAD

Makes 2 servings
Time: 10 minutes

Few leftovers are as desirable as cold crab, which is delicious on its own or with a squirt of lemon juice. You can make a crab salad using your favorite potato salad recipe, or with this one.

½ pound cold cooked crabmeat, picked over for cartilage
Several tablespoons Lime Mayonnaise (pages 230–231) or any mayonnaise spiked with lime juice to taste
1 shallot, minced
½ medium-size (or one very small) red or yellow bell pepper, seeded and minced
Salt and freshly ground black pepper to taste
1 teaspoon curry powder (optional)

Combine all the ingredients, taste and correct the seasoning, and serve with bread.

CRAB CAKES, VERSION I

Makes 4 servings
Time: 15 minutes, plus refrigeration time
These are very "crabby" crab cakes—not much filler, not much binder. They're delicate, rich, and flavorful.

1 pound fresh lump crabmeat, picked over for cartilage
1 large egg
¼ cup seeded and minced red bell pepper
½ cup minced scallion, both green and white parts
¼ cup mayonnaise
1 tablespoon Dijon mustard
Salt and freshly ground black pepper to taste
2 tablespoons unseasoned bread crumbs or as needed
1 cup flour for dredging
1 teaspoon curry powder
2 tablespoons peanut or vegetable oil
2 tablespoons butter or additional oil
Lemon wedges

Mix together the crabmeat, egg, bell pepper, scallions, mayonnaise, mustard, salt, and pepper. Add enough bread crumbs to bind the mixture just enough to form into cakes; start with 2 tablespoons and use more as needed. Refrigerate the mixture until ready to cook (it will be easier to shape if you refrigerate it for 30 minutes or more, but is ready to go when you finish mixing).

Season the flour with salt, pepper, and curry powder. Preheat a 12-inch skillet, preferably nonstick, over medium-high heat. Add the oil and butter and heat until the butter foam subsides. Shape the crabmeat mixture into four cakes, dredge each in the flour, and cook, adjusting the heat as necessary and turning once (very gently), until golden brown on both sides. Total cooking time will be about 10 minutes. Serve with lemon wedges.

CRAB CAKES, VERSION II

Makes 4 servings
Time: About 1 hour and 15 minutes
These are more traditional crab cakes, the kind you would have in many Maryland restaurants.

2 slices white bread
½ cup milk
1 pound fresh lump crabmeat, picked over for cartilage
¼ cup minced onion
¼ cup minced fresh parsley
1 teaspoon Worcestershire or high-quality soy sauce
Salt and freshly ground black pepper to taste
¼ cup (½ stick) butter

Soak the white bread in the milk until softened, about 5 minutes. Add it to a bowl along with all the remaining ingredients except the butter. Shape into 4 large or 8 small patties and refrigerate for 1 hour or more.

Heat the butter over medium-high heat in a 12-inch skillet. When the foam subsides, cook the crab cakes until lightly browned on both sides, turning once, very gently. Total cooking time will be about 12 minutes.

ALTERNATIVE FISH FOR THIS RECIPE:

Poached cod or salt cod; haddock, halibut, pollock, tilefish, turbot, weakfish, or whiting; chopped clams, crawfish, lobster, scallops, shrimp, or a combination.

STIR-FRIED CRABMEAT WITH DRIED MUSHROOMS

Makes 2 main course servings
Time: 20 minutes

A wonderful quick lunch or late-night snack. Mushrooms and crab have an almost mystical affinity.

¼ cup dried mushrooms: black trumpet, shiitake, or cèpe (porcini)
2 tablespoons peanut or vegetable oil
1 tablespoon minced garlic
1 teaspoon peeled and minced fresh ginger
1 cup cooked lump crabmeat (about ½ pound), picked over for cartilage
¼ teaspoon chili-garlic paste (available in Asian markets; optional)
1 tablespoon rice or distilled vinegar
1 tablespoon high-quality soy sauce
1 teaspoon sesame oil

Soak the mushrooms in warm to hot water to cover until softened, 10 to 15 minutes. Lift them from the water and chop. Strain the soaking liquid through a double thickness of paper towels and set aside. Heat a wok over high heat until smoking. Add the oil, then the garlic and ginger. Stir-fry for 15 seconds, then add the crabmeat. Cook for 30 seconds, then add the mushrooms. Cook for 30 seconds, then add ½ cup of the reserved mushroom liquid. Simmer for 1 minute; add the chili paste, vinegar, and soy sauce. Cook for 30 seconds, turn off the heat, add the sesame oil, stir, and serve over white rice.

STIR-FRIED CRABMEAT WITH SCALLIONS:
Substitute 1 cup scallions, cut into 1-inch lengths, for the mushrooms. Garnish with minced scallions.

STIR-FRIED CRABMEAT WITH TOMATOES AND CILANTRO:
Substitute 1 cup chopped fresh tomatoes for the mushrooms; add ¼ cup minced cilantro (fresh coriander) just before the sesame oil.

STIR-FRIED CRABMEAT WITH MUSHROOMS AND PORK:
Add ¼ pound minced pork before adding the crab, and stir-fry until it loses its color.

PASTA WITH CRABMEAT, EGGPLANT, AND TOMATO

Makes 4 servings
Time: 45 minutes

Meat from snow crab, rock crab, or blue crab, depending on what you can find, is all equally good here. And despite the relatively small amount of crabmeat in this sauce, and despite the presence of other strong flavors, the taste of crab dominates the dish. It's wonderful, and almost as good without the eggplant.

1 pound fresh tiny eggplant (4 to 6 eggplant)
¼ cup olive oil or more
2 cloves garlic, lightly crushed and peeled
3 dried hot red peppers
2 cups chopped tomatoes, fresh (or drained if canned)
2 tablespoons chopped fresh basil
1 pound large pasta, such as rigatoni
1 cup crabmeat (about ½ pound), picked over for cartilage
Salt and freshly ground black pepper to taste
½ cup chopped fresh parsley

Set a large pot of water to boil and salt it well. Peel the eggplant if you like it that way, then slice off the ends and cut each into three or four long slices. Heat the olive oil in a 12-inch nonstick skillet over medium heat. When it begins to shimmer, add the eggplant, a slice or two at a time, making sure not to add too much at once. Don't crowd the eggplant. As each piece browns, turn it; when it browns on the other side, remove it from the pan and place it on paper towels to drain. Continue until all the eggplant is done, adding more oil if necessary.

Add the garlic and red peppers to the oil remaining in the pan and cook, stirring, over medium-high heat until the garlic is fairly brown. Remove the garlic and peppers with a slotted spoon and add the tomatoes. Cook over medium heat until they begin to liquefy, add the basil, and reduce the heat to a simmer. Begin cooking the pasta. When the pasta is just about done, add the crabmeat, salt, pepper, cooked eggplant, and half the parsley to the sauce.

Drain the pasta, toss it with the sauce, and garnish with the remaining parsley.

ALTERNATIVE FISH FOR THIS RECIPE: Shrimp.

LINGUINE WITH CRABMEAT AND GARLIC

Makes 3 to 4 servings
Time: 30 minutes

½ cup fruity olive oil
1 tablespoon minced garlic
1 dried hot red pepper or to taste
1 cup lump crabmeat (about ½ pound), picked over for cartilage
Salt and freshly ground black pepper to taste
½ cup dry white wine
½ cup minced fresh parsley
1 pound linguine or spaghetti

Set a large pot of water to boil and salt it well. In a small saucepan, warm the olive oil, garlic, and pepper over low heat until the garlic turns golden brown. Add the crab, salt, pepper, and wine, and simmer until reduced slightly. Add half the parsley, cook another minute, and turn off the heat.

Cook the pasta according to the package instructions. When it is just about done, reheat the crab sauce. Drain the pasta, toss with the sauce, and top with the remaining parsley.

CRABMEAT NORFOLK STYLE

Makes 4 servings
Time: 10 minutes

An old-fashioned, minimalist treat from a city where crab is a staple. It's usually served over rice; I prefer it as an appetizer, with nothing but a little extra Tabasco or vinegar.

¼ cup (½ stick) butter
1 pound lump crabmeat, picked over for cartilage
¼ cup white or sherry wine vinegar
Several drops Tabasco or other hot pepper sauce
Salt and freshly ground black pepper to taste

Melt the butter in a 10-inch skillet over medium heat. Add the crabmeat, vinegar, Tabasco, salt, and pepper, and cook until the crab is hot, about 4 minutes. Serve immediately, passing vinegar and Tabasco at the table.

GRILLED SOFT-SHELL CRABS WITH BUTTER AND HOT SAUCE

Makes 2 to 4 servings
Time: 10 minutes (with cleaned soft-shells) plus time to build a fire

There's nothing easier or better than this, unless you opt—as I sometimes do—to grill over a wood fire. This is one instance in which it's really worth it; the wood flavor adds a great deal to the crisp claws of soft-shells. And you might as well grill some corn while you're at it—their seasons coincide.

4 to 8 soft-shell crabs, depending on size and appetite, cleaned (page 106)
¼ cup (½ stick) butter
Salt to taste
Juice of ½ lemon
Several drops of hot pepper sauce or to taste

Build a wood fire, preheat a gas grill, or start a charcoal one; the fire should be past its peak before grilling, as soft-shell crabs burn easily. Melt the butter and add salt, lemon juice, and hot sauce to taste. Grill the crabs about 4 inches from the source of heat, turning and brushing frequently; don't worry about burned claw-tips—they're inevitable. Total cooking time will be 6 to 10 minutes; the crabs are done when they're bright red and firm; don't overcook.

ALTERNATIVE FISH FOR THIS RECIPE:
Shrimp (leave the shells on) or squid (cleaned but left whole, and grilled very briefly over high heat).

SAUTÉED SOFT-SHELL CRABS, VERSION I

Makes 2 to 4 servings
Time: 20 minutes, using cleaned soft-shells

Some people deep-fry soft-shells, but I think nothing beats this simple breading, which has the added advantage of being easier and far less messy. If you want to serve the crabs as an appetizer, for up to eight people, just quarter them with a sharp knife as soon as they are cooked.

¼ cup (½ stick) butter, olive oil, or a combination
4 soft-shell crabs, cleaned (page 106)
Flour for dredging
1 large egg lightly beaten with 1 tablespoon water
Unseasoned bread crumbs for dredging, seasoned with salt and freshly ground black pepper
Lemon wedges

Heat a 12-inch nonstick skillet over medium heat for 3 or 4 minutes. Melt the butter in the skillet and, when the foam subsides, raise the heat to medium-high. Dredge a crab in the flour, dip it in the egg, then dredge it in the bread crumbs. Place it in the skillet and repeat the process (depending upon the size of your crabs, you may have to cook in batches). Cook until golden brown on one side, then turn and cook until golden brown on the other, about 4 minutes per side. Serve immediately, with lemon wedges.

SAUTÉED SOFT-SHELL CRABS WITH CAPONATA:
Cook the crabs only 2 minutes per side. Add 2 cups warm eggplant caponata (pages 60–61) to the skillet and complete the cooking by bringing the sauce to a simmer, then cooking 3 more minutes.

SAUTÉED SOFT-SHELL CRABS, VERSION II

Makes 2 to 4 servings
Time: 25 minutes, using cleaned soft-shells
This is more elegant and more time-consuming than the previous recipe; less common, too.

½ cup sliced blanched almonds
¼ cup flour
Salt and freshly ground black pepper to taste
1 large egg
5 tablespoons olive oil
4 large soft-shell crabs, cleaned (page 106)
1 tablespoon balsamic vinegar
1 sprig fresh tarragon, minced
1 teaspoon minced shallot

Toast the almonds by shaking them in a dry skillet over medium heat until they are light brown and fragrant. Reserve 1 tablespoon and grind the rest in a food processor, coffee grinder, or mortar and pestle. Combine with the flour, salt, and pepper. Beat the egg in a small bowl.

Heat a 12-inch nonstick skillet over medium-high heat for 3 to 4 minutes. Add 2 tablespoons of the olive oil and heat until it shimmers. Dip each of the crabs in the egg, then dredge in the almond-flour mixture. Cook until golden, adjusting the heat as necessary and turning once, about 6 to 8 minutes total. While the crabs are cooking, combine the remaining olive oil with the vinegar, tarragon, and shallot; mix well. Serve the crabs with a few drops of the vinaigrette on each; garnish with the reserved almonds.

SAUTÉED SOFT-SHELL CRABS, VERSION III

Makes 2 to 4 servings
Time: 30 minutes, using cleaned soft-shells

Flour for dredging
Salt and freshly ground black pepper to taste
½ cup (1 stick) butter
4 large soft-shell crabs, cleaned (page 106)
Dash cayenne pepper
Juice of 2 limes

Heat a 12-inch nonstick skillet over medium-high heat for 3 to 4 minutes. Season the flour with salt and pepper. When the skillet is hot, put in about ¼ cup of the butter. Just as the foam begins to subside, dredge the crabs, add them to the pan, and raise the heat to high. Cook until golden, adjusting the heat as necessary and turning once, about 6 to 8 minutes total. Remove the crabs and lower the heat to medium. Add the remaining butter and the cayenne and cook until the butter melts. Add the lime juice, stir to blend and heat through, and pour over the crabs.

SAUTÉED SOFT-SHELL CRABS WITH SHALLOTS AND CAPERS:

After the second addition of butter, add 2 tablespoons minced shallots; cook, stirring, about 2 minutes over medium-high heat, then add ½ cup dry white wine. Reduce by half, stirring; add salt and pepper to taste, ¼ cup capers, drained of their brine, and ¼ cup minced fresh parsley. Pour this sauce over the crabs and garnish with additional parsley. Serve with lemon wedges.

STIR-FRIED SOFT-SHELL CRABS

Makes 2 servings
Time: 30 minutes, using cleaned soft-shells
Really, the only way to cook soft-shells in a wok is by deep-frying, but you can sauté them in a skillet and finish the sauce with Chinese ingredients. The results are far less trouble and equally satisfying. Here is one possibility; you can use the same method for stir-frying soft-shells with almost any combination of ingredients you like.

2 large soft-shell crabs, or 4 small ones, depending on size, cleaned (page 106)
¼ cup peanut oil
1 tablespoon minced garlic
2 scallions, minced

1 tablespoon peeled and minced fresh ginger

2 dried hot red peppers

½ cup any fish or chicken stock (pages 40–41) or water

2 tablespoons fermented black beans, soaked in 2 tablespoons dry sherry for 10 minutes (available in Asian markets)

1 teaspoon sugar

1 tablespoon high-quality soy sauce

Preheat a 10- or 12-inch nonstick skillet over low to medium heat. Dry the crabs well, then sauté them in 2 tablespoons of the oil for 3 to 4 minutes per side. Remove and keep warm in a low oven.

Stir-fry the garlic, scallions, ginger, and peppers over high heat for 30 seconds. Add the stock, black beans, sherry, and sugar; cook for 30 seconds. Add the soy sauce, stir, and turn off the heat. Top the crabs with sauce and serve immediately.

CRAYFISH

Latin name(s): Several species of *Astacus* and *Cambarus*.
Other common names: Crawfish.
Common forms: Whole, live; whole, frozen; cooked (and sometimes peeled), refrigerated or frozen.
General description: A freshwater lobsterlike creature ranging, usually, from four to eight inches long. The meat is like that of shrimp in appearance and use.
For other recipes see: Lobster, and especially shrimp.
Buying tips: Like other live shellfish, such as lobster and crab, crayfish should be quite active.

There are many places in the world where people go wild over crayfish. They're especially beloved on the Gulf Coast (where they're always called crawfish, and are farm-raised in great number) and in Scandinavia, where crayfish pig-outs are an annual event.

Personally (and my Louisiana friends declare this is a genetic deficiency found in Northerners), I prefer shrimp to crayfish, and not only because shrimp are more widely available and generally cheaper; I find them tastier as well. Nevertheless, a great old crayfish boil is a hoot.

Crayfish are usually sold whole. To clean before or after cooking, just twist the tail off the head and peel and, if you like, devein the tail. Exceptionally large crayfish, which are quite rare in this country, have edible claw meat as well. Where tail and thorax meet is an orange or creamy white fat (the heptopancreas) that you can remove with a small knife or spoon; it's good in sauces, rice dishes such as jambalaya, or anything else to which you want to lend a crayfish flavor.

CRAYFISH BOIL LOUISIANA STYLE

Makes 2 to 3 servings
Time: 30 minutes, plus cooling time
One person—on a roll—can consume this many crayfish easily. You can make this more of a full meal by adding potatoes, corn, and/or whole small onions to the boil.

4 quarts Court Bouillon (page 41) or a mixture
  of 8 parts water to 1 part white vinegar
1 bay leaf
1 teaspoon dried thyme
Several black peppercorns
2 cloves garlic, crushed and peeled
Several coriander seeds
3 whole cloves
3 dried red peppers
Salt to taste
3 pounds whole crayfish
Tabasco or other hot red pepper sauce
Lemon wedges
Freshly ground black pepper to taste

Bring the liquid to a boil and add the bay leaf, thyme, peppercorns, garlic, coriander, cloves, pep-

114

pers, and plenty of salt. Simmer for 10 minutes over medium heat. Add the crayfish. Simmer for 5 minutes, then turn off the heat and let the crayfish cool in the liquid. Remove them with a slotted spoon, sprinkle with more salt, and serve, passing hot sauce, lemon wedges, and black pepper at the table.

ALTERNATIVE FISH FOR THIS RECIPE:

Blue crabs (3 or 4 per person) or whole shrimp (½ pound or more per person).

CRAYFISH IN CREAM SAUCE:

Cook the crayfish (or shrimp) as instructed above. Cool, remove the meat and fat, reserve the fat, and chop the tails. Strain the cooking liquid and reduce it over high heat to 1 cup (this could take a while). Melt 2 tablespoons butter in a 2-quart saucepan; add 2 tablespoons flour and cook over medium heat, stirring, for about 5 minutes, until lightly browned. Whisk in the reserved liquid and cook, stirring, until thick. Add the crayfish fat, 1 cup heavy, light, or sour cream, about ½ cup snipped fresh dill, and ½ teaspoon cayenne pepper. Season with salt and pepper, stir in the crayfish meat, and serve over white rice.

CRAYFISH ETOUFFE:

Cook the crayfish (or shrimp) as instructed above. Cool, remove the meat and fat, reserve the fat, and leave the tails whole. Strain the liquid and reduce it over high heat to 1 ½ cups (this could take a while). Heat 3 tablespoons vegetable oil in a 10- or 12-inch skillet; add 3 tablespoons flour and cook, stirring almost constantly, until the flour browns, about 15 minutes. Add ½ cup seeded and minced red bell pepper, ½ cup minced onion, and 1 tablespoon minced garlic; stir to combine. Whisk in the reserved liquid and cook, stirring, until thick. Add the crayfish fat. In another saucepan, melt 3 tablespoons butter over medium heat. Add the tails, ½ cup minced scallions (green and white parts), the juice of 1 lemon, ½ teaspoon cayenne pepper, salt, and freshly ground black pepper; cook 3 minutes, or until the crayfish are opaque. Add to the sauce and serve.

CRAYFISH CURRY

Makes 4 servings
Time: 1 hour

4 pounds fresh crayfish or more
2 quarts Court Bouillon (page 41) or a mixture of 8 parts water to 1 part white vinegar
1 bay leaf
½ teaspoon dried thyme
1 teaspoon whole peppercorns
2 cloves garlic, crushed and peeled
Several coriander seeds
3 whole cloves
5 dried red peppers
Salt and freshly ground black pepper to taste
1 cup dried unsweetened grated coconut
1 cup boiling water
3 tablespoons peanut or vegetable oil
1 tablespoon minced garlic
½ cup minced cilantro (fresh coriander)
½ cup whole unsalted roasted cashews

Shell the crayfish, reserving the heads and shell. Bring the liquid to a boil and add the heads and shells, along with the bay leaf, thyme, peppercorns, garlic, coriander, cloves, 2 of the red peppers, and plenty of salt and pepper. Simmer, uncovered, for 20 minutes. Strain the liquid, return it to the pan, and reduce it over high heat to about 1 cup. Set aside.

Place the coconut in a blender and cover it with the boiling water. Cover the blender and, holding the top on with a folded towel to reduce the possibilities of scalding, blend for 20 seconds or so. Let the mixture sit for a few minutes, then strain, pressing to extract as much liquid as possible.

Heat a 12-inch nonstick skillet over medium-high heat for 3 to 4 minutes. Add the oil and, when it shimmers, turn the heat to high and add the garlic and crayfish tails. Cook, stirring, over high heat for about a minute. Add the reserved stock and cook until it reduces by about half; add the coconut milk, lower the heat to medium, and cook, stirring, for about 3 minutes. Add half the cilantro, taste for seasoning, and add the cashews. Stir and serve immediately, over white rice, garnished with the remaining cilantro.

ALTERNATIVE FISH FOR THIS RECIPE: Shrimp.

BUTTER-GRILLED CRAYFISH

Makes 4 servings
Time: 30 minutes

At least 4 pounds fresh crayfish
½ cup (1 stick) unsalted butter
2 tablespoons minced shallots
½ cup minced fresh parsley
½ cup fresh bread crumbs, lightly toasted
Salt and freshly ground black pepper to taste

Cut the crayfish in half lengthwise; leave the shells and heads on. Spread in a baking pan, meat side up. Preheat the broiler.

Dot the crayfish with the butter, then sprinkle with the shallots, parsley, bread crumbs, salt, and pepper. Broil about 6 inches from the heat source until the bread crumbs brown lightly, about 6 to 8 minutes. Serve immediately.

ALTERNATIVE FISH FOR THIS RECIPE: Lobster (small ones), scallops (large ones), or shrimp (large ones).

CROAKER

Latin name(s): *Micropogonias undulatus* and other species.
Other common names: Hardhead, jewfish, blackmouth, drum.
Common forms: Whole, beheaded, and (rarely) steaks and fillets.
General description: A medium-size panfish which runs to two feet but is rarely seen above one foot these days; weight averages a pound, but sometimes is significantly larger, up to three or four pounds.
For other recipes see: Butterfish, mullet, porgy (especially), sea bass, spot, weakfish, small whiting.
Buying tips: As with any whole fish, croaker should be buried in ice (with ice separating individual fish), and have red gills, bright skin, and no bruising. The smell should be sweet.

Croaker is one of a large group of fish known as drums, which also includes the red drum (or redfish, stocks of which were depleted by the Cajun craze), the spot, and the weakfish. Its name comes from its ability to make a loud drumming (or croaking) noise. Because croaker is considered a panfish, many people automatically dust it with cornmeal and pan-fry it. You can, of course, do this (see Pan-fried Butterfish, page 65, for a recipe), but, as these recipes demonstrate, you need not stop there.

SAUTÉED CROAKER

Makes 2 servings
Time: 30 minutes

2 tablespoons fresh lemon juice
2 tablespoons dry white wine
1 teaspoon fennel seeds
¼ cup olive oil
2 cloves garlic, smashed and peeled
½ cup minced fresh basil
2 croaker, 1 pound or more each, skin on, scaled and gutted
Salt and freshly ground black pepper to taste

Mix together the lemon juice, wine, fennel seeds, half the olive oil, the garlic, and half the basil. Marinate the fish in this mixture for about 15 minutes, turning once or twice.

Heat a 12-inch nonstick skillet over medium-high heat for 3 to 4 minutes. Add the remaining olive oil; remove the fish from the marinade and dry with paper towels. Cook about 4 minutes on each side, until the fish is lightly browned and cooked through. (The fish is done when the interior is free of blood.) Sprinkle with salt and pepper, garnish with the remaining basil, and serve.
ALTERNATIVE FISH FOR THIS RECIPE:
Butterfish, mullet, porgy, sea bass, spot, weakfish, or small whiting.

SAUTÉED CROAKER WITH
VINEGAR AND GARLIC

Makes 4 servings
Time: 30 minutes

4 croaker, 1 pound or more each, skin on,
   scaled and gutted
Salt and freshly ground black pepper to taste
Flour for dusting
¼ cup olive oil
1 tablespoon minced garlic
1 tablespoon minced fresh rosemary or thyme
½ cup good vinegar, balsamic, sherry, or wine
½ cup fish (pages 40–41) or chicken stock
   (page 40) or dry white wine

Rinse and dry the croaker while you heat a 12-inch nonstick skillet over medium-high heat. Sprinkle the fish with salt and pepper and dust lightly with flour. Put the olive oil in the skillet and, when it is hot (a pinch of flour will sizzle), add the fish to the pan. Sear it over high heat and, after about 4 minutes, add half the garlic. Turn the fish and cook on the other side until done (the interior will be free of blood), about 4 minutes. Remove the fish to a plate. Add the remaining garlic to the pan, along with the rosemary and vinegar; cook for 1 minute or so, stirring. Stir in the stock, let it bubble away for about 30 seconds, spoon over the fish, and serve.

ALTERNATIVE FISH FOR THIS RECIPE:
   Butterfish, mullet, porgy, sea bass, spot, weakfish, or small whiting.

CUNNER

Latin name(s): *Tautogolabrus adspersus.*
Other common names: Perch, sea perch, blue perch, nipper, bergall.
Common forms: Whole fish and fillets.
General description: Once popular and now rarely seen, this usually smaller version of the blackfish can be treated in the same fashion.
For recipes see: Blackfish.
Buying tips: Unlike blackfish—to which it is otherwise similar—the cunner can be bought with the skin on.

CUSK

Latin name(s): *Brosme brosme.*
Other common names: Tusk, European cusk, brosmius.
Common forms: Fillets.
General description: A codlike fish from northern waters, usually a bit oilier than other white-fleshed fish but otherwise similar.
For recipes see: Cod and other white-fleshed fillets: Blackfish, dogfish, grouper, ocean perch, pollock, rockfish, sea bass, red snapper, tilefish, turbot, weakfish, wolffish.
Buying tips: Most important: Unlike many fish sold as cod substitutes (for example, ocean pout), cusk is definitely worth buying. Treat as you would cod.

DOGFISH

Scientific name: *Squalus acanthias* and others.
Other common names: Sand shark, nurse shark, grayfish, rock salmon, rock cod, etc.
Common forms: Skinless, bone-free fillets, up to a pound in weight.
General description: White, firm fillet, best for sautéing, broiling, and poaching.
For other recipes see: Blackfish, catfish, cod, grouper, ocean perch, pollock, sea bass, red snapper, tilefish, turbot, wolffish.
Buying tips: The best dogfish is always iced immediately after the catch, and fillets are kept ice cold from processor to retailer. Well-handled dogfish has little aroma, or may be slightly sweet-smelling; stick to those, rather than trying to deal with the stink of ammonia.

A small shark, as unlike mako as you can imagine, with pearly white flesh and a fillet that looks like young cod (hence "rock cod") but with a firmer texture. Dogfish is not yet popular: Recreational fishermen throw it back, and commercial fishermen sell it to processors, who in turn freeze it before shipping it to Europe, where it's appreciated.

Dogfish was once passed off as cod, but it really isn't that close. Like all sharks, it is built around cartilage, so its fillets are always completely bone-free. Dogfish fillets are longer and narrower than those of any other white-fleshed fish; they generally weigh a third of a pound or more, and are always skinless.

In the past, Americans enjoyed dogfish, often without knowing it. During the lean years of World War I, the government promoted it as a good protein source. But the market diminished in the prosperity of the 1920s. Later, dogfish were fished for their livers, which are extremely high in vitamin A; the meat was passed on to fish retailers, to be sold as "grayfish" or "whitefish." Although the practice was perhaps deceptive, consumption rose once again, which is not surprising: dogfish tastes good. It's a staple in England's fish and chips houses.

Like mako, dogfish must be handled properly. Because sharks (which have evolved little in the past 200 million years or so) have a primitive waste disposal system, improper handling results in the rapid development of ammonia. Although this is not necessarily a sign of spoilage (and can even be remedied by a short soak in milk, lemon juice, or vinegar), it is a rather piercing signal that the fish is not top quality.

BROILED DOGFISH WITH DILL BUTTER

Makes 4 servings
Time: 15 minutes
Quick and easy as this is, it's an impressive preparation, and a delicious one. Mix the dill with olive oil if you're trying to avoid saturated fats.

⅓ cup (about ⅔ stick) butter
1 clove garlic, finely minced
¼ cup minced fresh dill
1 to 1 ½ pounds dogfish fillets
Salt and freshly ground black pepper to taste
1 tablespoon vegetable oil, if necessary

Preheat the broiler. Put the butter, garlic, and dill in a blender or food processor and process until smooth; or mince the dill finely and use a fork to cream it with the butter and garlic. Season the fillets with salt and pepper, then spread them in a shallow nonstick baking pan (if you don't have a nonstick pan, brush a little oil on the bottom of any baking pan). Dot them with about two thirds of the dill butter.

Broil the fillets 3 to 6 inches from the heat source until brown, about 4 to 5 minutes. Remove them from the oven, spread them with the remaining dill butter, and serve immediately.

ALTERNATIVE FISH FOR THIS RECIPE:

This all-purpose recipe can be used for fillets of virtually any fish; adjust the cooking time according to the thickness of the fillet. Substitute any compound butter (page 44) for the dill butter if you like.

SESAME-CRUSTED DOGFISH FILLETS

Makes 4 servings
Time: 20 minutes

Unlike most white fillets, dogfish does not flake easily when cooked. This makes it ideal for sautéing. Lightly battered, rolled in toasted sesame seeds, and served with an Asian dipping sauce, it's sensational.

1 cup sesame seeds
3 tablespoons high-quality soy sauce
1 tablespoon white or rice vinegar
1 teaspoon sesame oil
1 teaspoon hot oil, Tabasco sauce, chili-garlic paste (available in Asian markets), or to taste (optional)
1 to 1 ½ pounds dogfish fillets
3 tablespoons peanut or vegetable oil
Flour for dredging

1 large egg, lightly beaten with 1 tablespoon water

Toast the sesame seeds in a dry skillet over medium heat (or in a microwave on high power) until they begin to pop, 3 to 5 minutes. Put them in a shallow bowl. Mix the soy sauce, vinegar, sesame oil, and hot oil together; set aside. Cut the long, thin fillets into two or three pieces each.

Heat a 12-inch nonstick skillet over medium-high heat for 3 to 4 minutes, then add the peanut oil. When the oil is good and hot (a pinch of flour will sizzle), dredge the fish pieces, one by one, in the flour; dip them in the egg, roll them in the sesame seeds, then gently place them in the skillet. Cook until nicely browned, 3 minutes or so per side. Serve immediately, with rice and the dipping sauce.

ALTERNATIVE FISH FOR THIS RECIPE:

Blackfish, grouper, monkfish, Atlantic pollock, rockfish, red snapper, striped bass, tilefish, or wolffish. Adjust cooking time accordingly.

BROILED DOGFISH WITH ONIONS, BACON, AND TOMATOES

Makes 4 servings
Time: 30 minutes

You can increase the amount of tomatoes in this recipe and top not only the fish but a batch of pasta with the sauce.

2 slices bacon, minced
1 medium-size onion, chopped
2 cups chopped fresh, ripe tomatoes (canned are fine; drain first)
1 tablespoon minced fresh basil
½ cup minced fresh parsley
Salt and freshly ground black pepper to taste
1 to 1 ½ pounds dogfish fillets, cut in half
2 tablespoons olive oil

Cook the bacon, stirring, over medium heat until it begins to crisp; remove it with a slotted spoon. Cook the onion in the bacon fat, stirring occasionally, until they soften, about 5 minutes. Add the tomatoes and cook, stirring occasionally, until they begin to liquefy, 3 to 5 minutes. Add the basil and half the parsley, stir, taste for salt and pepper, and turn off the heat. Preheat the broiler.

Brush a shallow baking pan with half the olive oil and lay the fillets in the pan. Brush them with the remaining oil, sprinkle with salt and pepper, and place under the broiler. Broil for 2 minutes; the fillets will not begin to brown. Spoon the tomato mixture onto the fillets and return to the broiler. Broil 2 more minutes and serve, garnished with the remaining parsley.

ALTERNATIVE FISH FOR THIS RECIPE:

Blackfish, cod, grouper, haddock, mackerel, Atlantic or Pacific pollock, rockfish, sablefish, red snapper, striped bass, tilefish, or wolffish. Adjust cooking time accordingly.

FISH AND CHIPS

Makes 4 servings
Time: 90 minutes, with some down time
This is the classic English takeout food. It's not elegant, but it is fun. It takes some time, however, and batches must be kept small. See the general guidelines for frying fish, pages 31–36.

The traditional accompaniment is malt vinegar, but lemon quarters are also excellent. For a change, try a mixture of 3 parts soy sauce, 1 part vinegar, a splash of sesame oil, and a few drops of chili oil.

1 cup unbleached all-purpose flour, plus more
   for dredging
1 teaspoon baking powder
1 cup water
1 large egg (optional)

2 large potatoes, peeled
Vegetable oil for deep-frying
Salt to taste
½ teaspoon freshly ground black pepper or to
   taste
1 to 1 ½ pounds dogfish fillets

Put the 1 cup flour and the baking powder in a bowl and mix. Add the water and beat well; then add the egg and beat until smooth. Let sit for a half hour or an hour, while you get the other food ready (drinking a glass or two of beer would be appropriate).

Cut the potatoes into long, thin strips, and soak the strips in water, changing the water once or twice.

Heat 3 inches or more of oil in a large pot or electric deep-fryer, until it is 350°F to 375°F. (If you don't have a thermostat or a frying thermometer, drop a small piece of bread in the oil; it should sink, then rise to the top and begin bubbling away.) Fry about half of the potatoes (remember that crowding is the enemy of crispness) until golden. Place chips on a baking tray lined with paper towels and keep them warm in a low oven.

To make the fish, first beat the batter again, adding the salt and pepper as you do so. Cut each long fillet into three- or four-inch lengths and dredge in flour, shaking off the excess. Dip into the batter, allowing excess batter to drip off. Then fry, 3 or 4 pieces at a time. When they puff and turn golden, they're ready. As you eat them, fry more chips or fish.

ALTERNATIVE FISH FOR THIS RECIPE:

Blackfish, catfish, cod, haddock, Pacific pollock, or wolffish.

SPICY DOGFISH WITH
CRISP ONIONS

Makes 4 servings
Time: 30 minutes
You'll need two sauté pans for this dish.

2 large yellow onions
6 tablespoons peanut or vegetable oil
1 teaspoon minced garlic
1 teaspoon turmeric
¼ teaspoon cayenne pepper
1 teaspoon coarse salt
1 ½ to 2 pounds dogfish fillets
Minced cilantro (fresh coriander) for garnish

Peel the onions, cut them in half along their axis, and slice them into half-moons. Heat 2 tablespoons of the oil in a large skillet over medium heat. Turn the heat to high and cook the onions, stirring, until they are dark brown and begin to crisp. Turn the heat to low while you prepare the fish.

Heat a 12-inch nonstick skillet over medium-high heat. Mix together the garlic, turmeric, cayenne, and salt, and rub this mixture into the fillets. Add the remaining oil to the skillet and turn the heat to high. Cook the fish about 3 minutes per side, turning once. Serve, topped with the crispy onions and garnished with cilantro.

ALTERNATIVE FISH FOR THIS RECIPE:
Fillets of any white-fleshed fish.

DOGFISH POACHED IN
GINGER SAUCE

Makes 4 servings
Time: 30 minutes
Don't hesitate to make this dish even if you don't have stock; it will still have plenty of flavor.

2 tablespoons peanut oil
1 clove garlic, minced
5 tablespoons peeled and very finely minced fresh ginger
½ cup Fast Fish Stock (page 40), Quickest Chicken Stock (page 40), or water
¼ cup high-quality soy sauce
¼ cup dry white wine
Salt and freshly ground black pepper to taste
1 to 1 ½ pounds dogfish fillets, cut into 2 or 3 pieces each

In a large skillet, warm the peanut oil over medium heat, then add the garlic and half the ginger; stir once or twice. When the garlic begins to color, add the liquids; raise the heat to high and reduce by about half. Season with salt and pepper. Lay the fillets in the liquid, cover, and poach until the fillets are white and opaque throughout, about 5 minutes. Garnish with the reserved ginger and serve immediately, over white rice.

ALTERNATIVE FISH FOR THIS RECIPE:
Blackfish, grouper, Atlantic pollock, rockfish, red snapper, striped bass, tilefish, or wolffish. Cooking times will vary slightly with the thickness of the fillets.

EEL

Latin name(s): *Anguilla rostrata*.
Other common names: American eel.
Common forms: Whole, usually live, sometimes gutted, filleted, and/or frozen.
General description: Long, slender fish, as large as twenty pounds; market size is usually two to eight pounds.
For other recipes see: Virtually none; eel is unique in shape and texture.
Buying tips: Buy eels live, from someone who is able and willing to kill and skin them for you. From that point on they are easy to deal with; once cooked, the rich, delicious meat comes off the central bone easily. Frozen eels have already been skinned.

"For twenty-three centuries man speculated on the origin of the eel," wrote A. J. McClane. These freshwater creatures showed no signs of mating, spawning, or raising young; what could be more mysterious? No wonder people thought they were monsters; their snakelike appearance, slimy skin, and ability to survive for long periods of time out of water didn't help their reputation.

It was not until this century when a Danish scientist discovered that eels—both European and American—were born, mated, and died in the Sargasso Sea, east of Florida. The transparent babies drift and swim toward Europe and the Americas (a three-year trip eastward, a mere year westward), during which they gain color and enter fresh water as elvers. There they live until maturity, at which point they depart to make the journey back to the Sargasso.

Most eels are caught during their freshwater phase, although there have been periods during which the arriving elvers were popular in the United States, sautéed as cakes (see Sartagnado, page 344, for a similar preparation) when they were in season each spring. Europeans still enjoy elvers, and angulas—the Spanish word for elvers—are a delicacy in Catalonia, where they are baked in a bath of olive oil and garlic until they turn a lovely lavender.

Mature eels remain a part of our national menu, especially at Christmastime when they are in demand, largely by Italians and other European immigrants. Because they are best sold live and skinned just before cooking (not an easy task), they are not likely to ever become a mass-market food in the United States. This is unfortunate, because few fish make better eating.

STEWED EEL, WITH VARIATIONS

Makes 4 servings
Time: 60 minutes or less

2 tablespoons olive oil
1 cup chopped onion
1 tablespoon minced garlic
1 medium-size carrot, peeled and chopped
Salt and freshly ground black pepper to taste
1 ½ pounds eel, cut into bite-size chunks
1 bay leaf

½ teaspoon dried thyme or 2 sprigs fresh
1 tablespoon flour
½ cup minced fresh parsley
1 medium-size ripe, fresh tomato, chopped
1 cup any chicken or fish stock (pages 40–41)
Juice of ½ lemon

Heat the oil in a skillet that can later be covered. Cook the onion, garlic, and carrot over medium-high heat until softened, stirring occasionally, about 10 minutes. Season with salt and pepper and stir. Add the eel and cook, stirring, for 2 to 3 minutes. Add the bay leaf, thyme, flour, and half the parsley; stir until the flour disappears. Add the tomato and stock, stir, cover, reduce the heat to low, and simmer until the eel is tender, 10 to 20 minutes. Sprinkle with the lemon juice and garnish with the remaining parsley. Serve immediately.

Eel in Red Wine:

Sauté the vegetables in half butter and half oil. Substitute 2 cups dry red wine for the stock and let it bubble away for 1 to 2 minutes before covering the skillet. Finish the dish by stirring in 2 tablespoons butter, a bit at a time (omit the lemon juice). (You can also stew eel in white wine: substitute sage for thyme if you do.)

Eel in Cider:

Start by sautéing ¼ pound minced bacon until crisp. Remove with a slotted spoon and drain on paper towels; sauté the vegetables in the remaining fat. Use 2 cups dry cider and 1 tablespoon cider or sherry vinegar in place of the tomato and stock. Let it bubble away for 1 to 2 minutes before covering the skillet. Finish the dish by stirring in 1 tablespoon butter (omit the lemon juice); garnish with the reserved bacon and parsley. (You can enhance this dish by soaking 6 to 10 prunes in some of the cider before adding it; add the prunes along with the cider and proceed as above.)

Curried Eel:

Stir 1 tablespoon curry powder into the vegetable mixture before adding the eel. Omit the thyme and substitute cilantro (fresh coriander) for the parsley. Add ½ cup dry white wine and 1 tablespoon white wine vinegar along with the stock; let bubble away for 1 to 2 minutes before covering the skillet. Finish as above.

Eel in Herbs:

Omit the bay leaf. Use 1 teaspoon each chopped fresh thyme and sage, 1 tablespoon chopped fresh chervil or dill, or any assortment of fresh herbs you like. Cook as directed.

SAUTÉED EEL

Makes 4 servings
Time: 30 minutes
Because it's rich and fatty, eel is delicious when treated simply.

2 cups flour for dredging
Salt and freshly ground black pepper to taste
2 pounds eel, cut into 2-inch pieces
½ to 1 cup olive oil, butter, or a combination
20 sprigs fresh parsley
2 lemons, quartered

Heat a 12-inch nonstick skillet over medium-high heat for 3 to 4 minutes. Place the flour in a bag, season it liberally, and shake the eel pieces, a few at a time, until they are well coated with flour. Add ½ cup of the oil to the pan and, when it is hot (a pinch of flour will sizzle) add the eel, a few pieces at a time; don't crowd. Brown the pieces well on all sides for a total of about 10 minutes; the meat will start to come away from the bone. Keep done pieces warm in a low oven, add oil to the pan as necessary, and complete the cooking. When the eel is done, cook the parsley in the same pan, stirring briefly; use it to garnish the eel. Serve with lemon wedges.

SAUTÉED EEL WITH BACON:

Serve with broiled or sautéed bacon, 1 or 2 pieces per person. You can also deep-fry the parsley; drop a couple of well-dried sprigs at a time into hot oil and fry for a few seconds, until darkened and crisp.

EEL WITH PASTA:

Cook as instructed in the main recipe, using a minimum of oil. When the eel is fully cooked, remove it from the bone and cut it into small pieces. Heat ½ cup olive oil over medium heat. Add 1 tablespoon minced garlic and 2 dried hot red peppers and cook, stirring, until the garlic is lightly colored. Remove the peppers. Cook 1 pound linguine according to the package instructions; toss with the garlicky oil, the eel pieces, and about ½ cup minced fresh parsley.

POACHED AND SAUTÉED EEL

Makes 4 servings
Time: 30 minutes
An extra step for extra tenderness and flavor.

2 pounds eel, cut into 2-inch pieces
2 cups dry white wine or as needed
1 onion, cut in half
1 bay leaf
Several sprigs fresh thyme or about ½ teaspoon
  dried
Flour for dredging
1 large egg, lightly beaten
Unseasoned bread crumbs for dredging
½ cup olive oil
20 sprigs fresh parsley
2 lemons, quartered

Simmer the eel in the wine to cover, along with the onion, bay leaf, and thyme, for about 10 minutes. Drain the eel (you can reserve the wine for finishing sauces if you like), then dredge it in the flour. Dip in the beaten egg, then roll in bread crumbs, patting to help the crumbs adhere. Sauté in olive oil until lightly browned and serve with parsley and lemon.

GRILLED OR BROILED EEL

Makes 4 servings
Time: 15 minutes or more

2 pounds eel, cut into 2-inch pieces
2 tablespoons olive oil
Salt and freshly ground black pepper to taste
2 lemons, quartered, *or* 1 to 2 teaspoons balsamic or sherry vinegar

Start a charcoal fire or preheat a gas grill or broiler. Skewer the eel pieces, rub them with the oil, and sprinkle with salt and pepper. Grill or broil about 4 to 6 inches from the heat source, about 4 minutes per side; eel is done when it begins to separate from the bone. Serve immediately with lemon wedges or brushed with the vinegar.

MARINATED EEL WITH HERBS:

Marinate the eel for about 1 hour in about ½ cup olive oil, ½ cup fresh lemon juice, and a handful of fresh herbs such as sage or rosemary. Skewer the eel and grill it, basting frequently with the marinade.

FLATFISH

Latin name(s): Bothidae and Pleuronectidae families.
Other common names: Flounders, dabs, plaices, and soles of all types.
Common forms: Whole or dressed fish, fillets (very common and usually skinned).
General description: From stark white to grayish fillets, usually under a half pound each, although they can be larger (some whole flatfish weigh ten pounds). One of the world's most popular fish: the annual catch is around 1 million tons. Whole fish are flat, with both eyes on the usually dark-colored top, and lighter (sometimes white) skin on bottom; the skin is edible and delicious.
For other recipes see: Blackfish, butterfish, catfish, cod, dogfish, grouper, haddock, halibut, mackerel, ocean perch, pollock, porgy, rockfish, sea bass, red snapper, tilefish, turbot, weakfish, whiting, wolffish.
Buying tips: Although some flatfish are better to eat than others—there are those with soft, virtually tasteless flesh—all are fine-grained and mild-flavored, and can be used interchangeably. Given a choice among flatfish, I'd make my decision based on freshness rather than species. Fillets, whether white, pearly, or gray, should glisten and smell of seawater. Whole fish should look firm and unbruised, with red gills and no off odors.

It's best to think of all the flounders, soles, dabs, and plaices as one type of fish. Unfortunately, we don't have the true Dover sole on our shores, and the East and West Coast fish called soles are, to the unpracticed eye, indistinguishable from flounders. By the time flatfish are filleted—as most in our markets are—even the experts have trouble telling them apart. So it does little good to recommend one over the other; although there are superior species, they're all worth eating.

Flatfish (including the larger halibut and turbot, which have their own entries) are distinguished by their eyes (which are on top of their heads); by their swimming style (on their sides); and by their protective coloring, which allows them to hide from both their enemies and their prey by burying themselves in the sand. There are more than a dozen flatfish caught off our shores, with the following common names among them: Dover (Pacific), petrale, lemon, gray, English, rock, and sand sole; blackback (winter), fluke (summer),

witch, southern, starry, rusty, and yellowtail flounder; and dab, sand dab, and plaice.

The thin, delicate fillets of flatfish are ideal for quick meals, especially if you're only serving two people (because the fillets are so thin, a quarter pound of them takes up a lot of space in skillet or baking pan). They must be cooked very, very quickly, usually for less than five minutes; the fish becomes white and opaque when done, and begins to flake and fall apart soon thereafter. I undercook flatfish fillets slightly; they invariably finish cooking between stove and table.

SIMMERED FLATFISH FOR TWO

Time: 15 minutes
This is a traditional Japanese method of preparing small whole fish. It works especially well with flounder and, with plain steamed rice, makes a wonderful lunch. The best way to eat it is to simply

pick at the fish with a pair of chopsticks and, ultimately, your fingers.

1 clove garlic, crushed and peeled
2 thin peeled slices fresh ginger or ½ teaspoon ground
¼ cup high-quality soy sauce
1 teaspoon sesame oil
1 teaspoon rice or other vinegar
1 whole flatfish, 1 to 1 ½ pounds, scaled and gutted

If you are making rice, start with that (the flounder only takes about 12 minutes from start to finish). Place all the ingredients except the flounder in a 10- or 12-inch nonstick sauté pan (one for which you have a cover) and bring to a boil. Lower the heat to a simmer, add the fish, and cover. Cook until the fish is done (it will just barely flake when prodded with a knife or fork), about 10 minutes. Serve, with the sauce, immediately.

PAN-GRILLED FLATFISH

Makes 2 servings
Time: 15 minutes
Although true Dover sole is almost never seen in our markets, many whole flatfish—such as petrale sole on the West Coast and fluke on the East—cook up just as nicely. Only attempt this dish when the fish is spanking fresh; get it from a boat or recreational fisherman if you can, and clean it yourself if you must (see below for directions). Once cleaned, cooking is the easy part; you can make as many of these as you have sauté pans, but you must figure only one fish per pan.

2 whole flatfish, about 1 ¼ pounds each
Coarse salt
1 teaspoon butter
½ lime or lemon

Heat two 10- or 12-inch nonstick sauté pans over medium-high heat while you ready the fish. Scale the fish according to the general directions on page 19 (the white side of flatfish have tiny scales which can be ignored, but it only takes a minute to remove them). Behead them, cutting at an angle from just behind the top of the head to behind the gill cover and on down. Remove the guts—most of them will come out with the head, but you can easily take out the rest with your fingers. Rinse and dry thoroughly.

Sprinkle the sauté pans with a thin layer of coarse salt. Turn heat to high. Using a sharp knife, slash both sides of each fish three times, about ⅛ inch deep. Place each fish on the salt, dark side down and cook (using an exhaust fan if you have one), shaking the pan once or twice, for 4 to 5 minutes. Turn and cook 3 to 4 minutes on the other side; you might make a small cut to see whether the fish is cooked through to the bone (the flesh will be opaque and tender), but, inevitably, it will be. Rub with a little butter and serve immediately, with a wedge of lime or lemon.

BROILED FLATFISH WITH MUSTARD AND THYME

Makes 4 servings
Time: 15 minutes
The sugar in this simple sauce provides a welcome sweetness and helps the coating color nicely. As you can see from the number of variations, this is a basic technique; use it to prepare flatfish with any dry topping or sauce that you like.

2 pounds flatfish fillets
1 tablespoon olive oil or melted butter
⅓ cup Dijon mustard
1 tablespoon sugar
1 teaspoon minced fresh thyme
1 tablespoon fresh lemon juice
Salt and freshly ground black pepper to taste

Preheat the broiler. Lay the fillets on a cookie sheet or broiling pan and brush with the oil. Mix together the sauce ingredients and spread thinly over the fish. Broil about 4 to 6 inches from the heat source, until lightly browned, 4 to 5 minutes. (You can also bake the fish here, or in any of the variations, at 450°F until it turns a flat white, about 6 minutes.) Remove from the broiler before the fillets flake when lightly touched. Serve immediately.

ALTERNATIVE FISH FOR THIS RECIPE:

Fillets of blackfish, catfish, cod, dogfish, grouper, haddock, ocean perch, pollock, rockfish, red snapper, tilefish, turbot, weakfish, or wolffish. Adjust the cooking times accordingly.

BROILED FLATFISH WITH LEMON AND DILL:

Dot the fillets with 2 tablespoons softened butter and sprinkle with minced fresh or dried dill. Broil as directed above and serve with lemon wedges. Alternatively, brush the fillets with olive oil, sprinkle with the dill, and make a sauce of 3 parts olive oil to 1 part fresh lemon juice, salt, pepper, and 2 tablespoons of minced dill.

BROILED FLATFISH WITH GARLIC AND MARJORAM:

Combine 1 tablespoon minced fresh marjoram (or oregano) or 1 teaspoon dried with 1 teaspoon minced garlic, ½ cup olive oil, ¼ cup fresh lemon juice, ¼ cup minced fresh parsley, salt, and pepper. Spoon some of this over the fish before broiling, and pass the rest at the table.

BROILED FLATFISH WITH SPICY TOMATO SAUCE:

Combine 2 cups chopped tomatoes (drained if canned) with ½ teaspoon cayenne pepper, ¼ cup fresh lime juice, ¼ cup minced cilantro (fresh coriander), and salt to taste. Spoon some of this over the fish before broiling, and pass the rest at the table.

BROILED FLATFISH WITH NUT SAUCE:

Heat 2 tablespoons olive oil over medium-high heat, add 1 cup chopped onion, and cook, stirring, until soft. Add 1 teaspoon minced garlic and ½ cup chopped walnuts or pecans, or whole pine nuts. Cook, stirring, for 1 minute, then add 1 cup chopped tomatoes (drained if canned). Season with salt and pepper and cook over high heat, stirring occasionally, until fairly thick, about 5 minutes. Spoon this over the fish before broiling.

BROILED FLATFISH WITH MUSHROOMS:

Soak about 1 ounce dried porcini (cèpes) in warm water to cover until softened, about 10 minutes. Drain and strain the soaking liquid through a double thickness of paper towels; set aside. Cut off the hard parts of the mushrooms; mince the rest. Melt 3 tablespoon butter over medium-high heat; add the the cèpes along with 1 cup chopped domestic mushrooms and cook, stirring, until the mushrooms soften. Stir in 1 tablespoon minced shallot and 2 tablespoons minced fresh parsley. Cook 1 more minute, then add the strained soaking liquid. Season with salt and pepper, then simmer until some of the liquid has evaporated. Spoon this over the fish before broiling.

BROILED FLATFISH WITH GARLIC SAUCE:

Simmer 15 cloves peeled garlic in 1 cup milk over medium-low heat for 10 minutes; add salt, pepper, ¼ cup minced fresh basil, ¼ cup olive oil, and ¼ cup minced fresh parsley and simmer for 5 more minutes. Puree in a blender; check the seasonings. Spoon some of this over the fish before broiling, and pass the rest at the table.

BROILED FLATFISH WITH GINGER-CILANTRO SAUCE:

Combine the juice of ½ lemon, 1 minced clove garlic, 3 tablespoons minced cilantro (fresh coriander), 1 tablespoon peeled and minced fresh ginger, and salt and pepper to taste. Spread this over the fish before broiling.

FLATFISH FILLETS EN PAPILLOTE ASIAN STYLE

Makes 4 servings
Time: 20 minutes

You can assemble these little packages ahead of time; cooking takes just a few minutes. See Red Snapper Fillets en Papillote (page 288) for variations.

1 ¼ to 1 ½ pounds flatfish fillets
24 snow peas, trimmed
1 tablespoon peeled and minced fresh ginger
2 tablespoons minced scallions, green and white parts
1 tablespoon sesame oil
¼ cup high-quality soy sauce
1 tablespoon rice or other mild vinegar

Preheat the oven to 400°F. Place each fillet on a piece of aluminum foil large enough to enclose it along with some air space. Top each fillet with 3 snow peas, some minced ginger, and some scallion. Mix together the sesame oil, soy sauce, and vinegar and drizzle over each of the fillets. Close up the packages and place them all on a baking sheet or in a baking pan. Bake until steaming hot, 6 to 8 minutes. Open each envelope carefully, remove two fillets to each of four plates (these do well atop white rice), and drizzle with a little of the cooking liquid.

ALTERNATIVE FISH FOR THIS RECIPE:

Fillets of blackfish, catfish, cod, dogfish, grouper, haddock, ocean perch, pollock, rockfish, red snapper, tilefish, turbot, weakfish, or wolffish. Adjust the cooking times accordingly.

SWEET-AND-SOUR FLATFISH

Makes 8 appetizer servings
Time: 12 to 24 hours

An escabèche-style dish in which the fish is marinated after it is cooked.

2 pounds flatfish fillets
Salt and freshly ground black pepper to taste
¼ to ½ cup olive oil
Flour for dredging
2 large Spanish onions, very thinly sliced
½ cup sherry or balsamic vinegar
1 cup dry white wine
1 cup water
¼ cup raisins
2 bay leaves
¼ cup pine nuts

Preheat a 12-inch nonstick skillet over medium-high heat for 5 minutes or so. Season the fillets with salt and pepper. Add ¼ cup oil to the pan. Dredge as many fillets in the flour as will fit comfortably in the skillet, shaking to remove excess flour. Cook until golden brown on both sides, about 5 minutes total. As the fillets finish, transfer them to an earthenware or porcelain dish and cook the remaining fillets. Add more oil if necessary.

When you've finished cooking the fish, cook the onions in the same oil over low heat until quite soft, 20 to 30 minutes. Add the vinegar and turn up the heat to medium-high, cooking and stirring until the liquid is almost evaporated, 5 to 7 minutes. Stir in the wine, water, and raisins and simmer over low heat for about 10 minutes.

Sprinkle the bay leaves and pine nuts over the cooked fish; pour over the cooking liquid. Cover with aluminum foil and marinate, refrigerated, for 12 to 24 hours. Bring to room temperature and serve.

ALTERNATIVE FISH FOR THIS RECIPE:

Fillets of striped bass, catfish, dogfish, mackerel, rockfish, red snapper, or weakfish. Adjust the cooking times accordingly.

BASIC FLATFISH MEUNIÈRE

Makes 2 servings
Time: 20 minutes

This classic preparation for fillets of sole works equally well for any other flatfish. Serve hot, hot, hot.

Salt and freshly ground black pepper to taste
½ to ¾ pound flatfish fillets
1 tablespoon olive or vegetable oil
¼ cup (½ stick) butter
Flour for dredging
Juice of ½ lemon
Chopped fresh parsley for garnish
2 lemon wedges

Heat two plates in a low oven. Season the fillets. Heat a 12-inch nonstick skillet over medium-high heat for 3 to 4 minutes and add the oil and half the butter. When the butter foam subsides, dredge the fillets, one by one, in the flour, shaking off any excess, and add them to the pan. Cook until golden on each side, 4 to 5 minutes total. Remove to the warm serving plates. Reduce the heat to medium and add the remaining butter to the pan; cook until the butter foams, 1 or 2 minutes. Add the lemon juice, and stir, scraping the bottom of the pan as you do so; pour the sauce over the fillets. Sprinkle with the parsley and serve immediately with the lemon wedges.

ALTERNATIVE FISH FOR THIS RECIPE:

Fillets of blackfish, catfish, cod, dogfish, grouper, haddock, ocean perch, pollock, rockfish, red snapper, tilefish, turbot, weakfish, or wolffish. Adjust the cooking times accordingly.

FLATFISH WITH CAPERS:

Add 1 tablespoon capers, rinsed, to the skillet along with the lemon juice (you can also add a couple of minced anchovies if you like). Cook 30 seconds, then pour over the fillets.

FLATFISH WITH PINE NUTS:

Begin by sautéing ½ cup chopped onion and 1 teaspoon minced garlic in 2 tablespoons olive oil over medium-high heat until soft. Remove the onion mixture with a slotted spoon; add 2 tablespoons butter, then dredge the fillets in flour and cook as directed above. Season with salt, pepper, and the juice of ½ lemon; remove the fillets to a plate in a warm oven. Add ½ cup pine nuts and ½ cup any fish or chicken stock (pages 40–41) to the skillet, along with the onions. Cook for 2 minutes and spoon over the fish. Serve immediately.

SAUTÉED FLATFISH WITH NOODLES AND BROTH

Makes 2 servings
Time: 30 minutes
This is flatfish cooked meunière style, but served in an Asian broth with udon noodles; linguine may be substituted.

2 cups any chicken or fish stock (pages 40–41)
2 tablespoons shoyu (Japanese soy sauce; available in Asian markets and health food stores)
1 tablespoon mirin (sweet rice wine; available in Asian markets and health food stores)
6 ounces udon noodles (available in Asian markets and health food stores)
Flour for dredging
Salt and freshly ground black pepper to taste
3 tablespoons peanut or vegetable oil
½ pound flatfish fillets
Minced scallions, both green and white parts, or cilantro (fresh coriander) for garnish

Set a pot of water to boil for the noodles, and begin to preheat a 12-inch nonstick skillet over medium-high heat. Warm the stock with the soy sauce and mirin and keep it warm. Begin to cook the noodles according to the package instructions. Season the flour with salt and pepper, add the peanut oil the pan, and, when the oil is hot (a pinch of flour will sizzle), dredge the fillets in the flour, shaking off any excess flour, and cook them about 2 minutes per side, until just beginning to brown. Drain the noodles. Place a portion of noodles in each of two large bowls, add a cup of the broth, and top with a portion of fish. Garnish with the scallions and serve.

ALTERNATIVE FISH FOR THIS RECIPE:
Fillets of blackfish, catfish, cod, dogfish, grouper, haddock, ocean perch, pollock, rockfish, red snapper, tilefish, turbot, weakfish, or wolffish. Adjust the cooking times accordingly.

FLATFISH WITH CREAM AND GRAPES

Makes 2 servings
Time: 20 minutes
Here flatfish are sautéed far more gently than in a meunière, with classic and elegant results. You can use almost any white wine in this dish, but the ones noted here will make a pleasantly subtle difference, and you'll enjoy drinking them with the fish. Ask in any decent wine store for a Kabinett-level Moselle or similar American wine, such as a Riesling.

3 tablespoons butter
2 tablespoons minced shallot
3/4 pound flatfish fillets
1/2 cup fruity white wine
1/2 cup heavy cream
Salt and freshly ground black pepper to taste
1/2 cup seedless green grapes

Melt the butter in a 12-inch nonstick skillet over medium heat. Add the shallot and cook, stirring, until soft; add the fish and cook gently, still over medium heat, about 2 minutes per side, until white. Remove the fish to a plate and keep warm in a low oven. Add the wine to the skillet, turn the heat to high, and reduce by half. Lower the heat to medium and add the cream; cook, stirring, for about 5 minutes. Add salt and pepper and taste the sauce for seasoning. Add the grapes and let them

heat through for 30 or 60 seconds; spoon over the fillets. Serve immediately, with white rice.

ALTERNATIVE FISH FOR THIS RECIPE:
Fillets of blackfish, catfish, cod, dogfish, grouper, haddock, ocean perch, pollock, rockfish, red snapper, tilefish, turbot, weakfish, or wolffish. Adjust the cooking times accordingly.

RAW FLATFISH SALAD

Makes 6 appetizer servings
Time: 1 hour, mostly resting time
This variation on seviche, and the one for sea bass on page 255, can be made with almost any thin fillet; I suggest making it only when you're by the seashore and can buy fish straight from the boat, or nearly so. Even then, make sure the fish has been iced from the moment of capture (this is not so much an issue of safety but one of peak flavor).

1 pound flatfish fillets, cut into 1/2-inch dice
1/2 teaspoon coriander seeds
1 teaspoon salt
2 tablespoons flavorful olive oil
1/2 cup fresh lemon juice
1/4 teaspoon minced garlic
Pinch cayenne pepper
Lettuce leaves
Chopped fresh mint or cilantro (fresh coriander)

Combine the fish with the coriander seeds, salt, olive oil, lemon juice, garlic, and cayenne. Mix gently, cover, and refrigerate for about 1 hour. Serve on a bed of lettuce, garnished with mint.

ALTERNATIVE FISH FOR THIS RECIPE:
Thin fillets of butterfish, mackerel, ocean perch, pompano, porgy, salmon, cut scallops (page 244), trout, weakfish, or wolffish.

GROUPER

Latin names(s): Various species, but especially *Mycteroperca* and *Epinephelus*.

Other common names: Sand perch, rock cod, coney, sea bass, jewfish.

Common forms: Whole fish (usually no more than five or ten pounds in the market, although much larger fish are caught), skinless fillets (up to two or three pounds), and (rarely) steaks.

General description: White, firm fillet; an excellent all-purpose fish with an extremely pleasing, meaty texture and mild flavor.

For other recipes see: Blackfish, carp, cod, dogfish, haddock, halibut, mahi-mahi, mako, monkfish, ocean perch, pollock, rockfish, sablefish, sea bass, red snapper, striped bass, tilefish, or wolffish.

Buying tips: Fillets should be stark white, with no graying or browning, and smell of seawater. Whole grouper can be of almost any color, but should be in good shape, attractive and unbruised. Grouper of ten pounds or more, and grouper roe (which you will rarely see) should be avoided, as both have been implicated in ciguatera poisoning (page 16).

To say that there are many kinds of grouper is an understatement; there are hundreds of species, and we commonly see a dozen or more, all from warm Atlantic, Pacific, and Caribbean waters. In good fish markets, on a good day, you might see five different species. For culinary purposes, they're pretty much equivalent.

Grouper can grow to several hundred pounds, but it's the smaller fish, up to ten pounds or so, that make it to market. Like red snapper, tilefish, striped bass—to which it is related—and other high quality white-fleshed ocean fish, grouper has big taste and firm, lobsterlike texture. Filleted, it is perfectly boneless and firm enough to deep fry and even grill; cubed, it can be kebabed or used in chowders or stews. Heads and skeletons make good stock.

BAKED WHOLE GROUPER WITH POTATOES, ONIONS, AND FRESH HERBS

Makes 6 to 8 servings
Time: 60 minutes

I like this best with a bunch of rosemary branches, but you can use whatever herb you find in your supermarket or garden. With the variations, this is one of the most basic of all fish recipes, and can be used with almost any whole, white-fleshed round-fish and many large fish steaks.

One 5-pound grouper, scaled and gutted with
   head on
Salt
4 cloves garlic, cut into slivers
¼ cup olive or peanut oil
1 lemon, thinly sliced
20 or more sprigs fresh thyme, rosemary, parsley, sage, and/or basil
12 to 15 small new potatoes, washed well
12 to 15 small onions, peeled
3 to 5 carrots, cut into chunks
1 cup dry white wine or any fish stock (pages
   40–41)
Salt and freshly ground black pepper to taste

Rinse the fish well. Cut 3 or 4 gashes on each side
of the fish, from top to bottom. Salt the gashes,
and salt the fish's cavity as well. Let it sit while you
prepare the other ingredients, and preheat the oven
to 450°F.

Push half the garlic slivers into the gashes. Rub
the fish with a little of the olive oil, and pour the
rest onto the bottom of a large baking pan. Spread
the lemon slices over the bottom of the pan and
top it with most of the herbs. Lay the fish over the
herbs, then spread the potatoes, onions, carrots,
and remaining garlic around the fish. Pour the
wine over all, and sprinkle with salt and pepper.
Top with the remaining herbs.

Cover with aluminum foil and bake, undisturbed, until the vegetables are nearly tender, 30 to
40 minutes. Uncover and continue to bake, shaking the pan occasionally, until the potatoes are nice
and soft and the fish is cooked through, 10 to 20
minutes more. (Look at one of the gashes in the
thickest part of the fish; the meat will appear
opaque clear down to the central bone.) If the pan
is drying out, add a little more wine, stock, or
water.

To serve, remove the grouper's skin (it's not
especially good), scoop the flesh from the fish with
a spoon, and top with some vegetables and sauce.

ALTERNATIVE FISH FOR THIS RECIPE:

You need a good whole fish for this, such as
carp, red snapper, striped bass, or tilefish.

BAKED WHOLE GROUPER WITH TOMATOES
AND PERSILLADE:

Add 2 cups chopped tomatoes (canned are fine;
don't bother to drain them) to the baking pan.
Toward the end of baking, mix together 1 cup
minced fresh parsley and ½ cup plain bread
crumbs. Spread this mixture over the fish and continue baking until it browns lightly.

BAKED WHOLE GROUPER WITH FENNEL AND
MUSHROOMS:

Substitute several stalks of fresh fennel for the
herbs; omit the potatoes and carrots. Add about 1
pound mushrooms (fresh cèpes, if available, or
other "wild" mushrooms, or a mixture of wild and
domestic mushrooms, or domestic mushrooms
with some reconstituted dried cèpes mixed in) and
1 cup chopped tomatoes (canned are fine, but
drain them first). When you uncover the fish, top it
with fennel tops and a sprinkling of chopped scallions, both green and white parts.

BAKED WHOLE GROUPER WITH CUMIN AND
LEMON:

Rub the fish with 1 tablespoon ground cumin
after rubbing it with the olive oil. Use cilantro
(fresh coriander) sprigs under and over the fish.
Omit the potatoes and carrots; add several
unpeeled cloves garlic. When you uncover the fish,
add 1 cup chopped tomatoes (canned are fine, but
drain them first) and a sprinkling of about ¼ cup
minced cilantro (fresh coriander). Garnish with
minced cilantro and sprinkle with fresh lemon juice
before serving.

WHOLE BRAISED GROUPER WITH
HOT-AND-SOUR SAUCE
....

Makes 2 to 4 servings
Time: 30 minutes

This is the kind of dish for which many Chinese restaurants charge a premium, as though it were difficult to make. It isn't. It is, however, a real treat. Be sure to bring the whole fish to the table before removing the skin—it looks great, and you'll want to pick at the bones.

One 2- to 3-pound grouper, gutted and scaled, with head on
3 tablespoons dry sherry
1 tablespoon fermented black beans (available in Asian markets)
1 cup any chicken or fish stock (pages 40–41)
2 dried shiitake (black) mushrooms
½ cup peanut oil
Flour for dredging
1 large onion, sliced
Salt
2 teaspoons minced garlic
1 tablespoon peeled and minced fresh ginger
½ teaspoon cayenne pepper or to taste
2 tablespoons high-quality soy sauce
¼ cup rice or distilled vinegar
1 teaspoon sesame oil
Minced scallions, both green and white parts, for garnish

Check to make sure the fish will fit in your 12-inch sauté pan. If not, cut off its head (page 20). Make 3 shallow cuts, from top to bottom, on each side of the fish. Rinse it with 2 tablespoons of the sherry and set aside.

Soak the black beans in the remaining sherry. Heat the stock and soak the mushrooms in it.

Preheat the 12-inch sauté pan over medium-high heat for 3 to 5 minutes. Add the peanut oil; when a pinch of flour sizzles in it, you can begin to cook. Dredge the grouper in the flour and gently place it in the oil. Raise the heat to high until the oil sizzles loudly, then back off on the heat a little bit to avoid burning the oil or flour. Cook until golden brown, 3 to 5 minutes, then turn the fish carefully and brown the other side. Remove the fish to a plate.

Remove the mushrooms from the stock, rinse, and thinly slice them. Pour the stock through a double thickness of paper towels to remove any sand deposits. Set both aside.

Pour off most of the oil from the pan you cooked the fish in, return the pan to the stove over high heat, and add the onion. Sprinkle with salt and cook, stirring, for 2 to 3 minutes. Add the garlic, ginger, and cayenne; cook another couple of minutes, until the onion softens a bit. Add the mushrooms to the pan; then add the black beans along with the sherry. Stir, then add the soy sauce, vinegar, and stock. Bring to a boil, cook 1 minute, then lower the heat and return the grouper to the pan. Cover and cook gently until the grouper is cooked through (peek in one of the slashes; the meat should be opaque clear to the bone), about 10 minutes.

Remove the grouper to a platter, reduce the braising liquid if it looks thin, add the sesame oil, and spoon the sauce and the onions over and around the fish. Garnish with the scallions. To serve, peel back the skin (grouper skin is not delicious), spoon the meat from the bone, and serve immediately, with plenty of white rice.

ALTERNATIVE FISH FOR THIS RECIPE:

Whole specimens of any firm-fleshed fish: Carp, rockfish, sea bass, red snapper, striped bass, or tilefish. Adjust cooking times accordingly.

GROUPER SANDWICH
WITH SPINACH

Makes 2 servings
Time: 30 minutes

Proof positive that fish is indeed portable; I've eaten this sandwich on the train, in the car, and at picnics, and have relished it each time. Although I like it served hot, I think it improves with a few hours' aging, as the bread softens and the flavors mingle.

½ pound fresh spinach
¾ pound grouper fillets
3 tablespoons olive oil
Bread crumbs for dredging
2 cloves garlic, minced
French or Italian bread or rolls
Salt and freshly ground black pepper to taste
Fresh lemon juice to taste

Wash the spinach well. Place it in a covered pot and steam it with the water remaining on its leaves until it is tender, 5 to 10 minutes. Plunge it into cold water for a moment, place it in a colander, and let it drain. Rinse the grouper and dry it between paper towels.

Preheat a 10- or 12-inch nonstick skillet over medium-high heat for 3 to 4 minutes. Add 2 tablespoons of the oil, dredge the grouper in the bread crumbs, and cook it until the crumbs brown nicely, 3 or 4 minutes per side. Drain the fish on paper towels and wipe the pan clean.

Chop the spinach and add the remaining olive oil to the pan in which you cooked the fish; add the garlic and, immediately, the spinach. Cook over medium-high heat, tossing frequently, until hot, just 1 or 2 minutes.

Put the grouper on the bread or rolls and top with the spinach. Drizzle with lemon juice and sprinkle with salt and pepper. Serve immediately, or wrap in aluminum foil and serve cold or at room temperature.

Alternative fish for this recipe:

Blackfish, dogfish, Atlantic pollock, rockfish, red snapper, striped bass, tilefish, or wolffish. Cooking time will vary slightly with the thickness of the fillets.

Grilled Grouper over Spinach:

Prepare the spinach as directed above. Then brush the grouper with olive oil and grill it, or cook it as above; serve the grouper on the spinach, with lemon wedges.

GRILLED GROUPER STEAKS

Makes 4 servings
Time: 30 minutes

Large grouper can be made into steaks, which are firm enough to grill with no trouble.

½ cup olive oil
1 large onion, roughly chopped
4 cloves garlic, chopped
2 teaspoons peeled and grated fresh ginger or 1 teaspoon dried
¼ teaspoon cayenne pepper or to taste
Juice of 1 lemon
Salt to taste
Four 1-inch-thick grouper steaks

Put all the ingredients except the fish in a food processor or blender and process until nearly smooth. Pour this mixture over the grouper and marinate while you start a charcoal fire or preheat a gas grill or broiler.

Cook the grouper over white-hot coals, basting frequently with the sauce. Turn once. Steaks will be ready in 8 to 10 minutes. To check, use a thin-bladed knife to pry a little of the flesh away from the bone and peek inside; the flesh should be opaque throughout.

Alternative fish for this recipe:

This is an uncomplicated, simple recipe, but few

other steaks stand up to the grill as well as grouper: Try bonito (if you can find it), mahi-mahi, mako shark, monkfish (whole tails), striped bass, or swordfish.

FILLETED GROUPER WITH PASTA AND TOMATOES

Makes 4 servings
Time: 40 minutes

I emphatically believe that fish and cheese do not belong on the table at the same time. This is one of the exceptions, a fishy pasta sauce with a tomato-y fish, and a great way to cook two courses at the same time. It's also one of those all-purpose recipes, useful for almost any fin- or shellfish you have in the house.

3 tablespoons olive oil
2 dried hot peppers or to taste
2 cloves garlic, peeled and lightly crushed
2 cups chopped seeded and peeled tomatoes, fresh or canned
1 teaspoon dried rosemary
Salt and freshly ground black pepper to taste
1 large or 2 small grouper fillets, about 1 pound total
1 pound spaghetti, linguine, or capellini
½ cup minced fresh parsley
Freshly grated Parmesan

Preheat the oven to 300°F and set a large pot of water to boil for the pasta. Heat the oil in a large skillet over medium-high heat. Add the peppers and garlic and cook, stirring, until the garlic becomes brown (this is a somewhat strong-tasting sauce). Remove and discard the peppers and garlic and add the tomatoes. Cook, stirring, until the tomatoes begin to liquefy, about 5 minutes; add the rosemary, salt, and pepper. Cook another 5 minutes, then gently place the fillets in the sauce. Cover the skillet.

Cook, over medium heat, until the fillets are almost done, 5 to 8 minutes, depending on their size (they will be pasty white and offer little resistance to a thin-bladed knife). Remove them carefully and place them in the oven. Cook the pasta; stir most of the parsley into the sauce. Dress the pasta with sauce and cheese; garnish the fish with the remaining parsley. Serve the pasta first, then the fish at room temperature; or serve them together.

ALTERNATIVE FISH FOR THIS RECIPE:

Fillets of blackfish, dogfish, Atlantic pollock, rockfish, red snapper, tilefish, or wolffish; steaks of halibut, striped bass, or tilefish.

RISOTTO WITH GROUPER AND CHIVES

Makes 4 appetizer or light main course servings
Time: 45 minutes

This isn't a true risotto (see Risotto with Shrimp and Greens, page 268, if you're looking for one), but it takes a little less work and gives good results.

5 tablespoons butter
1 small onion, minced
½ cup minced carrot
1 tablespoon olive oil
1 or 2 grouper fillets, about 1 pound total, cut into bite-size pieces
1 cup arborio or other short-grain rice
3 ½ cups any fish or chicken stock (pages 40–41)
Salt and freshly ground black pepper to taste
¼ cup freshly minced chives

In a 6- or 8-cup saucepan over medium heat, melt 2 tablespoons of the butter and slowly cook the onion and carrot, stirring occasionally, until soft.

Meanwhile, heat a 12-inch nonstick skillet over high heat. Add the oil and 1 tablespoon of the butter, then cook the fish, stirring occasionally, until lightly browned on all sides. Remove to a plate.

When the carrot and onion are tender, add the rice and stir to coat with butter. Add the stock, all at once, season with salt and pepper, and simmer, uncovered, over medium heat, stirring occasionally. When all the liquid has been absorbed—15 to 20 minutes—stir in the sautéed grouper (along with any liquid that has accumulated around it), the chives, and the remaining butter. Cook over low heat, stirring, for 3 minutes, and serve immediately.

ALTERNATIVE FISH FOR THIS RECIPE:

Any white fish or shellfish that will hold up to this treatment: Blackfish, eel, monkfish, red snapper, striped bass, or wolffish; clams, oysters, scallops, shrimp, snails, or squid. Adjust cooking times accordingly; the shellfish, especially, will need only a minute or two of browning in the oil/butter combination.

PAN-FRIED GROUPER WITH SOUTHWESTERN TOMATO SAUCE

Makes 4 servings
Time: 30 minutes

1 tablespoon cumin seeds
½ cup plus 2 tablespoons peanut or vegetable oil
2 cloves garlic, crushed and peeled
3 cups ripe or canned tomatoes, chopped and drained briefly
¼ teaspoon cayenne pepper or to taste
1 tablespoon balsamic or sherry wine vinegar
1 teaspoon minced garlic
Salt and freshly ground black pepper to taste
1 tablespoon ground cumin
1 or 2 grouper fillets, about 1 ½ pounds, cut into serving pieces
1 cup unbleached all-purpose flour
¼ cup minced cilantro (fresh coriander)

Toast the cumin seeds in a dry 10-inch skillet over medium heat until fragrant, about 3 minutes. Add the 2 tablespoons of oil and the crushed garlic; raise the heat to medium-high and cook until the garlic is golden brown. Add the tomatoes and cayenne, reduce the heat to medium, and cook about 10 minutes, stirring occasionally. Add the vinegar, minced garlic, salt, and pepper, and cook 5 minutes more, stirring occasionally. Taste for seasoning and reduce the heat to low.

Preheat a 10-inch nonstick skillet over medium-high heat for 3 to 4 minutes. Mix together the flour, ground cumin, and some salt and pepper. Add the ½ cup of oil to the skillet and when it is hot (a pinch of flour will sizzle) raise the heat to high, dredge the grouper fillets one by one in the flour, and put them in the skillet. Cook until golden brown, 3 to 4 minutes per side. Drain the fish on paper towels and serve, napped with the tomato sauce and garnished with cilantro.

ALTERNATIVE FISH FOR THIS RECIPE:

Almost any thick fillet works nicely here: Blackfish, cod, dogfish, monkfish, pollock, rockfish, red snapper, striped bass, tilefish, or wolffish.

GROUPER IN YELLOW CURRY

Makes 4 servings
Time: 45 minutes

1 cup unsweetened shredded coconut
2 cups boiling water
5 tablespoons peanut or vegetable oil
1 pound grouper fillets, cut into chunks
Flour for dredging
2 cups sliced onion
1 teaspoon turmeric
¼ teaspoon cayenne pepper
½ teaspoon ground coriander
¼ teaspoon freshly ground black pepper

Salt to taste
2 tablespoons fresh lemon juice
Minced cilantro (fresh coriander) for garnish

Put the coconut in a blender. Cover with water, blend (hold the cover on tight with a towel while the machine is on for extra safety), and let rest for a few minutes.

Heat 3 tablespoons of the oil in a 12-inch skillet over medium-high heat until it is hot (a pinch of flour will sizzle). Dredge the grouper chunks lightly in the flour and cook quickly over high heat until lightly browned, 3 to 4 minutes. Remove the fish with a slotted spoon and set aside.

Add the remaining oil to the pan and cook the onion over medium heat, stirring occasionally, until very soft and beginning to turn brown, about 10 minutes. Stir in the turmeric, cayenne, coriander, pepper, and salt. Cook for about 2 minutes.

Strain the coconut milk and add the liquid to the onion mixture; bring to a boil over medium-high heat and reduce by about a third. Add the fish, reduce the heat to medium, and cook for about 5 minutes. Add the lemon juice, taste and correct the seasonings, garnish with cilantro, and serve.

ALTERNATIVE FISH FOR THIS RECIPE:

Chunks of blackfish, dogfish, halibut, mahi-mahi, mako shark, monkfish, pollock, rockfish, red snapper, striped bass, tilefish, or wolffish.

HADDOCK

Latin name(s): *Melanogrammus aeglefinus*.
Other common names: Scrod (or schrod), a market name used also for cod and sometimes pollock.
Common forms: Almost exclusively skin-on fillets (easily recognized by the black lateral line and distinctive "thumbprint" above the pectoral fin); white flesh much like that of cod.
General description: Codlike white fillet of mild flavor and good texture.
For other recipes see: Blackfish, cod (especially), dogfish, flatfish, grouper, halibut, mackerel, monkfish, ocean perch, pollock, rockfish, sea bass, red snapper, tilefish, turbot, weakfish, wolffish.
Buying tips: As for any white-fleshed fillet: Avoid fish that appears dried out or has browning. Gaping should be minimal and smell should be fresh. Haddock is almost always sold with skin on.

Smaller than cod (few top five pounds), haddock is often substituted for its slightly more famous relative. There is little difference. As with cod, overfishing has made haddock more expensive and harder to find in recent years.

GRILLED HADDOCK "SANDWICH" WITH PICKLED ONIONS

Makes 4 servings
Time: 12 hours, including marinating time for the onions; 20 minutes cooking time
It's difficult to grill lean, tender white-fleshed fish, but it's far from impossible. Here, the haddock's skin is left intact, and layers of pickled onions add further protection. A grilling basket (page 26) is essential here.

1 large Spanish onion, thinly sliced and separated into rings
¼ cup sugar
⅓ cup distilled vinegar
⅓ cup water
1 tablespoon olive oil
1 teaspoon salt (optional)

2 haddock fillets, about 1 pound each, skin on (it is helpful if the fillets are roughly the same shape and ideal if they are from the same fish)
Salt and freshly ground black pepper to taste

Make the pickled onions 12 to 24 hours in advance: Mix together the onion rings, sugar, vinegar, water, olive oil, and salt. Stir, cover, and refrigerate. Stir every few hours.

When you're ready to cook, start a charcoal fire or preheat a gas grill. Sprinkle the fillets with salt and pepper. Oil a fish basket unless it is coated with nonstick material. Layer the bottom of the basket with about a third of the onions, making the rough shape of the fillets. Place a fillet, skin side down, on top of the onion slices; cover the fillet with another handful of onions, then make a sandwich, using the second fillet, skin side up. Place the remaining onions on the skin of the second fillet, and cover it tightly with the top half of the basket.

Grill the sandwich about 5 to 8 minutes per side; it's fine if some of the onion rings burn a little. The fish is done when a thin-bladed knife passes through the sandwich with little resistance. Carefully remove the top half of the grill, cut the sandwich into slices, and serve. The interior onion slices

---

should be barely warm, and the fish will be cooked through and tender.

ALTERNATIVE FISH FOR THIS RECIPE:

It's best to make this with fish that retains its skin, but not essential. Try it with paired fillets of blackfish, grouper, mackerel, ocean perch, pollock, rockfish, red snapper, or wolffish. Adjust cooking times accordingly.

ROAST HADDOCK FILLETS WITH SESAME SAUCE

Makes 4 servings
Time: 30 minutes

½ cup sesame seeds
2 tablespoons fresh lemon juice
½ cup olive oil
¼ teaspoon cayenne pepper
2 cloves garlic, peeled
1 medium-size onion, peeled and quartered
½ cup cilantro (fresh coriander) leaves
Salt and freshly ground black pepper to taste
1 to 1 ½ pounds haddock fillets
1 lemon, quartered

Toast the sesame seeds: Place them in a medium-size sauté pan and cook over medium heat, shaking the pan occasionally, until they darken and begin to pop. Remove from the heat and set 2 tablespoons aside.

Preheat the oven to 450°F. Place the sesame seeds in a food processor with the lemon juice and process for 15 seconds. Add the olive oil, cayenne, garlic, onion, and half the cilantro; process until smooth. Season with salt and pepper.

Brush a baking pan with a bit of oil and lay the fillets in it; spread with the sesame paste. Bake until the blade of a knife pierces the fillets easily, about 10 minutes. Garnish the fish with the reserved sesame seeds and lemon and serve immediately.

ALTERNATIVE FISH FOR THIS RECIPE:

Fillets of cod, dogfish, flatfish, grouper, halibut, ocean perch, pollock, rockfish, sea bass, red snapper, tilefish, turbot, weakfish, or wolffish. Adjust the cooking time accordingly.

HADDOCK AND WINTER VEGETABLES

Makes 4 to 6 servings
Time: 1 hour
This casserole is best made with the Flavorful Fish and Vegetable Stock on page 40.

3 tablespoons butter, softened
1 tablespoon minced garlic
½ pound carrots, cut into rounds
½ pound celery, cut into ½-inch dice
½ pound potatoes, peeled and cut into ½-inch dice
1 large onion, sliced into rings
1 ½ pounds haddock fillets, cut roughly into 1-inch pieces
Salt and freshly ground black pepper to taste
2 cups chicken or fish stock (pages 40–41), a mixture of wine and water, or water

Preheat the oven to 375°F. Spread some of the butter on the bottom of a baking dish or casserole. Sprinkle the minced garlic on it, then top with about half each of the carrots, celery, potatoes, onion, and fish. Season with salt and pepper, spread with a little more of the butter, and make another layer of vegetables and fish. Sprinkle with a little more salt and pepper, pour the stock over all, and dot with the remaining butter. Cover and bake until the potatoes are cooked through, 45 minutes or so.

ALTERNATIVE FISH FOR THIS RECIPE:

Blackfish, cod, dogfish, flatfish, grouper, pollock, rockfish, sea bass, red snapper, tilefish, turbot, weakfish, or wolffish. Adjust the cooking time accordingly.

HAKE

Latin name(s): Urophycis, various species.
Other common names: Whiting, red hake, ling, cod, white hake, silver hake, black hake.
Common forms: Whole fish, fillets, steaks.
General description: One of the most confusing names in fish. Most are whiting or forms of cod. Usually decent white fish whatever it is.
For recipes see: Cod, whiting, or other white fish such as dogfish, flatfish, ocean perch, pollock, rockfish, sea bass, red snapper, tilefish, weakfish, or wolffish.
Buying tips: May be soft- or firm-fleshed, but always white. Avoid browning, graying; smell for freshness.

HALIBUT

Latin name(s): *Hippoglossus hippoglossus* (Atlantic), *Hippoglossus stenolepis* (Pacific).
Other common names: Greenland halibut, California halibut.
Common forms: Steaks are most common; smaller fish are sometimes filleted or sold whole, headless and dressed.
General description: The largest of the flatfish, with fine-textured, extremely lean white meat that can be on the dry side.
For other recipes see: Catfish, cod, dogfish, flatfish, grouper, haddock, monkfish, ocean perch, pollock, rockfish, salmon, skate, red snapper, swordfish, turbot (a close relative), weakfish, whiting, wolffish.
Buying tips: Steaks should have glistening, stark-white flesh. Browning or gaping are bad signs; the smell should be of seawater.

By far the largest flatfish—the record fish weighed seven hundred pounds, and two-hundred-pound specimens are not uncommon—the Atlantic halibut has, over the past decade, become increasingly rare and consequently more expensive. Fortunately, there is some indication that populations are recovering. In any case, the more plentiful Pacific halibut is equally good. (So-called California, Greenland, and black halibut are usually inferior.)

The flesh of halibut is firm, tight-grained, and flavorful, but it has a tendency to dry out. So although it can be grilled, broiled, roasted, or sautéed, I really believe it is at its best when poached, braised, or steamed, and have skewed the following recipes in that direction. Steaks are sold with skin on, and usually should be cooked that way (although the first recipe below "fillets" the steaks), as the skin helps the fish retain its shape. The skin is edible.

SIMMERED HALIBUT WITH CÈPES, SHALLOTS, AND TOMATOES

Makes 4 main course or 8 appetizer servings
Time: 40 minutes

This classic and easily varied halibut preparation cries out for bread, but it is also nice on top of a bed of rice. This is a fine dish for a dinner party; you can make the sauce in the morning and finish the cooking in less than 15 minutes at night.

2 large halibut steaks, about 1 pound each
1 ½ cups water
1 bay leaf
10 black peppercorns
2 cloves garlic, crushed and peeled
½ ounce dried cèpes (porcini)
⅓ cup olive oil
4 large shallots, minced
½ cup dry white wine
2 or 3 sprigs fresh tarragon or ¼ teaspoon dried
Salt and freshly ground black pepper to taste
1 cup roughly chopped fresh or canned plum tomatoes (drained if canned)
½ lemon (optional)

Using a sharp, thin-bladed knife, cut each of the four sections out of the two halibut steaks; this is much easier than it sounds and quite self-evident. You will have eight small fillets; refrigerate them until ready to use. Combine the trimmings with the water, bay leaf, peppercorns, and garlic. Bring to a boil and simmer gently over medium-low heat for about 10 minutes. Strain; you should have about 1 ½ cups of stock.

Soak the cèpes in ½ cup of the stock. Heat the olive oil in a 10- or 12-inch sauté pan (one you can cover) over medium heat. Add the shallots and cook, stirring occasionally, until softened. Drain and chop the cèpes (strain the soaking liquid through a double thickness of paper towels and set aside), and add them to the shallots. Cook 1 minute. Add the wine, tarragon, mushroom soaking liquid, and the balance of the fish stock and raise the heat to high.

Reduce the sauce by about half, taste for salt and pepper, and add the tomatoes. Cook over medium-high heat for another 2 to 3 minutes, stirring occasionally (you may prepare the dish ahead up to this point). Add the halibut fillets to the pan, cover, and simmer gently for about 5 minutes; halibut is extremely delicate, so be careful not to overcook—as soon as a thin-bladed knife meets no resistance, the fish is done. As a general guideline, figure 8 minutes per inch of thickness.

Remove the fish to a warm platter and check the sauce for salt. If it seems to lack acidity, add a few drops of lemon juice. Reduce the sauce a little further if it is thin, then pour it over the halibut and serve.

ALTERNATIVE FISH FOR THIS RECIPE:

Thick fillets or steaks of cod, grouper, haddock, pollock, rockfish, red snapper, or turbot. Adjust the cooking times accordingly.

HALIBUT IN CREAM:

Omit the tomatoes and lemon juice; finish the sauce by adding ½ to 1 cup heavy or light cream or half-and-half and boiling to reduce slightly before adding the fillets to the pan. Cook gently, over quite low heat.

HALIBUT WITH LEEKS AND CREAM:

Add 1 cup chopped well-cleaned leeks (white part only) along with the shallots. Finish with cream as in variation above.

SICILIAN HALIBUT:

Add 4 to 6 minced anchovy fillets, ½ cup pitted black oil-cured olives, ½ teaspoon fennel seeds, and one medium-size onion, sliced, along with the shallots. Finish as directed in the original recipe.

HALIBUT WITH GREEN SAUCE:

Omit the tomatoes. Serve the halibut with parsley pesto (see Broiled Pollock with Parsley Pesto, page 208) or Green Tomato Salsa (page 219), passing either at the table.

RAITO
(Stewed Halibut and Vegetables in Red Wine)

Makes 4 servings
Time: 60 to 90 minutes

One 1 ½-pound halibut steak, 1 inch thick or more
¼ cup olive oil
Flour for dredging
2 large onions, roughly chopped
3 medium-size carrots, roughly chopped
2 or 3 sprigs fresh thyme, tarragon, or rosemary or ½ teaspoon dried
3 cloves garlic, peeled and lightly crushed
2 cups good fruity red wine
4 plum tomatoes, fresh or canned (drained if canned), chopped
2 bay leaves
Salt and freshly ground black pepper to taste
Chopped fresh parsley for garnish

Heat a 10- or 12-inch ovenproof nonstick skillet for 3 to 4 minutes over medium-high heat. Dry the halibut with paper towels; add 2 tablespoons of the oil to the skillet. Toss a pinch of the dredging flour into the oil; when it sizzles, the oil is ready. Dredge the fish, shake off the excess flour, and brown it quickly, raising the heat to high, 2 to 3 minutes per side. Remove it to a plate and set aside.

Wipe out the pan and add the remaining oil, then the onions, carrots, and thyme. Cook over medium heat, stirring occasionally, until the onions soften and just begin to brown, 10 to 15 minutes. Add the garlic and sprinkle with 1 tablespoon of the dredging flour; stir and cook another minute or two. Add the wine, tomatoes, and bay leaves and simmer over medium to medium-low heat until most of the liquid is evaporated, 30 to 40 minutes.

Preheat the oven to 400°F. Taste for salt and pepper, then nestle the fish in the sauce, spooning some of it over the top of the fish. Bake until fish is just done (a thin knife inserted between bone and meat will show that the flesh is opaque), about 10 minutes. Garnish with the parsley and serve immediately, with lots of crusty bread.

ALTERNATIVE FISH FOR THIS RECIPE:

Thick fillets or steaks of cod, grouper, haddock, pollock, rockfish, red snapper, or turbot. Adjust the cooking times accordingly.

POACHED HALIBUT WITH VEGETABLES

Makes 4 servings
Time: 30 minutes

2 cups any chicken or fish stock (pages 40–41)
3 tablespoons butter
2 medium-size carrots, finely diced
2 medium-size onions, finely diced
2 stalks celery, finely diced
1 clove garlic, minced
2 halibut steaks, ¾ to 1 pound each
Salt and freshly ground black pepper to taste

Bring the stock to a boil and keep it warm. In the smallest skillet or casserole that will later hold both the fish steaks, melt the butter over medium heat; add all the vegetables and cook over low heat, stirring occasionally, until they wilt, 5 to 10 minutes. Place the fish steaks atop the vegetables, season with salt and pepper, and add stock to cover. Simmer over medium-low heat until the halibut is done, about 10 to 12 minutes (a thin knife inserted between bone and meat should show that the flesh is opaque). Remove the steaks with a slotted spoon and serve, topped with vegetables and a little of the broth.

ALTERNATIVE FISH FOR THIS RECIPE:

Any white-fleshed steak, including cod, hake, grouper, red snapper, and tilefish. Adjust the cooking times accordingly. (This recipe is also suitable for darker fleshed fish such as mahi-mahi, but for those I prefer the similar but heartier Vietnamese-style Soup on page 167.)

POACHED HALIBUT WITH MUSTARD SAUCE

Makes 4 servings
Time: 30 minutes
This is a Dutch recipe, wonderful with any North Atlantic white fish.

About 4 cups Court Bouillon (page 41), Fast Fish Stock (page 40), or a mixture of 8 parts water to 1 part white vinegar
1 ½ pounds halibut steaks
1 tablespoon butter
1 tablespoon unbleached all-purpose white flour
Salt and freshly ground black pepper to taste
1 tablespoon Dijon mustard
Minced fresh parsley for garnish

In a skillet just large enough to hold the halibut, bring 4 cups of the the court bouillon to a simmer. Add the steaks and enough additional court bouillon or water to cover. Poach over medium-low heat until the fish is cooked through (peek between bone and flesh with a thin-bladed knife; the flesh should be opaque). Remove the fish with a slotted spoon to a platter; keep warm.

Melt the butter in a small saucepan over medium heat; add the flour and cook, stirring, until the mixture turns nut brown, about 3 to 4 minutes. Strain a cup of the court bouillon used for the poaching into the mixture, stirring constantly to eliminate lumps, and cook until thickened, 4 to 5 minutes. Season with salt and pepper and add the mustard. Serve the halibut topped with the sauce and minced parsley. Boiled potatoes are the ideal accompaniment.

ALTERNATIVE FISH FOR THIS RECIPE:

Steaks or fillets of cod, haddock, Atlantic pollock, tilefish, or weakfish. Adjust the cooking times accordingly, and be especially careful not to overcook fillets.

VARIATION:

Poach the halibut and serve with red pepper relish (see Grilled Blackfish with Cumin-scented Red Pepper Relish, page 55) or salsa fresca (see Sautéed Pollock with Salsa Fresca, page 209).

STEAMED HALIBUT WITH GINGER, SESAME OIL, AND GARLIC

Makes 2 servings
Time: 20 minutes
This is a Malaysian recipe, brought home for me by my good friend John Willoughby.

2 tablespoons sesame seeds
¼ cup peeled and minced fresh ginger
1 tablespoon rice or white wine vinegar

1 tablespoon high-quality soy sauce
2 halibut steaks, about 6 ounces each
1 tablespoon peanut oil
1 teaspoon minced garlic
1 teaspoon sesame oil

Toast the sesame seeds in a dry frying pan over medium heat, shaking occasionally, until they begin to pop. Mix them with the ginger, vinegar, and soy sauce. Spread this mixture on top of the steaks.

Steam the halibut on a rack over boiling water in a covered wok or large pot until just done; figure about 10 minutes per inch of thickness (a ¾-inch steak will take about 7 or 8 minutes), then, using a thin-bladed knife, peek between the bone and flesh to make sure the fish is opaque throughout.

While the fish is steaming, warm the peanut oil and garlic together over low heat, stirring once or twice, until the garlic is golden brown; add the sesame oil and heat 30 seconds more. When the fish is done, drizzle the oil over the steaks and serve immediately.

ALTERNATIVE FISH FOR THIS RECIPE:

Steaks of cod, mackerel, mako shark, red snapper, striped bass, or tilefish; fillets of blackfish, grouper, Atlantic pollock, red snapper, rockfish, tilefish, or wolffish. Adjust the cooking times accordingly, and be especially careful not to overcook fillets.

CURRIED HALIBUT

Makes 4 servings
Time: 30 minutes
This is a moist, garlicky curry; serve it with plenty of white rice.

5 tablespoons peanut or vegetable oil
2 large or 4 small halibut steaks, about 1 ½ to 2 pounds total
Flour for dredging

2 large onions, chopped
2 tablespoons minced garlic
1 tablespoon curry powder
1 cup chopped fresh or drained canned tomatoes
Salt and freshly ground black pepper to taste
1 cup plain yogurt
Minced cilantro (fresh coriander) for garnish

Heat 3 tablespoons of the oil over medium-high heat in a 10- or 12-inch nonstick skillet. When it is hot (a pinch of flour will sizzle), dredge the fish steaks in the flour and cook until golden on both sides, 3 to 4 minutes per side. Remove the fish and keep it warm.

Add the remaining oil to the pan and cook the onions over medium heat, stirring occasionally, until it wilts. Stir in the garlic and curry powder and cook 1 minute, stirring. Add the tomatoes, salt, and pepper, and cook over medium heat, stirring occasionally, until the tomatoes break down, about 5 minutes. Stir in the yogurt, then return the halibut to the pan. Cook until the steaks are cooked through (using a thin-bladed knife, peek between the bone and flesh; the meat should be opaque), about 5 minutes more. Garnish with cilantro and serve immediately.

ALTERNATIVE FISH FOR THIS RECIPE:
Steaks of cod, striped bass, or tilefish; thick fillets of blackfish, grouper, Atlantic pollock, or tilefish. Adjust the cooking times accordingly.

HALIBUT POACHED IN CIDER

Makes 4 servings
Time: 40 minutes
There are probably as many recipes for white-fleshed fish baked or poached in cider as there are fishermen in Western Europe, and most, quite frankly, are pretty dull. The addition of bacon,

apples, and vinegar makes this one special. Serve with boiled new potatoes and, of course, hard cider.

4 slices good bacon
1 cup sliced onion
4 crisp apples (such as Cortland or Granny Smith), peeled, cored, and sliced
2 cups hard cider
¼ cup cider or sherry wine vinegar
Salt and freshly ground black pepper to taste
1 ½ pounds halibut steaks, in 1 or 2 pieces
¼ cup snipped fresh chives

In a deep sauté pan or casserole that can later be covered, cook the bacon over medium-high heat until crisp. Remove the bacon to drain on paper towels; drain the pan of all but 3 tablespoons of fat. Add the onion and cook, stirring occasionally, until translucent, then add the apples and cook, stirring occasionally, about 5 more minutes; they should soften slightly but not begin to disintegrate. Add the cider and let it bubble away for 1 to 2 minutes. Add the vinegar and salt and pepper; cook 1 minute more. Taste for acidity and seasoning; add more vinegar, salt, or pepper as needed.

Rest the halibut on the onion mixture, lower the heat to medium-low, and cover the pan. Cook gently until the fish is done, 10 to 15 minutes (use a thin-bladed knife to peek between the bone and flesh; the flesh should be opaque). Crumble the bacon and sprinkle it, with the chives, over the fish. Serve immediately.

ALTERNATIVE FISH FOR THIS RECIPE:
Thick fillets or steaks of cod, tilefish, or turbot. Adjust the cooking times accordingly.

ROAST HALIBUT WITH BUTTER
AND BREAD CRUMBS

Makes 4 servings
Time: 25 minutes

It's not that you can't bake or broil halibut, it's that you must be extremely careful to prevent it from drying out. Butter affords some protection, as does the thickness of the fish itself; but neither is a guarantee. Watch this carefully.

½ cup (1 stick) butter, melted and seasoned
   with salt and pepper
1 cup fresh bread crumbs
1 large or 2 medium-size halibut steaks, total-
   ing about 1 ½ pounds or more
Salt and freshly ground black pepper to taste

Preheat the oven to 450°F. Pour about half the butter into the bottom of a baking dish and lay the fish on top of it. Drizzle with the rest of the butter and sprinkle the bread crumbs over all (don't worry if some of the bread crumbs miss the fish). Season well and place in the oven. Bake about 8 to 10 minutes, then check for doneness by peeking between the flesh and the bone with a thin-bladed knife; when there is just the tiniest bit of translucence remaining, remove the fish from the oven—it will finish cooking by the time you get it to the table. Serve with some of the pan juices spooned over the fish.

ALTERNATIVE FISH FOR THIS RECIPE:

Thick fillets or steaks of cod, grouper, haddock, pollock, rockfish, salmon, red snapper, turbot, or wolffish. Adjust the cooking times accordingly.

HERRING

Latin name(s): *Clupea harengus harengus* (Atlantic), *Clupea harengus pallasi* (Pacific).
Other common names: Sardine, common herring, California herring, etc.
Common forms: Whole.
General description: One of the great underappreciated dark-fleshed fish, herring is rarely available fresh in this country; most of it is smoked (kipper is smoked herring) or pickled. If you are lucky enough to find some, cook it using any mackerel or sardine recipe.
Buying tips: In this country, fresh herring that does make it to market is only rarely handled well; watch out for bruising, and make extra certain that the fish has no off odors.

JACK

Latin name(s): Various members of the Carangidae family.
Other common names: Yellow jack, green jack, crevalle jack, amberjack, black jack, bar jack, blue runner, etc.
Common forms: Whole fish, steaks, fillets.
General description: Dark-fleshed tropical fish (ours are found mostly in the Gulf of Mexico) that range from delicious to mediocre. If you are certain of the source—jacks require careful handling after capture—cook using any pompano recipe.
Buying tips: Jack has been implicated in cases of ciguatoxin (page 16), so avoid large fish or frequent repeated servings of fish from the same source.

JOHN DORY

Latin name(s): *Zeus faber*.
Other common names: St. Pierre.
Common forms: Whole fish, fillets.
General description: Medium-size fish widely cooked in Europe but rarely seen here, although there are some in the western Atlantic. Firm, white, good-tasting flesh; best cooked whole, as filleted yield is relatively low (although fillets are good) and bones add good flavor to stews and stocks (St. Pierre is often used in bouillabaisse).
For recipes see: Blackfish, catfish, cod, dogfish, grouper, haddock, monkfish, pollock, porgy, rockfish, sea bass, red snapper, tilefish, wolffish.
Buying tips: This funny-looking fish is most likely to arrive by plane from the eastern Atlantic, and, consequently, will be costly. Make sure it looks like it just came out of the water, with shiny, unbruised skin and red gills; the smell should be sweet.

KINGFISH

Latin name(s): *Menticirrhus saxatilis*; *Scomberomorus cavalla*.
Other common names: King whiting, king mackerel, cavalla.
Common forms: See below.
Buying tips: What can you say about a name that is used to describe a big whiting—which is a white-fleshed fish—and a large mackerel, often in the same markets? I can say this: If you are offered a "kingfish" with white flesh, see whiting; if you are offered one with dark flesh, see mackerel.

LOBSTER

Latin name(s): *Homarus americanus*.
Other common names: Florida, spiny, or rock lobster is a different species, with no claws. See below.
Common forms: Whole, live; cooked meat; frozen tails (usually of rock lobster).
General description: The beloved and familiar crustacean of the northeastern United States; Western Europe has a similar species (*Homarus gammarus*).
For other recipes see: Crab, crayfish, shrimp, squid.
Buying tips: Lobsters begin to die the minute they leave the sea; holding tanks just delay the process. As a Maine lobsterman I know says, "Just because it's alive doesn't mean it's fresh." Thus a live lobster on ice may actually taste fresher than one swimming in a tank. When you're buying lobster, lift each one (make sure its claws are pegged or banded); if it doesn't flip its tail and kick its legs, look for another.

Lobster—called the cardinal of the seas by French writer Jules Janin—is proof positive that simple foods are best. Lobster needs almost nothing— maybe a squirt of lemon. There have been times I thought I would never eat lobster in any other fashion; recipes just seem to complicate what is already perfect. But, if I manage to find a bunch of inexpensive lobsters two or three times during the course of a week, I start to play around a bit.

For the most part, though, I take my lobster boiled. A good, fresh one, not overcooked, makes butter and everything else superfluous. (Making certain lobster is fresh is not as easy as it seems— see Buying tips, above.)

There is another issue to be aware of when you're buying lobster, especially in the summer. Like blue crabs (page 105), lobsters grow by shedding, or molting, their shells and growing new ones. This usually happens in the summer. But soft-shell lobsters—or "shedders"—have a smaller meat-to-shell ratio than hard-shells, and they fill with water as you cook them. There are some people who believe that soft-shells—which you can identify just by squeezing the shell—have sweeter

meat (and I have had some wonderful ones), but I make a point of asking for hard-shelled lobsters in the summer.

The final point to consider in the market is size. Lobsters grow slowly—it takes them at least five years to reach a pound in size, and as many as twenty years to reach four pounds—and they have been overfished for decades. Consequently, there are more "chickens" (one-pounders), eighths (one and an eighth pounds), and quarters than there are larger lobsters. It is argued that big, heavy lobsters are less tender than these little ones. But in my experience, two people sharing a three-pound lobster will get more meat of equally high quality than if each has their own pound-and-a-half lobster; try it and you'll see. There's less work, less waste, and more meat hidden in those out-of-the-way places. And though it's unlikely that you'll ever see a six-foot lobster (they did exist in the New England area just two hundred years ago, when lobsters were so plentiful they were used as fertilizer), you can find a ten-pounder easily enough—the hard part is figuring out how to cook it.

Now, about boiling: Though steaming lobster is

You must kill lobsters before splitting them for grilling or cutting up for stir-frying. Here's how to kill and split a lobster:

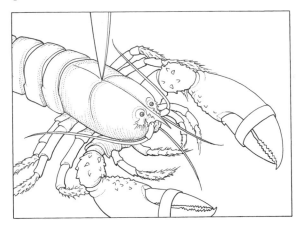

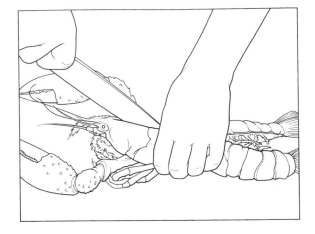

There is a cross-mark on the top of every lobster shell. Insert the point of a sharp, sturdy chef's knife into this.

Split the lobster from one end to the other.

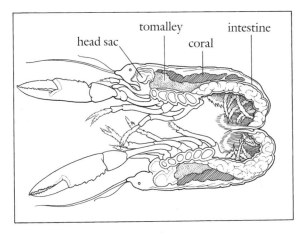

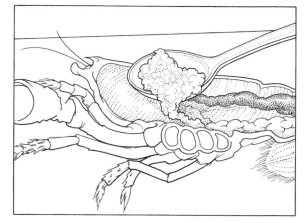

Here is what a split lobster will look like. You want to dispose of the head sac and, if you like, the slender intestine running along the meat. Remove the dark coral, present only in females, and reserve it for sauces.

You must also remove the runny, light green tomalley. It can be used in sauces or discarded.

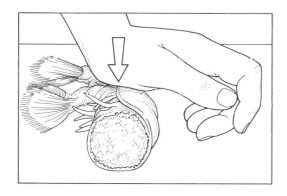

To extract the meat from the tail, roll it in the shell on a counter or other hard surface until the shell cracks.

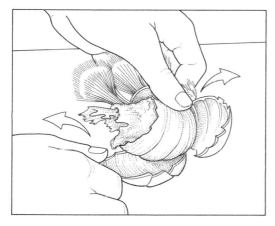

Extract the meat by peeling the shell as if it were that of a shrimp.

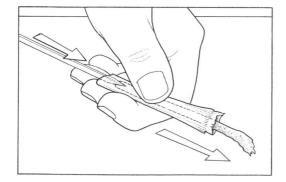

On larger lobsters, those more than two pounds, there is good meat in the small legs. Use a skewer to push the meat through the other side.

certainly acceptable, and much easier than bringing gallons of water to a boil, boiling is better, especially when you're cooking a bunch. Lobsters flavor the cooking water, which in turn flavors the lobsters. When you steam, all that flavor ends up underneath the lobster, making a great sauce base but not helping the lobster any. I've eaten lobster in places that boil them all day long, and there is no question that they taste best in the evening, thanks to the rich broth produced by their predeceased brothers and sisters.

For broiling, grilling, sautéing, and stir-frying, you'll need to kill the lobster before cooking; take heart, and see the illustrations on page 152.

There are very few parts of a lobster that you cannot eat. If you split the lobster for grilling (page 152), you can remove all of the inedibles before cooking. You can also remove the tomalley (the green, liverlike organ) and the coral (the black eggs, found in females only) to use in sauces. Otherwise, remove the stomach, intestine, and gills after boiling.

Finally, there is the spiny lobster, also called Florida lobster, rock lobster, or, in Florida, crawfish. These lobsters and their related species are found worldwide, and it is their tails which are frozen to become the ubiquitous "lobster tails." With no claws, these babies are far simpler to eat than northern lobsters. They're not bad at all, and can be used in virtually any recipe for lobster, shrimp, or crayfish. Simply boiled, however, they don't compare to *Homarus americanus*.

BASIC BOILED
OR STEAMED LOBSTER

Time: 30 minutes or less
For each person, you will need a lobster that weighs 1 ½ pounds or more; a 3-pound lobster is enough for two people. Steaming is a little easier and less

messy than boiling, especially if you're only cooking one or two lobsters.

If you have two lobsters or more, you'll need a very large pot. Bring lots of water to a boil—or just an inch if you choose to steam—and add salt, a couple of tablespoons or so (if you have access to clean seawater, that's a nice touch, as is steaming atop a pile of fresh seaweed; all of this seems to contribute, however subtly, to the flavor). Plunge the lobster(s) into the water.

As far as timing goes, cook a lobster about 8 minutes for its first pound—from the time the water returns to the boil—and then an additional 3 or 4 minutes per pound thereafter. Thus a 3-pounder should boil for about 15 minutes. How do you know when lobster is done? The meat becomes opaque and firm, and the coral, if there is any, turns, well, coral-colored (it stays black until it is cooked). None of this does you any good if the lobster is whole, since you can't see or feel the meat or the coral. One assurance: It's difficult to undercook a small lobster if you use the timing guidelines above (also, small lobsters are cooked by the time their shells turn red; this visual cue is not, however, reliable with lobsters over 1 ½ pounds or so). If you're boiling a larger one, insert an instant-read thermometer into the tail meat by sliding it in between the body and the tail joint; lobster is done at 140°F.

Remove the lobsters, which will be bright red, and let them sit for 5 minutes or so before serving (this allows some of the water to retreat into their meat, minimizing mess—which will be considerable in any case—and maximizing moistness). Poke a hole in the crosshatch on the top of the lobster's back (see illustration, page 152), and drain some of the water out. To eat, see illustrations. As an added refinement, you might also crack the claws (with a nutcracker, small hammer, or the back of a chef's knife) before bringing the lobster to the table.

The traditional accompaniment is drawn butter. But—given the richness of lobster meat—this is as archaic as serving steak with béarnaise. Try a squeeze of lemon over lobster meat; there is nothing better. But if drawn butter is your thing, just melt a stick of butter (usually enough for four people) over low heat. Divide it among small bowls.

STEAMED LOBSTER WITH GINGER-SOY DIPPING SAUCE

Makes 4 servings
Time: 30 minutes

4 or 5 scallions
1 tablespoon sherry
4 slices peeled fresh ginger, plus 1 teaspoon minced
4 cloves garlic: 2 crushed and peeled, 2 minced
¼ cup high-quality soy sauce
1 tablespoon peanut oil
4 lobsters, about 1 ¼ pounds each
1 teaspoon sesame oil

Cut the greens from half the scallions and put them in a pot large enough to hold the lobsters. Mince the remaining greens and set them aside. Chop about half of the white parts of the scallions and add them to the pot along with the sherry, the sliced ginger, the crushed garlic, half the soy sauce, and slightly less than 1 inch of water. Bring to a boil, add the lobsters, and cover.

While the lobsters cook, mince the remaining white parts of the scallions, and combine them in a small saucepan with the minced ginger, the minced garlic, the remaining soy sauce, and the peanut oil. Bring to a simmer over medium heat and cook about 2 minutes. When the lobsters are done (about 10 minutes), remove them to a platter and keep warm, either in a very low oven or by covering lightly with aluminum foil.

Strain the lobster cooking liquid into a second saucepan and reduce over high heat to about ½ cup; add the soy mixture and bring back to a boil.

Add the sesame oil and turn off the heat. Drizzle a little of this sauce over the lobsters, and garnish them with the remaining scallion greens. Divide the remaining sauce into dipping bowls and serve.

ALTERNATIVE FISH FOR THIS RECIPE:

Mussels or hard-shell clams; use even less water to start and adjust the cooking times accordingly.

GRILLED LOBSTER FOR FOUR

Time: 30 minutes

You can grill whole lobsters, but I can almost guarantee you that the claws will be dry and the tail underdone. It's better to split them, as illustrated on page 152, and remove the inedible parts. They will then grill evenly and quickly.

Start a charcoal fire or preheat a gas grill. Kill 4 lobsters as illustrated on page 152, cut them in half, and remove the stomach and intestine. The coral and tomalley may remain in the body; if you are preparing the recipe below, remove and reserve them. Grill the lobster for about 5 minutes on its back to firm up the meat. Sprinkle it with salt and pepper, turn it over, and grill for another 8 minutes or so. The meat is done when it is firm and white. Serve with lemon quarters or melted butter.

BROILED LOBSTER WITH HERB STUFFING

Makes 4 servings
Time: 30 minutes

I'm no fan of the stuffed lobster served in most restaurants, which is usually a soggy mess. With a full cup of fresh herbs, however, this is quite delicious.

4 lobsters, about 1 ¼ pounds each
1 clove garlic, peeled
1 cup fresh parsley, cilantro (fresh coriander),
   or basil leaves

Salt and freshly ground black pepper to taste
2 cups plain bread crumbs
¾ cup olive oil
2 tablespoons fresh lemon juice

Prepare the lobsters as described in the preceding recipe, setting aside the tomalley and coral; preheat the broiler and set the rack about 6 to 8 inches from the heat source.

In a food processor, mince the garlic, parsley, salt and pepper, bread crumbs, olive oil, lemon juice, and the tomalley and coral. Add a little additional olive oil or lemon juice if the mixture seems dry. Stuff the lobsters' body cavities with this mixture and broil until the tail meat is white and firm and the stuffing nicely browned. (If the lobster is browning too quickly, either move it farther from the heat source or turn off the broiler and turn the oven heat to 500°F to complete the cooking.)

A SIMPLIFIED VERSION OF JEAN-LOUIS GERIN'S LOBSTER SAUTÉ

Makes 4 servings
Time: 60 minutes

This dish, greatly modified for home kitchens (and with thanks and apologies to its creator), is straightforward, nice looking, and quite delicious. For the original, book a table at Restaurant Jean-Louis in Greenwich, Connecticut. It will make you gasp.

One 2- to 2 ½-pound lobster
1 pound waxy potatoes (3 or 4 medium-size)
¼ cup (½ stick) butter
Salt and freshly ground black pepper to taste
4 to 6 cups mixed greens, washed and dried
1 tablespoon olive oil, plus extra for the
   dressing
1 shallot, minced
Juice of 1 or 2 lemons

Steam the lobster in 2 inches of boiling water for 20 to 25 minutes. Be careful not to overcook it (in fact, slight undercooking is fine). Remove it from the cooking water and allow the water to continue to simmer. Quickly break off the claws and tail and return the body to the pot; cover and simmer over medium heat while you continue to work.

Remove the meat from the claws and tail as soon as they are cool enough to handle. Return the shells to the simmering lobster stock and set the meat aside. Simmer the stock, covered, for another 10 minutes.

Meanwhile, preheat a 12-inch nonstick sauté pan over medium heat. Peel the potatoes and slice them thinly, about 1/8 inch thick. Place 3 tablespoons of the butter in the pan and, when it has melted and the foam subsided, arrange the potatoes in the butter in two layers. Sprinkle with salt and pepper and adjust the heat so the butter bubbles but does not burn. Press down on the potatoes occasionally, using a large spatula or, better still, the cover of a 10-inch sauté pan.

Cut a small slit down the middle of the back of the tail and remove the intestine. Cut the lobster meat into chunks, leaving the smaller claw whole for garnish. Arrange the greens on a platter.

In 15 to 20 minutes, when the potatoes are nicely browned, turn them (one piece is nice, but don't worry if they break) and continue to cook. Heat the oil in another sauté pan over medium heat. Add the shallot and cook, stirring occasionally, until it's fragrant, then raise the heat to high and add the lobster chunks. Cook quickly, tossing and stirring, until hot.

Dress the salad sparingly with olive oil and some lemon juice; it should be barely moist and you should just be able to taste the dressing. Spoon the lobster chunks over the greens. Working quickly, add the remaining butter to the sauté pan. Take 3/4 cup of the simmering stock and strain it into the pan. Reduce by half over high heat. Add lemon juice, tasting for acidity and salt; the sauce should be strong. Pour most of the sauce over the lobster, then slide the potatoes on top. Drizzle the remaining sauce on top, and finish with the reserved lobster claw. Serve immediately.

STIR-FRIED LOBSTER WITH SCALLIONS AND BLACK BEANS

Makes 4 to 6 servings
Time: 40 minutes

Here's a way to enjoy lobster without spending a fortune on it. Three 1 1/4-pound lobsters in a stir-fry can easily serve four or more people, depending on the side dishes (serve lots of rice; this sauce is wonderful). I like a little cayenne in this recipe, but some people feel it detracts from the flavor of the lobster; decide for yourself. Eat this messy dish with fingers, chopsticks, and forks.

Three 1 1/4-pound lobsters or slightly larger
1 tablespoon fermented black beans (available in Asian markets)
2 tablespoons dry sherry
2 tablespoons peanut oil
1 teaspoon minced garlic
1 teaspoon peeled and minced fresh ginger
1/2 teaspoon cayenne pepper or to taste (optional)
1/2 cup any chicken or fish stock (pages 40–41)
1 tablespoon high-quality soy sauce
1 teaspoon sesame oil
1 cup chopped scallions, with some of the greens, or 1 cup chopped fresh chives

Assemble all the ingredients and start cooking your rice before killing the lobsters. Begin warming a wok over low heat while you kill the lobsters as illustrated on page 152. Soak the black beans in the sherry. Remove the small legs of the lobster, then reserve the bodies for another use (you can freeze them if you want to make stock later). Cut the tails crosswise into three or four sections each, and separate the claws at the joints. Smack each of the claw pieces gently with a hammer or the back of a large knife to crack the shell in a couple of places. You will have a couple dozen pieces altogether.

When you're ready, raise the heat under the wok to high and add the peanut oil, then the garlic and ginger. Stir-fry for 15 seconds, then put in the lobster pieces. Stir and cook for 1 or 2 minutes; add the cayenne. Add the black beans with the sherry, the stock, and soy sauce; stir and cover. Cook until all the lobster pieces are bright red, about 5 minutes.

Uncover and, with the heat still on high, add almost all of the scallions (reserve a little for garnish). Stir and cook until nicely blended, 1 minute or so. Turn off the heat, drizzle the sesame oil on top, and garnish with the rest of the scallions before serving.

ALTERNATIVE FISH FOR THIS RECIPE:

Hard-shell clams or mussels (cook until they open); soft-shell crabs (cut into pieces); shrimp; cleaned squid (add the squid last and cook very briefly). Adjust the cooking times accordingly.

STIR-FRY WITH LOBSTER MEAT

Makes 2 servings
Time: 20 minutes
If you have a leftover tail or two from a lobster feast (hey, stranger things have been known to happen), try this stir-fry. The sweet, rich flavor of the lobster really shines here.

1 large Spanish onion, halved and cut into half rings
2 tablespoons peanut oil
1 medium-size carrot, diced
1 tablespoon minced garlic
1 teaspoon peeled and minced fresh ginger
½ to 1 cup diced cooked lobster meat
2 tablespoons dry sherry
1 tablespoon high-quality soy sauce
¼ teaspoon hot oil, chili-garlic paste (available in Asian markets), or other fiery seasoning, or to taste
Salt and freshly ground black pepper to taste
⅓ to ½ cup any fish or chicken stock (pages 40–41) or water

Heat a wok over high heat until smoking. Cook half the onion, dry, until somewhat wilted, about 5 minutes, stirring occasionally. Remove and repeat with the other half of the onion.

Add the oil to the wok and cook the carrot, stirring, until it starts to brown, about 3 minutes. Remove with a slotted spoon and mix with the onion. Add the garlic and ginger to the oil, stir once, and add the lobster. Stir-fry for about 1 minute, then return the onion-carrot mixture to the wok. Add the sherry and soy sauce and let bubble away for a minute. Add the hot oil, stir, and season with salt and pepper. Add a little stock, stir, cook for 1 minute, add a little more stock or water if the mixture looks dry, and serve, with white rice.

ALTERNATIVE FISH FOR THIS RECIPE:
Cooked crab or crayfish; uncooked shrimp.

LOBSTER BISQUE

Makes 4 servings
Time: 60 minutes
With apologies to Julia Child, whose lobster bisque in *Mastering the Art of French Cooking* is the paradigm. This is somewhat simpler and much faster. Make it the day after a lobster feast and you may find yourself begging in fish markets for free lobster bodies.

¼ cup (½ stick) butter

1 medium-size onion, peeled and chopped

1 clove garlic, peeled and chopped

1 medium-size carrot, chopped

1 bay leaf

Several sprigs fresh thyme or ½ teaspoon dried

4 to 8 lobster bodies, cooked or uncooked, with as many shells as you can find, plus coral, tomalley, and any stray bits of meat you might find

1 cup dry white wine

1 cup chopped tomatoes, fresh or canned (drained if canned)

6 cups any chicken or fish stock (pages 40–41) or strained liquid reserved from boiling lobsters

1 cup heavy cream

Minced fresh parsley for garnish

Salt and freshly ground black pepper to taste

Melt 2 tablespoons of the butter over medium heat in a large saucepan or casserole; add the onion, garlic, carrot, bay leaf, and thyme and cook, stirring occasionally, until the onion softens. Add the lobster bodies and, if they are uncooked, cook, stirring, until they turn red (if they're already cooked, cook, stirring, about 5 minutes). Add the wine and tomatoes, bring to a gentle boil, lower the heat to medium, cover, and simmer for 10 minutes. Add the stock, raise the heat until the liquid boils, then return it to medium, cover, and simmer another 20 minutes. Remove the bay leaf and thyme sprigs. Remove the lobster shells, crack them if necessary, and pick off any meat you find. Return the meat to the soup.

Place the soup, in batches if necessary, in a blender or food processor, and process until smooth. (You can refrigerate the soup at this point until you're ready to serve it.) Return the soup to the pot and bring to a boil. Add the remaining butter, in bits, until it melts. Add the cream and any lobster meat and heat through. Check for seasoning, sprinkle with the parsley, season with salt and pepper, and serve.

LOBSTER SPREAD

Makes 8 servings
Time: 10 minutes
A good way to use a small amount of leftover lobster.

2 cups roughly chopped cooked lobster meat

1 tablespoon fresh lemon or lime juice

¼ cup minced fresh parsley, basil, or cilantro (fresh coriander)

1 tablespoon finely minced onion

1 tablespoon capers

Mayonnaise (page 43) as needed

Salt and freshly ground black pepper to taste

Mix the first five ingredients together in a bowl. Add enough mayonnaise to bind. Season with salt and pepper, bearing in mind that capers are salty. Chill until ready to serve (this will keep overnight just fine). Serve with crackers or small pieces of toast.

ALTERNATIVE FISH FOR THIS RECIPE:
Cooked crabmeat, crayfish, or shrimp.

MACKEREL

Latin name(s): *Scomber scombrus*, *Scomberomorus maculatus* (Spanish mackerel), and others.
Other common names: Common or Atlantic mackerel, Spanish mackerel, cero, tinker mackerel, Pacific mackerel, king mackerel, sierra, etc.
Common forms: There are many different mackerel; common mackerel are usually no larger than two pounds, and may be sold whole or filleted; larger fish, such as Spanish mackerel, may be steaked or sold whole or filleted.
General description: Dark, rich fish, with no scales and good-tasting skin; the bones are easily removed, making mackerel the best fish on which to practice filleting.
For other recipes see: Bluefish, butterfish, mahi-mahi, pompano, sardine, striped bass, tuna.
Buying tips: Since the vivid colors of mackerel begin to fade after death, the freshest fish are bright and vivid. Mackerel on ice should appear to be almost alive; if they have a dull, dead look, you should turn your gaze elsewhere. Smell should be very fresh and clean.

Mackerel is one of the loveliest fish there is, one of the tastiest, cheapest, most versatile, and most plentiful. And it's scorned by nearly everyone, the symbol of stinkiness, a fish we think of as too strong-flavored, too oily, and too fishy.

But mackerel is fatty, rich-flavored, moist, and so sweet that it is almost requisite to cook it with acidic flavorings such as lemon or tomato. It is mackerel's fat that has given it and its many close cousins, such as Spanish mackerel, such a bad reputation. But sirloin steak's got a high fat content, too. And, unlike steak, mackerel is high in Omega-3s and low in cholesterol.

Even more than most fish, mackerel is best eaten when it is super-fresh. It does not freeze well, and its quality deteriorates rapidly once the fish is out of water. The English realized this three hundred years ago, when they made an exception to their blue laws and allowed mackerel to be hawked in the streets of London on Sunday, implicitly acknowledging that the fish would be nearly worthless by Monday.

Good icing techniques have made the rush to market a little less urgent, but mackerel still must be iced when it is caught and shipped without delay. Whether this has been done ought to be obvious at the fish counter (see Buying tips, above). Mackerel are gorgeous (the French *maquereau* also means pimp), an iridescent blue-green with vertical black stripes. They run in size from less than a pound ("tinker" mackerel) to two pounds or so; related species are usually larger. In most cases they are sold whole; since they have an uncomplicated bone structure and no scales, mackerel are easily cleaned or filleted by your fishmonger (or even yourself).

The English prefer mackerel smoked, the Japanese and French pickle it, and the Greeks dry it in the wind. All of these excellent treatments are rather old-fashioned ways of preserving a fragile fish. I like to broil whole mackerel, or grill it (its high oil content keeps it moist and discourages sticking), or pan-roast it with just a little fat and a little liquid; fillets are terrific poached or broiled.

LIME-BROILED MACKEREL
WITH HERBS

....

Makes 4 servings
Time: 30 minutes

You can never go wrong if you combine mackerel with herbs and an acidic ingredient like citrus.

3 tablespoons olive oil
Zest and juice of 1 lime
3 tablespoons chopped fresh herbs: parsley, thyme, rosemary, tarragon, chives, chervil, etc.
Salt and freshly ground black pepper
4 mackerel fillets, skin on, 4 to 6 ounces each

Mix together the oil, lime zest and juice, herbs, salt, and pepper, and toss with the fillet. Let sit for 10 minutes, no longer.

Preheat the broiler. Broil the mackerel skin side down, about 4 inches from the source of heat, for about 5 minutes (use a thin-bladed knife to check the interior of the fillets; they will be opaque and tender when done). Brush the fillets once or twice with the marinade while cooking.

ALTERNATIVE FISH FOR THIS RECIPE:
Fillets of bluefish, mahi-mahi, or pompano.
MACKEREL WITH TOMATO, GINGER, AND GARLIC:

Marinate the fish in a combination of 1 cup chopped fresh tomatoes, 1 tablespoon peeled and minced fresh ginger, 1 tablespoon minced garlic, and ¼ teaspoon cayenne pepper (or to taste). Broil as directed above. Garnish, after broiling, with chopped cilantro (fresh coriander).

GRILLED MACKEREL WITH BACON

....

Makes 2 servings
Time: 20 minutes

This dish is deceptive; with only two ingredients, the preparation time is nil. But you must be very careful when grilling if you are to cook the mackerel through without burning the bacon. A grilling basket is essential here.

2 whole mackerel, gutted, with heads on, about 1 pound each
4 slices good bacon

Start a charcoal fire or preheat a gas grill or broiler. Rinse and dry the fish. Cut off their belly flaps, the limp section of skin and bone that remains after they've been gutted. Leave the heads on if they will fit in your basket that way; otherwise remove them. Wrap each fish with 2 pieces of bacon (or lay 1 strip of bacon along each side of the fish) and place in the basket. Grill or broil over low to medium heat, 4 to 6 inches from the heat source, turning frequently, until the bacon is slightly crisp and the mackerel are cooked through (the flesh will be opaque and tender when done). Total cooking time will be 10 to 15 minutes.

ALTERNATIVE FISH FOR THIS RECIPE:
Pompano.

BROILED MACKEREL FILLETS
WITH MUSTARD BUTTER

....

Makes 2 servings
Time: 15 minutes

3 tablespoons butter
1 tablespoon Dijon mustard
1 teaspoon fresh lemon juice
Dash cayenne pepper
Salt and freshly ground black pepper to taste
½ cup chopped fresh parsley
Two ¾- to 1-pound mackerel, filleted, skin on

Use 1 tablespoon of the butter to grease the bottom of a baking pan; preheat the broiler. Cream the remaining butter with the mustard, lemon juice, cayenne, salt, pepper, and half the parsley. Spread the fillets with about half this mixture and broil, about 4 inches from the source of heat, for about 5 minutes (use a thin-bladed knife to check the interior of the fillets; they will be tender and opaque when done). Brush the cooked fillets with the remaining mustard butter and sprinkle with the remaining parsley.

ALTERNATIVE FISH FOR THIS RECIPE: Bluefish or mahi-mahi.

MACKEREL WITH ORANGE SAUCE

Makes 2 servings
Time: 20 to 40 minutes

Another recipe that demonstrates the affinity between mackerel and acidic ingredients. Feel free to substitute any other citrus fruit, or a combination, for the oranges.

2 tablespoons olive oil
¼ cup freshly squeezed orange juice
1 ½ teaspoons chopped fresh thyme or a pinch dried
Salt and freshly ground black pepper to taste
4 mackerel fillets, a total of about 1 pound, skin on
2 oranges, segmented, or peeled and thinly sliced

Mix the olive oil, orange juice, thyme, salt, and pepper together in a shallow bowl. Add the mackerel and, if time allows, let rest for 20 minutes or so. Preheat the broiler.

Place the fish in a broiling or baking pan and brush with the marinade. Broil about 6 inches from the heat source, basting once or twice, for 5 to 8 minutes, until the fish is lightly brown on top and almost cooked through (it will be tender and opaque throughout). Top with the oranges, baste once more, and broil another minute. Serve immediately.

ALTERNATIVE FISH FOR THIS RECIPE: Steaks or fillets of blackfish, bluefish, grouper,

swordfish, or tuna. Adjust the cooking time accordingly.

ROASTED MACKEREL WITH ONIONS AND LEMON

Makes 4 servings
Time: 30 minutes

¼ cup (½ stick) butter
1 large onion, chopped
1 teaspoon minced garlic
1 medium-size shallot, minced
½ cup minced fresh herbs: parsley, tarragon, chives, thyme, and/or chervil
4 medium-size mackerel, about ¾ pound each, cleaned, gutted, beheaded, belly flaps removed
Salt and freshly ground black pepper to taste
2 lemons, cut into thin slices
Juice of ½ lemon

Preheat the oven to 450°F. Melt 1 tablespoon of the butter in a medium-size skillet or saucepan over medium heat; cook the onion slowly, stirring occasionally, until softened but not browned. Mix together the garlic, shallot, and herbs and stuff the cavities of the fish with this mixture. Sprinkle the fish with salt and pepper. Melt the remaining butter.

Lay the onions and a few of the lemon slices on the bottom of a baking dish large enough to hold the fish. Place the fish atop the onions, drizzle with the melted butter and lemon juice, and top with the remaining lemon slices. Roast, uncovered, until done (the interior cavity of the mackerel will have the barest trace of pink), about 15 minutes. Serve immediately, spooning the pan juices over the fish and rice or boiled or baked potatoes.

SIMPLE SAUTÉED MACKEREL

Makes 2 servings
Time: 20 minutes
Despite its simplicity, this dish has a wonderful balance of flavors. Whole mackerel is easy to cook and easy to eat.

2 mackerel, about 1 pound each, gutted
3 tablespoons olive oil
Salt and freshly ground black pepper
1 meaty plum tomato, minced
2 tablespoon minced fresh parsley
Juice of 2 limes

The mackerel may be cooked with heads on or off. Cut off their belly flaps, the limp section of skin and bone that remains after they've been gutted. Wash and dry them well. Heat the olive oil over medium heat in a 10- or 12-inch nonstick skillet. When it is hot but not smoking, add the mackerel. Cook over medium to medium-high heat, turning frequently and adding salt and pepper to each side. When nicely browned, about 10 to 15 minutes later, the fish are done (there will be the barest trace of redness in the body cavity). Remove the fish to a platter.

Over medium heat, add the tomato to the same skillet. Stir once or twice, then add the parsley and lime juice. Cook, stirring, for 30 seconds or so. Pour the sauce over the mackerel and serve at once.

ALTERNATIVE FISH FOR THIS RECIPE:
Whole small bluefish, butterfish, or pompano.

SALTED AND LIGHTLY PICKLED MACKEREL

Makes 4 servings
Time: About 70 minutes
This is not a real pickle, but a warm dish with a strong vinegar flavor.

4 mackerel fillets, about 1 pound total, skin on
1 tablespoon salt
2 tablespoons peanut or vegetable oil
2 tablespoons white wine vinegar
¼ teaspoon cayenne pepper or to taste
1 tablespoon minced garlic
1 tablespoon peeled and minced fresh ginger
Minced cilantro (fresh coriander) for garnish

Rub the fillets with the salt and let sit for 30 minutes. Rinse briefly and dry. Mix together the oil, vinegar, cayenne, garlic, and ginger and marinate the fish in this mixture for another 30 minutes.

Toward the end of the marinating time, preheat the broiler. Broil the fish about 6 inches from the heat source for 5 to 6 minutes, until just lightly browned (the thinnest end of the smallest fillet should just flake when prodded with a fork or knife, and the fish should all be opaque). Garnish with the cilantro and serve immediately or at room temperature.

ALTERNATIVE FISH FOR THIS RECIPE:
Spanking fresh fillets of bluefish or mahi-mahi.

SAUTÉED MACKEREL WITH GARLIC AND ROSEMARY

Makes 2 servings
Time: 30 minutes
Another simple recipe that displays the wonderful affinity mackerel has for strong flavors. You can make this with fillets, too; just reduce the cooking time accordingly.

3 tablespoons olive oil
One 1 ½- to 2-pound mackerel, gutted and belly flaps removed
Flour for dredging
3 cloves garlic, peeled
2 sprigs fresh rosemary
1 lemon

Salt and freshly ground black pepper
½ cup red wine
1 teaspoon balsamic vinegar

The mackerel can be cooked with its head on or off; you can also cut it in half, right down the middle, if it is too long to fit in the skillet. Preheat a 12-inch nonstick skillet over medium heat for 3 or 4 minutes, then add the olive oil. Dredge the mackerel lightly in the flour and, when the oil is hot (a pinch of flour will sizzle) place the fish in the pan. Crush one of the garlic cloves and add it to the pan with one of the sprigs of rosemary. Regulate the heat so the mackerel cooks in a lively fashion but does not burn. Meanwhile, mince the other two garlic cloves and cut three slices from the lemon; squeeze the juice from the rest of the lemon.

Sprinkle the fish with salt and pepper, turn it when it has browned on one side, then season the other side. Cook until the belly cavity has just the barest trace of red remaining, about 4 to 5 minutes per side. Remove it to a platter and keep warm in a low oven. Remove the garlic and rosemary from the skillet and discard. Pour the wine and vinegar in the skillet and stir with a wooden spoon over medium-high heat; add the minced garlic and remaining sprig of rosemary and stir.

Decorate the fish with the lemon slices, then remove the rosemary from the skillet—it should have cooked only for a minute—and place it atop the lemon. Add the lemon juice to the sauce, along with any liquid that has accumulated around the mackerel, stir once, and pour over the fish.

ALTERNATIVE FISH FOR THIS RECIPE:
Whole small bluefish, butterfish, or pompano; fillets of bluefish or mahi-mahi.

HOT-SMOKED MACKEREL

Makes 4 servings
Time: 90 minutes
Please read the general guidelines for smoking fish, page 30. You can use this recipe for any dark-fleshed fish.

2 handfuls hardwood chips (about 1 ½ cups)
¼ cup coarse salt
¼ cup sugar
4 mackerel fillets, about 1 pound, skin on
2 tablespoons freshly ground black pepper
1 tablespoon Dijon mustard
2 tablespoons fresh lemon juice

Soak the wood chips in water to cover for at least 1 hour, and as long as 24 hours. Mix together the salt and sugar and sprinkle the fish on both sides. Let sit for 30 to 40 minutes, refrigerated if the room is especially warm. Mix together the pepper, mustard, and lemon juice and rub into the fillets; marinate for another 30 minutes.

Smoke according to the directions on page 31.

MACKEREL FILLETS SIMMERED IN SOY SAUCE

Makes 4 servings
Time: 20 minutes
Sauce for rice and delicious fish in one pot, in 20 minutes, with seven ingredients? No problem.

½ cup high-quality soy sauce
½ cup water
⅓ cup dry sherry
2 tablespoons rice or white wine vinegar
5 or 6 thin slices peeled fresh ginger
3 or 4 cloves garlic, crushed
4 mackerel fillets, about 1 pound total, skin on

In a 12-inch skillet with a cover, mix together all the ingredients except the fish. Bring to a boil and simmer over medium heat for about 5 minutes, uncovered. Add the fish, skin side down, cover, and simmer until the fish is cooked through (the thinnest end of the smallest fillet should just flake when prodded with a fork or knife, and the fish should all be opaque), 7 to 10 minutes. To serve, spoon a fillet and some sauce onto a mound of white rice.

ALTERNATIVE FISH FOR THIS RECIPE:

Many fish can be cooked this way (including whole flatfish, see page 127)—fillets of blackfish, catfish, dogfish, grouper, Atlantic pollock, red snapper, striped bass, tilefish, or wolffish. You can also use steaks of swordfish, salmon, cod, halibut, or marlin. Adjust the cooking time accordingly.

MACKEREL POACHED IN RED WINE WITH JUNIPER BERRIES

Makes 4 servings
Time: 40 minutes

This is a luxurious, wintry dish, seemingly quite rich but with no added fat whatsoever. You won't regret cooking it in—or serving it with—a high-quality red wine.

1 cup good dry red wine
1 cup any fish or chicken stock (pages 40–41) or an additional cup of wine
¼ cup minced shallots
1 tablespoon juniper berries
1 cup minced fresh parsley
Salt and freshly ground black pepper to taste
4 mackerel fillets, about 1 pound total, skin on

In a steep-sided skillet big enough to hold the fish in one layer, boil the wine and stock until the combination is reduced by about half, about 10 minutes. Add the shallots, juniper berries, half the

parsley, and the salt and pepper and simmer 5 minutes over medium-low heat. Add the mackerel fillets, cover, and simmer until they are just done, 5 to 7 minutes (the thinnest end of the smallest fillet should just flake when prodded with a fork or knife, and the fish should all be opaque). Scoop out the fillets with a spatula and place on a warm serving platter. Reduce the sauce over high heat until there is barely ½ cup remaining; spoon a little over each fillet and serve, with white rice or crusty bread.

ALTERNATIVE FISH FOR THIS RECIPE:

Fillets of bluefish or mahi-mahi. Adjust cooking time accordingly.

SPANISH MACKEREL CAKES WITH SPICY SAUCE

Makes 4 servings
Time: 30 minutes

Somewhat firmer than smaller mackerel, Spanish is the species of choice for Thai-style fish cakes.

1 pound Spanish mackerel fillets (or steaks, meat taken off the bone)
1 egg, beaten
2 tablespoons all-purpose flour, plus some for dredging
1 teaspoon minced garlic
1 teaspoon peeled and minced ginger
2 tablespoons minced scallion
¼ cup minced cilantro (fresh coriander)
Salt and freshly ground black pepper to taste
⅓ cup plus 1 tablespoon peanut oil
1 tablespoon high-quality soy sauce
Lime wedges or Spicy Pepper Sauce for Fried Fish (page 42)

Chop the fish by hand or pulse it several times in a food processor until it is minced but not pureed. Mix or gently process it with the egg, flour, garlic, ginger, scallion, cilantro, salt, pepper, the table-spoon of peanut oil, and the soy sauce. If the mixture seems dry, add a little more soy sauce or water. Shape the mixture into patties and, if time permits, refrigerate for ½ hour.

When you're ready to cook, preheat a 12-inch nonstick skillet over medium-high heat for 4 to 5 minutes. Add the peanut oil and, when it is hot (a pinch of flour will sizzle), dredge the cakes and sauté over medium-high heat until nicely browned on both sides, about 10 minutes total. Serve hot or at room temperature, with lime wedges or spicy pepper sauce.

MAHI-MAHI

Latin name(s): *Coryphaena hippurus*.
Other common names: Dolphinfish, dorada.
Common forms: Steaks, fillets, whole fish.
General description: Brightly colored warm-water fish with dark meat that turns white after cooking. Good flavor and texture.
For other recipes see: Blackfish, bluefish, grouper, mackerel, mako, pollock, pompano, rockfish, red snapper, striped bass, swordfish, tuna.
Buying tips: Look for flesh of bright, consistent color; mahi-mahi begins to get brown and streaky as it ages.

First things first: Mahi-mahi, often called dolphinfish, is not a mammal. Not even close. Don't worry about it for a second.

Mahi-mahi is found in most of the world's warm waters; it was first imported to the U.S. mainland from Hawaii, but is now caught off the Florida and California coasts. It is almost always skinned before cooking, and, if not, should be skinned before eating; the skin is tough and tasteless.

Like mako shark, mahi-mahi is a decent alternative to the ever-popular and overfished swordfish. But, like mako, it lacks the full flavor and incomparable juiciness of sword. What it has is good, grillable texture and decent flavor. Overall, though, I think this is one fish that benefits from being cooked with many other flavorful ingredients; my recipes reflect this prejudice.

PAN BAGNA WITH MAHI-MAHI

Makes 4 servings
Time: 60 minutes, plus resting time
Pan bagna—which translates as "bathed bread"—is not only one of the most beautiful sandwiches you've ever seen, it is ideal for picnics: The longer it sits, the better it gets. View this recipe, if you will, as a general set of guidelines rather than as a firm formula; you can make it with whatever you have on hand (including leftover grilled fish). Just make sure to weight it for a while to allow the flavors to mingle and the bread to soften.

1 small eggplant or zucchini
Salt
½ to ¾ pound skinless mahi-mahi, in one small steak no more than ½ inch thick
Extra virgin olive oil as needed
1 or 2 medium to large red bell peppers or 2 canned red peppers (often called pimentos)
One 8- to 10-inch round, crusty loaf of bread
1 teaspoon capers or to taste
6 to 8 good black or green olives, pitted
4 to 6 anchovy fillets or to taste
4 canned or bottled artichoke hearts, rinsed
2 or 3 thick slices fresh tomato
Chopped fresh parsley and/or basil
Freshly ground black pepper to taste
Juice of ½ lemon

Rinse the eggplant or zucchini and slice it lengthwise; place in a colander and salt liberally. Let sit for 30 to 45 minutes; rinse and dry. Meanwhile, preheat a gas grill or start a charcoal fire; the heat should be moderate. At the same time, marinate the fish in 2 tablespoons of oil.

Grill the fish for 2 to 3 minutes per side (peek in between the flakes with a thin-bladed knife; mahi-mahi is white when done). At the same time, oil the eggplant lightly and grill it until lightly browned on both sides. Grill the red peppers until the skin blackens and blisters all around. When the peppers are cool enough to handle, peel and core them; cut into strips.

Cut the bread in half, horizontally. Remove some of the white crumb from each half to make the bread somewhat hollow. Then build the sandwich, placing the mahi-mahi, eggplant, pepper strips, capers, olives, anchovies, artichoke hearts, tomato, herbs, salt, and pepper. Drizzle liberally with more olive oil and sprinkle with lemon juice.

Close the sandwich and wrap it well in aluminum foil. Place it on a plate, with another plate on top, and weight the second plate with whatever is handy—rocks, bricks, gallon jugs of water, whatever. Use a lot of weight—15 pounds or more. Let the sandwich sit overnight, refrigerated if the room is warm. When you're ready to eat, unwrap the sandwich and cut it into wedges.

ALTERNATIVE FISH FOR THIS RECIPE:

Steaks or thick fillets of bluefish, mackerel, mako shark, swordfish, or tuna. Adjust the cooking times accordingly and be sure to remove all bones.

VIETNAMESE-STYLE SOUP WITH MAHI-MAHI

Makes 4 servings
Time: 30 minutes
This soup simmers with a couple of dried red peppers, enough to give it some bite. Some Vietnamese chefs, however, would serve a few small, minced fresh jalapeños as an optional garnish.

4 cups any fish or chicken stock (pages 40–41)
1 clove garlic, peeled and crushed
2 dried hot peppers
1 pound skinless mahi-mahi fillet or steak
One 4-ounce package cellophane noodles (bean threads; available in Asian markets)
1 cup chopped watercress or bean sprouts
1 tablespoon fish sauce (available in Asian markets; optional)
1 tablespoon high-quality soy sauce (use more if you have no fish sauce)
1 lime
3 scallions, minced, green and white parts

Simmer the stock with the garlic and hot peppers. Set aside about 2 ounces of the mahi-mahi and cut the rest into ½-inch cubes. Soak the cellophane noodles in warm water to cover.

Add the cubed fish to the simmering stock. Cut the remaining fish into tiny julienne strips. When the cellophane noodles are soft—it only takes a few minutes—cut the long strips into more manageable pieces with a scissors. Divide the noodles, julienned fish, and watercress into four serving bowls. Add the fish sauce, soy sauce, and the juice of half the lime to the stock; remove the garlic clove and hot peppers. Make sure the stock is very hot.

Ladle the stock and cubed fish into the bowls, top with the minced scallions, and serve with the remaining half lime, cut into wedges.

ALTERNATIVE FISH FOR THIS RECIPE:

Bluefish, mackerel, mako shark, pompano, swordfish, or tuna. Adjust the cooking times accordingly.

BLASTED MAHI-MAHI WITH SOY AND LIME

Makes 2 servings
Time: 30 minutes

This is what you might call blackened fish, an overused term if ever there was one. There's no trick to it, except to keep the windows open and the exhaust fan on high; this is a smoky preparation.

1 tablespoon high-quality soy sauce
2 tablespoons fresh lime juice
2 skinless mahi-mahi steaks, about 6 ounces each
Freshly ground black pepper to taste

Heat a 12-inch nonstick skillet over high heat for 10 minutes; it will smoke. Combine the soy sauce with 1 ½ tablespoons of the lime juice. Place the steaks in the pan, season with pepper, and cook until browned on one side, about 3 minutes; turn and brown on the other side. Turn off the heat, then add the soy-lime mixture and turn the fish in it a couple of times, until the liquid evaporates, which will happen almost instantly. Sprinkle with the remaining lime and serve immediately.

ALTERNATIVE FISH FOR THIS RECIPE:

Any steak of bluefish, mackerel, mako shark, swordfish, or tuna. Adjust the cooking times accordingly.

GRILLED MAHI-MAHI WITH CUMIN-RED PEPPER BUTTER

Makes 4 servings
Time: 45 minutes

1 medium-size red bell pepper
1 teaspoon ground cumin
⅓ cup any fish or chicken stock (pages 40–41) or dry white wine
Salt and freshly ground black pepper to taste

¼ cup (½ stick) butter, slightly softened
4 skinless mahi-mahi steaks, about 6 ounces each
2 tablespoons olive oil

Roast the red pepper over a charcoal fire, the flame of a gas stove, or under the broiler until blackened all over. Meanwhile, toast the cumin in a small saucepan for 1 minute over medium heat; add the stock and reduce to 1 tablespoon.

When it is cool enough to handle, remove the skin, seeds, and ribs from the pepper. Pound with a pestle in a mortar or puree in a food processor or blender. Cream together with the salt, pepper, butter, and cumin. Refrigerate, covered, until ready to use.

Prepare a charcoal or gas grill; the fire should be medium-hot. Brush the fish with the olive oil, season with salt and pepper, and grill until nicely browned on both sides and just done in the center, about 8 minutes total (peek in between the flakes with a thin-bladed knife; mahi-mahi is white when done). Top each steak with 1 tablespoon of the compound butter and serve.

ALTERNATIVE FISH FOR THIS RECIPE:

Bluefish, mackerel, mako shark, pompano, swordfish, or tuna. Adjust the cooking times accordingly.

GRILLED MAHI-MAHI WITH ORANGE-SOY BUTTER:

Melt 6 tablespoons (¾ stick) butter; add ½ cup fresh orange juice and ¼ cup soy sauce; heat through, then cool slightly. Marinate the mahi-mahi in this mixture while you preheat the grill. Grill about 4 minutes per side, basting with the marinade.

GRILLED MAHI-MAHI WITH TAPENADE:

Chop together 3 cloves garlic, 10 pitted calamata or other good large black olives, and 3 anchovy fillets. Stir together with about ¼ cup olive oil. Brush on the fish as it grills.

SPICE-CURED MAHI-MAHI

Makes 6 to 8 servings
Time: 1 hour plus 1 day resting time
This is great for sandwiches or salad niçoise or, for that matter, Pan Bagna (page 166).

2 tablespoons minced garlic
2 tablespoons salt
2 tablespoons freshly ground black pepper
1 tablespoon ground cumin
2 tablespoons high-quality soy sauce
One 2-pound piece mahi-mahi, in a single steak or fillet
Anchovy Mayonnaise (pages 336–337)
Lemon wedges

Make a paste of the garlic, salt, pepper, cumin, and soy sauce, using a mortar and pestle, food processor, or a knife; rub it all over the mahi-mahi. Wrap the fish in plastic wrap and refrigerate for at least 1 day.

Start a charcoal fire or preheat a gas grill; the fire should be rather low. Grill the mahi-mahi until done (peek in between the flakes with a thin bladed knife; mahi-mahi is white when cooked), about 8 minutes per side. Cool. Slice thinly and serve with the mayonnaise and lemon wedges.

ALTERNATIVE FISH FOR THIS RECIPE:

Swordfish or tuna. Adjust the cooking times accordingly.

MAKO SHARK

Latin name(s): *Isurus oxyrhynchus*.
Other common names: Bonito shark, shark.
Common forms: Steaks, fillets, chunks, usually with tough, inedible skin removed.
General description: Ivory-pink meat that makes a good substitute for swordfish; increasingly available and fairly inexpensive.
For other recipes see: Blackfish, bluefish, dogfish, grouper, mackerel, monkfish, pollock, pompano, rockfish, red snapper, swordfish (especially), tuna, wolffish.
Buying tips: Color varies, but should be ivory-pink rather than brownish; dark red sections are more strongly flavored, so you may want to look for pieces where their proportion is minimal. Smell is important: A whiff of ammonia is unacceptable (see below).

Mako shark sales tripled in the years immediately following the appearance of the movie *Jaws*, and they haven't slowed much. It isn't surprising—there are three hundred or so shark species worldwide, with a large number off both American coasts, and mako is among the best to eat (dogfish, which has completely different flesh, is also a shark).

Shark is a useful fish: Its oil was once used as a substitute for whale oil in lubrication and lamp fuel, and its liver was used as a primary source of vitamin A through the 1940s, when synthetic vitamins were developed. Shark skin is still sometimes used as leather and sandpaper (don't try to eat it).

But until the 1980s little undisguised shark made it to the table. Mako shark, especially, was sometimes sold as swordfish, which it resembles in texture and color, though not in appearance (it lacks the whorls so evident in swordfish steaks) or taste (some people prefer mako; others, myself included, prefer swordfish).

Now shark is served routinely in restaurants and offered in supermarkets. Most is called mako; not all of it is. Most of the fish comes from the Southeast, and might be black-tip, dusky, silky, lemon, bull, tiger, or hammerhead shark. All of this explains the variability you see in the color and texture of "mako." It doesn't matter that much; most of these sharks are just as good as mako for eating.

What matters most to us, as consumers, is not what kind of shark we're eating—it's unlikely we'll be able to determine that with any kind of frequency—but how fresh it is. When you have old or mishandled shark, you know it, and few foods are as unappetizing.

With its primitive kidney system, shark maintains a high proportion of nitrogen compounds in its blood. When these break down, the first sign is the unappealing smell of ammonia. But good handling of the fish, which must begin the moment it's caught and continue until you serve it, can prevent any trace of ammonia from appearing. So when you buy shark, smell it. Under no circumstances should you perceive the smell of ammonia, a sure indication of age or poor handling.

Good mako is pretty close to tasteless, sort of like the white meat of most chicken. And, like chicken, it takes well to marinating, grilling, and spicy flavors.

MARINATED AND GRILLED MAKO
WITH VINEGAR AND HOT SAUCE

Makes 4 servings
Time: 30 minutes, plus marinating time
Shark, like chicken, it is a wonderful carrier of other flavors. Don't be afraid to douse it with spice.

1 cup distilled vinegar
1 teaspoon freshly ground black pepper
Salt to taste
1 teaspoon chili-garlic sauce (available in Asian markets; you can substitute any good hot sauce)
1 tablespoon plus 1 teaspoon minced garlic
1 ½ pounds skinless shark fillets or steaks
1 large sweet onion, cut in half and sliced
2 tablespoons minced cilantro (fresh coriander)
2 tablespoons olive oil

Combine the first four ingredients plus 1 tablespoon of the garlic. Place the shark in a shallow bowl and scatter the onions over it; pour the marinade over all. It should come at least halfway up the sides; if it doesn't, add a little water. Refrigerate, turning occasionally, for as little as 2 or as many as 12 hours.

When ready to cook, start a charcoal fire or preheat a gas grill or the broiler; the heat should be fairly intense. Remove the onions from the marinade and drain them. Heat an 8- or 10-inch nonstick skillet over high heat. Score the flesh of the shark in a crosshatch pattern (as you would do to the skin of a baked ham). Combine the remaining garlic, the cilantro, and salt, and rub it into the slits. Grill or broil the shark about 6 or 8 inches from the heat source, about 5 minutes per side, turning once (peek into the steak, using a thin-bladed knife; all translucence will be gone when the shark is done). Meanwhile, add the olive oil to the skillet; when it is hot, add the onions. Cook them, stirring occasionally, until soft, about 5 to 8 minutes. Serve the shark topped with the onions.

ALTERNATIVE FISH FOR THIS RECIPE: Mahi-mahi. Adjust cooking time accordingly.

BRAISED MAKO STEAKS
WITH LEMON PESTO

Makes 4 servings
Time: 40 minutes
This is about as elegant as shark gets.

2 tablespoons olive oil
2 tablespoons butter
4 skinless mako steaks, about 6 ounces each
Flour for dredging
Salt and freshly ground black pepper to taste
1 medium-size onion, chopped
1 medium-size red bell pepper, seeded and chopped
1 bay leaf
10 fresh basil leaves, minced
1 teaspoon minced garlic
1 cup chopped tomatoes, fresh or canned (drained if canned)
½ cup dry white wine
Zest of 2 lemons
3 cloves garlic, peeled
1 cup packed fresh basil leaves
½ cup packed chopped fresh parsley

Heat a 12-inch nonstick skillet over medium-high heat. Add the olive oil and butter and when the butter foam subsides, dredge the shark steaks in the flour, shaking off any excess. Brown quickly on both sides, for just 2 to 3 minutes per side; season with salt and pepper and remove from the pan.

Add the onion and bell pepper to the pan and cook over medium heat, stirring occasionally, until the onion wilts. Add the bay leaf, minced basil, and minced garlic and cook 1 minute. Add the tomatoes and wine and cook over medium heat until the tomatoes break down and the sauce reduces slightly. Season the sauce with salt and pepper and return the shark steaks to the pan. Cook until the fish is done, about 6 to 8 minutes (it will be fairly tender, and all translucence gone).

Meanwhile, make the pesto: In a small food processor or blender, combine the lemon zest, garlic cloves, basil leaves, parsley, and a pinch of salt; process until finely minced, then check and correct seasoning if necessary. Serve the fish with a bit of sauce, passing the pesto at the table.

ALTERNATIVE FISH FOR THIS RECIPE:
Steaks of blackfish, grouper, or swordfish. Adjust the cooking times accordingly.

MAKO KEBABS WITH BLACK BEANS AND RICE

Makes 4 servings
Time: 2 hours, including marinating and cooking beans
Another recipe that takes advantage of mako's meaty flavor and texture.

⅓ cup olive oil
2 tablespoons fresh lime juice
2 cloves garlic, peeled
3 slices peeled fresh ginger
Salt and freshly ground black pepper to taste
¼ cup loosely packed cilantro (fresh coriander) leaves, plus 2 tablespoons minced leaves for garnish
¼ teaspoon cayenne pepper
One 1-pound skinless shark fillet or steak, about 1 inch thick, cut into 1-inch cubes
1 cup short-grain rice

1 ½ cups water
3 cups well-seasoned cooked black beans (pages 156–157)
Lime quarters

Combine the first seven ingredients in a food processor and blend until smooth. Marinate the shark cubes in the mixture for about 1 hour. Rinse the rice well, then soak for 30 minutes in the water. Toward the end of the marinating time, start a gas or charcoal grill or preheat the broiler; the heat should be fairly high. Warm the beans and cook the rice over medium-high heat in its soaking water, covered, until nearly all the water is absorbed, about 8 minutes. Allow the rice to sit, covered.

Skewer the pieces of shark and grill until nicely browned on all sides, about 10 minutes. Add the remaining marinade to the beans. When the shark is cooked, place a mound of rice in the center of each plate, top with some black beans, and place a few cubes of shark around the mound. Garnish with the minced cilantro and serve with lime wedges.

ALTERNATIVE FISH FOR THIS RECIPE:
Swordfish (reduce the marinating time to 20 minutes and adjust the cooking time accordingly).

SKEWERED MAKO WITH CILANTRO:
Combine 1 cup cilantro (fresh coriander) leaves, ¼ cup olive oil, ¼ cup fresh lime juice, 1 scallion, the zest of 1 lime, and salt and pepper in a food processor or blender and puree. Marinate the shark cubes in this for 1 hour. Grill as instructed above and garnish with minced scallion or cilantro. This is good served with Avocado Salsa (page 43).

MONKFISH

Latin name(s): *Lophius piscatorius*, *L. americanus*.
Other common names: Goosefish, angler, allmouth, lotte (French).
Common forms: Skinned, deboned tails (almost always), whole (rarely).
General description: Wonderful white flesh with extremely firm texture; "poor man's lobster." Very versatile.
For other recipes see: Blackfish, carp, catfish, cod, dogfish, grouper, haddock, mako shark, octopus, pollock, rockfish, sablefish, scallops, shrimp, red snapper, squid, tilefish, wolffish.
Buying tips: Monkfish should appear moist; dryness is a sure sign of age, as, of course, are any off odors. Ask the fishmonger to remove any membrane that remains on the fillet, or you'll have to do it yourself (see below).

Generally considered one of the ugliest fish of the sea (Alan Davidson lists it under "Miscellaneous Uncouth Fish"), the monkfish is almost all head. And its head is almost all mouth. This allows it to eat a lot, which I suppose is what makes its meat rich. In any case, it's among the densest, meatiest of fish.

When monkfish are caught, they are usually cut in half; the tail end is kept and the head and body tossed overboard (monkfish heads make superior stock; buy them when you see them). The tail is then skinned, and usually filleted (if it hasn't been, it will take you just a second or two to remove the single bone that runs through it). A thin gray membrane may sometimes be left on the tail; cut and peel it off before cooking. And if any of the meat is grayish or tan, cut that off and discard it (it isn't bad, but it has a grainy texture that makes it less enjoyable than the white meat).

One of my favorite fish stories involves monkfish: Ten years ago, when monkfish was still considered trash, and cost eighty-nine cents a pound (if you could find it), I knew a fisherman who was selling his monkfish tails to a processor, who froze them and shipped them to Europe. I suggested he might sell them directly to a French restaurant from time to time to try to make more money. But his local French chef, as haughty as a caricature, said no: "I only buy my fish from France," he said. Turned out the chef was buying frozen lotte—that is, monkfish—from France. The French exporter, of course, was buying this frozen lotte from the United States!

Monkfish meat is among the best: Firm, tasty, and versatile. You can grill it, poach it, roast it, or sauté it and, using any of these methods, turn out some spectacular dishes. Even though monkfish has been discovered, and now costs three to four dollars a pound—and more—in most markets, it's a bargain when compared to almost any other animal.

GRILLED MONKFISH WITH CHERRY TOMATOES AND ASPARAGUS

Makes 2 servings
Time: About 60 minutes, including marinating
A wonderful summer dish, with the flavor of basil at the forefront. If asparagus season has passed you by, grill zucchini or eggplant (no parboiling needed).

1 pound fillet of monkfish tail, cut from the thick end if possible, in one piece, membranes removed
2 tablespoons olive oil
Juice of 1 lime
¼ teaspoon cayenne or crushed red pepper
1 tablespoon chopped fresh basil
Salt and freshly ground black pepper to taste
½ pound asparagus (6 to 18 spears, depending on thickness)
8 cherry tomatoes

Cut the monkfish into big chunks, about 2 inches thick. Soak for 30 minutes in a mixture of the olive oil, lime juice, cayenne, basil, salt, and pepper. Meanwhile, start a charcoal fire or preheat a gas grill—the fire should be quite hot. Peel the asparagus if necessary and parboil it for 2 to 4 minutes until it begins to become tender but is not cooked through, depending on thickness. Drain and cool quickly.

Skewer the tomatoes. Skewer the asparagus, using two skewers in parallel, one through the bud ends and one through the stalks (this facilitates turning). When ready to cook, skewer the monkfish, using two skewers.

Grill the monkfish over the hottest part of the fire, with the asparagus and tomatoes off to the side. Brush the vegetables with a little of the marinade as they cook. Turn the vegetables as soon as they brown slightly; turn the monkfish when it is good and browned, about 7 to 8 minutes. The vegetables will probably be done before the fish, in a total of 10 minutes or less; the monkfish will take a total of 15 to 18 minutes; it's done when quite firm to the touch and browned all over.

Remove the vegetables and fish from the skewers and serve all together on a platter.

ALTERNATIVE FISH FOR THIS RECIPE:
Big chunks of blackfish, grouper, mako shark, or swordfish. You can also use large shrimp or scallops. Adjust the cooking times accordingly.

MONKFISH SKEWERED WITH ONIONS AND MUSHROOMS:
Alternate the monkfish chunks on skewers with quartered onions, small mushrooms, bacon, bay leaves, and zucchini chunks.

MONKFISH IN THE STYLE OF VEAL

Makes 4 servings
Time: 40 to 50 minutes
When I first encountered monkfish, it cost less than a dollar a pound and was being sold in a New Haven Italian fish market as "veal of the sea." The owner routinely cut it into medallions (or even thin scallops), the idea being that you would cook it in any of the myriad of ways you would thin slices of veal. Though I've never seen this done anywhere else, it's a sound preparation, and one that can offer infinite variations; I give three here.

2 pounds fillet of monkfish tail, in one or two pieces, membranes removed
½ cup olive oil
2 cups drained canned plum tomatoes
2 large eggs, lightly beaten
Flour for dredging, liberally seasoned with salt and pepper
¼ cup chopped fresh basil
1 clove garlic, minced
Salt and freshly ground black pepper to taste
Minced fresh parsley for garnish

Cut the fish into ¾-inch-thick medallions (when it

narrows at the tail, leave a piece about 2 inches long) and set aside. In a medium-size saucepan, heat ¼ cup of the olive oil and add the tomatoes, crushing them with a fork, simmer over low heat while you cook the monkfish.

Heat a 12-inch nonstick skillet over medium-high heat for about 5 minutes. Add about ¼ cup of the oil and, one by one, dip the medallions in the egg and then the flour, shaking off any excess each time, then put them in the pan. You will probably need to cook the monkfish in two batches. Adjust the heat so that the fish sizzles but doesn't burn. Turn when the fish is brown on one side; then brown on the other. Monkfish is done when easily pierced with a fork (it is somewhat rubbery until then).

Keep the first batch of medallions warm in a low oven while you cook the remainder. Halfway through the second batch, add the basil and garlic to the tomato sauce and taste it for salt and pepper. When all the monkfish is cooked, arrange it on a platter and nap it lightly with the tomato sauce and minced parsley. Serve immediately.

ALTERNATIVE FISH FOR THIS RECIPE:

Thick slices of blackfish, grouper, Atlantic pollock, rockfish, red snapper, or wolffish. Adjust the cooking times accordingly.

SAUTÉED MONKFISH WITH LEMON:

Make no tomato sauce. Reduce ½ cup dry white wine by half in the skillet, then add the juice of 1 lemon. Pour the sauce over the cooked medallions and serve with more lemon. This is also good topped with ½ cup slivered almonds cooked briefly in a little butter or olive oil.

SAUTÉED MONKFISH WITH SPINACH:

Make no tomato sauce. Steam 1 pound fresh spinach, well washed and tough stems removed, with 1 minced garlic clove, then sprinkle with 1 teaspoon or more lemon juice. Arrange the cooked medallions on a bed of spinach and serve with more lemon.

SAUTÉED MONKFISH THAI STYLE:

Make no tomato sauce. When the monkfish is cooked, wipe out the pan and add 3 tablespoons peanut oil. Over medium-high heat, cook, stirring, 1 tablespoon minced garlic. When it colors, add 1 large onion, chopped, 2 tablespoons fish sauce (available in Asian markets; you may substitute soy sauce), 1 cup minced fresh basil, and 1 fresh jalapeño, seeded, deveined, and minced (or 1 tablespoon chili-garlic paste, available in Asian markets). Stir and cook for 2 minutes. Return the monkfish to the pan and reheat in the sauce. Serve over rice.

MONKFISH WITH FRESH TOMATOES AND CRISP POTATOES

Makes 4 servings
Time: 60 minutes

This combines the best features of several monkfish preparations I've had in Spain. It's a great textural combination, and the sauce is so creamy you'll want to eat it with a spoon.

About 1 pound waxy potatoes
½ cup olive oil, more or less
3 sprigs fresh rosemary or 1 teaspoon dried
Salt and freshly ground black pepper to taste
1 medium-size red bell pepper, seeded and thinly sliced
1 tablespoon balsamic or sherry wine vinegar
1 ¼ pounds fillet of monkfish tail, membranes removed, cut into 1 ½-inch chunks
Flour for dredging
2 cloves garlic, minced
1 large shallot, minced
½ cup any fish or chicken stock (pages 40–41), dry white wine, water, or a combination
3 good-size fresh ripe tomatoes, roughly chopped
½ cup minced fresh parsley

Heat a 10- or 12-inch nonstick skillet over medium-high heat while you wash and cut the potatoes into ½-inch dice (peeling is optional). Add 2 table-spoons of the oil. Add the potatoes and half the rosemary. Avoid crowding; you may have to do the potatoes in two batches. Adjust the heat so they don't burn but become brown and crisp on all sides; season well and keep warm when they're done.

Meanwhile, heat a second nonstick skillet over high heat. Sear the red pepper, shaking the pan occasionally. When it begins to blacken, add 1 tablespoon of the olive oil and cook another 1 or 2 minutes, just until the pepper begins to soften. Add the vinegar, toss for 30 seconds or so, and remove the pepper to a warm place. Wipe out the pan and place it back over medium-high heat.

Add 2 tablespoons of the olive oil to the pan and when it's hot (a pinch of flour will sizzle), begin dredging the monkfish chunks well in the flour, shaking any excess off them, and cooking them. Do not crowd; brown them well on all sides, adjusting the heat as necessary, and removing pieces as they are done and adding more. Use more olive oil if necessary. Season the monkfish well as it cooks.

When the monkfish is browned (it need not be fully cooked), set the heat to medium, add another 1 tablespoon of olive oil to the skillet, then add the garlic and shallot. Cook, stirring, for a minute or so. Add the stock, raise the heat to high, and reduce it by half. Add the tomatoes and remaining rosemary and cook until the tomatoes begin to break down. Add half the parsley and the fish chunks and cook over medium heat, spooning the sauce over the fish occasionally. Cook until the monkfish is cooked through (you will be able to pierce it easily with a fork), about 10 minutes.

Remove the monkfish and sauce to a shallow bowl, then top with the potatoes, peppers, and, finally, the remaining parsley. Serve immediately.

ALTERNATIVE FISH FOR THIS RECIPE:
Blackfish, grouper, mako shark, or swordfish.

You can also use large shrimp or scallops. Adjust the cooking times accordingly.

MONKFISH WITH BLACK PEPPER

Makes 4 servings
Time: 30 minutes

2 tablespoons olive oil
4 to 6 small fillets of monkfish tails, about 1 ½ pounds, membranes removed
Flour for dredging
½ cup dry white wine
1 cup Fast Fish Stock (page 40)
2 tablespoons minced shallots
¼ cup (½ stick) butter, softened
1 tablespoon cracked black pepper
2 tablespoons minced fresh parsley

Preheat the oven to 350°F. Heat a 12-inch nonstick skillet over medium-high heat for 4 to 5 minutes. Add the oil and when it is hot (a pinch of flour will sizzle), dredge the monkfish tails lightly in the flour, shaking off all the excess, and sear on all sides until lightly browned, about 12 minutes. Remove the monkfish to an ovenproof platter and place in the oven while you finish the sauce.

Add the wine to the pan and reduce over medium-high heat, stirring. Add the stock and shallots and cook down to about ½ cup. Lower the heat to a minimum and stir in the butter, 1 tablespoon at a time, until the sauce is smooth and thick. Add the pepper and parsley and stir. Pour in any juices that have accumulated around the monkfish. Spoon the sauce over the fish and serve immediately.

ALTERNATIVE FISH FOR THIS RECIPE:
This is best with monkfish, but it's not bad at all with strips cut from thick fillets or steaks of black-fish, grouper, or striped bass.

WHOLE MONKFISH TAILS ROASTED WITH HERBS

Makes 4 servings
Time: 45 minutes

Wilton's is a two-hundred-year-old oyster bar on Jermyn Street in London, where the waitresses wear white and the customers are almost all pompous men. It's one of the world's great fish restaurants, and one where the food is current, despite the stuffy atmosphere. Among the surprises on its menu the last time I was there was a monkfish dish similar to this one.

4 to 6 small fillets of monkfish tails, about 1 ½ pounds, membranes removed
½ cup chopped mixed fresh herbs: parsley, basil, chervil, tarragon, rosemary, chives, marjoram, sage, etc.
1 cup unbleached all-purpose flour
Salt and freshly ground black pepper to taste
3 tablespoons olive oil
1 cup any fish or chicken stock (pages 40–41), dry white wine, water, or a combination

Preheat the oven to 450°F. Rinse and dry the monkfish. Mix together the herbs, flour, salt, and pepper. Heat a flameproof baking dish over medium-high heat and add the olive oil. When it's good and hot (a pinch of flour will sizzle), dredge the fish tails in the flour mixture and brown for a couple of minutes on all sides. Add the stock and place in the oven.

Roast until the monkfish is tender, 20 to 30 minutes, turning once or twice. Remove the fish to a warm platter. If the pan juices are a little thin, reduce a bit; if they're too thick, add a little more stock or water and cook over medium heat for 1 to 2 minutes. Serve the fish, over rice or with bread, with the sauce spooned over.

ALTERNATIVE FISH FOR THIS RECIPE:
Thick fillets of blackfish, dogfish, grouper, Atlantic pollock, rockfish, red snapper, tilefish, or wolffish. Adjust cooking times accordingly.

GARLIC-STUDDED ROAST MONKFISH WITH SALSA FRESCA:
Sliver 1 or 2 cloves garlic and, using a thin-bladed knife, insert the slivers into the monkfish tails. Dredge in flour (the herbs are optional but still good) and cook as directed above. Serve with salsa fresca (from Sautéed Pollock with Salsa Fresca, page 209).

ROAST MONKFISH MOROCCAN STYLE

Makes 4 servings
Time: 40 minutes

4 to 6 small fillets of monkfish tails, about 1 ½ pounds, membranes removed
¼ cup minced fresh parsley
1 tablespoon minced garlic
¼ teaspoon cayenne pepper or to taste
1 tablespoon ground cumin
½ teaspoon ground coriander
Pinch ground cloves
¼ teaspoon ground cinnamon
¼ cup olive oil
2 cups chopped ripe or canned tomatoes, drained briefly
Salt and freshly ground black pepper to taste

Preheat the oven to 450°F. Rinse and dry the monkfish. Mix together the parsley, garlic, cayenne, cumin, coriander, cloves, and cinnamon (you can do this in a food processor and avoid mincing the garlic and parsley by hand; add a little olive oil or white wine if needed to process). Rub the monkfish all over with this mixture.

Spread half the olive oil on the bottom of a roasting pan. Place the monkfish in the pan, top with the tomatoes and the remaining olive oil, and roast until the monkfish is tender, 20 to 30 minutes, turning once or twice. Serve the fish, over rice or with bread, with the sauce spooned over it.

ALTERNATIVE FISH FOR THIS RECIPE:

Strips of blackfish, grouper, or striped bass, cut from steaks or thick fillets.

MONKFISH BAKED WITH APPLES AND ZUCCHINI

Makes 4 servings
Time: 60 minutes

¼ cup (½ stick) butter or olive oil
2 cups thinly sliced zucchini or yellow squash
1 cup cored, peeled, and thinly sliced crisp apple
1 cup sliced onion
1 teaspoon minced fresh thyme or ¼ teaspoon dried
Salt and freshly ground black pepper to taste
½ cup dry white wine
1 pound fillet of monkfish tail, membrane removed, cut into 1 ½-inch chunks

Preheat the oven to 375°F. Smear 1 tablespoon or so of the butter or oil onto the bottom of a baking dish. Layer the zucchini, apples, and onion in the dish, dot with a little more butter, and sprinkle with the thyme, salt, and pepper. Bake, uncovered, for about 30 minutes.

Remove from the oven and raise the heat to 450°F. Pour in the wine and place the monkfish atop the vegetables. Season with a little more salt and pepper, dot with the remaining butter, and roast until the monkfish is tender, 15 to 20 minutes. Serve immediately.

ALTERNATIVE FISH FOR THIS RECIPE:

Blackfish, catfish, dogfish, grouper, Atlantic pollock, rockfish, red snapper, or wolffish. Adjust the cooking times accordingly.

POACHED MONKFISH WITH LEMON SAUCE

Makes 4 servings
Time: 30 minutes

A more-or-less traditional Provençal preparation, one that must be served with good bread, or at least a sauce spoon.

¼ cup (½ stick) butter
2 leeks, washed well, trimmed of tough green parts, and diced
½ cup dry white wine
1 cup any fish or chicken stock (pages 40–41) or water
1 teaspoon minced fresh thyme or ½ teaspoon dried
1 ½ pounds fillet of monkfish tails, membranes removed, cut into medallions
1 tablespoon fresh lemon juice
Salt and freshly ground black pepper to taste

Melt half the butter in a 10- or 12-inch skillet over medium-high heat, then add the leeks and cook, stirring, until softened, about 5 minutes. Add the wine, stock, and thyme; bring to a boil and let bubble for 1 to 2 minutes. Add the monkfish, lower the heat to medium-low, cover, and simmer until it cooks through, 4 to 5 minutes. Remove the fish with a slotted spoon and keep warm.

Reduce the sauce over high heat until about ¾ cup remains; this will take 10 minutes or so. Add the lemon juice, then stir in the remaining butter, a bit at a time. Season with salt and pepper, return the monkfish medallions to the sauce to heat through, and serve immediately.

ALTERNATIVE FISH FOR THIS RECIPE:

Blackfish, grouper, scallops, shrimp, or wolffish. Adjust the cooking times accordingly.

MONKFISH POACHED IN BITTER GARLIC SAUCE

Makes 4 servings
Time: 40 minutes

Much has been made of the mellowness of slowly cooked garlic, but garlic takes on an entirely different character when cooked until it becomes dark brown; it becomes strong and bitter, not like raw garlic, but like nothing else. Powerful as this flavor is, it is also—like that of chiles—readily enjoyable.

1 whole head garlic
1 dried hot pepper
¼ cup olive oil
2 cups canned tomatoes, measured with about ½ cup of their juice
Salt and freshly ground black pepper to taste
½ cup minced fresh parsley
1 ½ to 2 pounds fillets of monkfish tails, membranes removed, cut into 1 ½-inch chunks

Split the garlic into cloves, peel them, and slice the cloves into slivers. Place them in a large skillet with the hot pepper and oil and turn the heat to medium. Cook, stirring only occasionally, until the garlic begins to sizzle; then cook it watchfully, until the garlic is dark brown but not burned, about 10 to 15 minutes. Turn off the heat and wait 3 minutes.

Cut up or crush the tomatoes and add them, along with their juice, to the garlic. Increase the heat to medium-high and cook until the sauce is fairly thick, about 10 minutes; add salt, pepper, and half the parsley. Add the monkfish and cook over medium-low heat, covered and stirring occasionally, until the monkfish is tender, about 10

minutes. Serve immediately, garnished with the remaining parsley.

ALTERNATIVE FISH FOR THIS RECIPE:
Blackfish, grouper, or mako shark. Adjust the cooking times accordingly.

DIJON WINTER VEGETABLE STEW WITH MONKFISH

Makes 6 to 8 servings
Time: 40 minutes

¼ cup (½ stick) butter
1 tablespoon vegetable or olive oil
3 cups ¼-inch-thick carrot slices
1 head cauliflower, broken into small florets
3 cups ¼-inch-thick yellow onion slices
3 cups ¼-inch-thick yellow squash slices
12 ounces small white mushrooms (or quartered larger mushrooms)
⅓ cup dry white wine
2 cups any fish or chicken stock (pages 40–41)
1 to 1 ½ pounds fillet of monkfish tails, membranes removed, cut into 1 ½-inch chunks
¼ cup Dijon mustard
½ cup light cream or half-and-half
Salt and freshly ground black pepper to taste
2 tablespoons fresh chopped dill or 1 tablespoon dried
1 cup fresh or defrosted frozen peas

Melt the butter and oil in a large, heavy casserole over medium heat just until the butter foams. Add the carrots and cook, stirring, for 2 to 3 minutes, then add the remaining vegetables except the peas, cooking, stirring occasionally, until the onions start to wilt, about 5 to 6 minutes more. Pour in the wine, raise the heat to high, and cook for 1 to 2 minutes. Add the stock and monkfish, cover, reduce the heat so the liquid just simmers, and cook until the vegetables and fish are tender, about 8 to 10 minutes.

Stir the mustard into the cream and add it to the stew along with the salt, pepper, dill, and peas. Stir to blend and continue to cook slowly over medium-low heat for another 2 to 3 minutes. Adjust the seasoning, adding more mustard if needed, and serve over rice or cooked pearled barley.

ALTERNATIVE FISH FOR THIS RECIPE:

Blackfish, grouper, Atlantic pollock, or wolffish. Adjust the cooking times accordingly.

CURRIED MONKFISH SOUP WITH TOMATOES AND DRIED APRICOTS

Makes 4 servings
Time: 30 minutes

An unusual but appropriate combination, this is not only great for cold winter nights, but can be chilled for serving in warm weather.

8 cups any fish or chicken stock (pages 40–41)
3 tablespoons butter
1 cup minced onion
1 teaspoon minced garlic
1 tablespoon curry powder
2 cups chopped drained canned or fresh tomatoes
½ cup minced dried apricots
Salt and freshly ground black pepper to taste
¼ teaspoon cayenne pepper or to taste (optional)
1 pound fillets of monkfish tails, membranes removed, cut into ½-inch pieces
½ cup heavy cream
Minced cilantro (fresh coriander) for garnish

Warm the stock and keep warm. In a casserole or large saucepan, melt the butter over medium heat. Add the onion and garlic and cook, stirring occasionally, until the onion wilts, 5 to 10 minutes. Add the curry powder and cook, stirring, for about 2 minutes. Add the stock and bring to a simmer. Add the tomatoes and apricots and simmer, stirring occasionally, for about 10 minutes. Season with salt and pepper; taste and correct the seasonings—add additional curry powder and the cayenne.

Add the monkfish and cook until it's done, about 8 to 10 minutes (remove a piece and cut it in half; it should be opaque and not at all rubbery). Add the cream and heat through (do not boil). Taste again for salt and pepper, garnish with the cilantro, and serve.

ALTERNATIVE FISH FOR THIS RECIPE:

Catfish, grouper, scallops, red snapper, or wolffish. Adjust the cooking times accordingly.

MULLET

Latin name(s): *Mugil cephalus*, etc.
Other common names: Striped mullet, white mullet, liza, fantail mullet, red mullet, etc.
Common forms: Whole fish, skin-on fillets.
General description: A popular fish for frying on the Gulf Coast. Must be perfectly fresh to be worth eating.
For other recipes see: Butterfish, croaker, mackerel, pompano, porgy, sea bass.
Buying tips: Personally, I only buy mullet when I'm in mullet country—the Gulf Coast. Otherwise, it's never quite fresh enough and its flavor, while not bad, is disappointing.

Generally speaking, mullet is not as good a fish as the other fish of its general size and type listed above. If you're on the Gulf Coast, and you get some just out of the water, by all means cook it. But don't go out of your way for it, especially if you're not in the South; its shelf life—the time it stays fresh once out of the water—is among the shortest of any saltwater fish. Mullet roe (which also deteriorates quickly) is delicious; most of it is flown to Japan.

Perhaps the most important thing to know about our mullet is that it is most decidedly *not* European mullet (*Mullus surmuletus*). When a recipe in a European (or even European-style) cookbook calls for mullet fillets, substitute ocean perch; when you're looking for whole "mullet," use croaker or porgy. All of these are superior to our mullet, and much more like the European mullet, which is also known as goatfish or rouget.

MULLET WITH ROASTED SUMMER VEGETABLES

Makes 2 servings
Time: 40 minutes
This recipe will work with almost any whole, good-flavored fish, and will appeal especially to gardeners (who will also know that the vegetable list can be varied according to their garden's production). The vegetables help keep the fish moist; the high heat makes cooking time relatively short. I serve this dish with rice or kasha, but good bread is a fine alternative.

2 cups diced eggplant, peeled if desired
2 cups diced zucchini
2 cups diced fresh tomatoes
1 cup chopped onion
1 cup snapped green beans
3 cloves garlic, minced
Salt and freshly ground black pepper to taste
Several sprigs fresh rosemary or 1 teaspoon dried
Several sprigs fresh parsley, plus minced parsley for garnish
¼ cup olive oil
One 1½- to 2-pound mullet, well scaled and gutted, with head on
1 teaspoon fresh lemon juice

Preheat the oven to 500°F while you chop the vegetables. Mix them together with the garlic, salt, pepper, rosemary, parsley, and olive oil in a baking dish that can later accommodate the fish. Roast about 20 minutes, stirring once or twice, until the tomatoes have dissolved, the sauce is bubbling, and the zucchini is fairly tender. Lay the fish atop the vegetables, spoon some of the vegetables over it, lower the heat to 450°F, and return the pan to the oven. Roast another 15 minutes (the stomach cavity of the fish will become white), basting the fish once or twice. Spoon the fish and vegetables onto plates, sprinkle with the lemon juice, and serve.

ALTERNATIVE FISH FOR THIS RECIPE:

Use any whole fish of 1 ½ to 3 pounds, such as croaker, small red snapper or rockfish, sea bass, spot, small tilefish, or whiting, and adjust the cooking times accordingly.

FRIED MULLET

Makes 4 servings
Time: 30 minutes

This recipes come from the Buggy Bayou Mullet Festival, an annual event held in Niceville (no kidding), Florida, and undoubtedly the best place in the country to eat mullet. They also smoke mullet at the festival; you can do that using the recipe for Hot-smoked Mackerel, page 163; season with a little melted butter, lemon juice, and Worcestershire sauce.

2 pounds mullet fillets
Cornmeal for dredging
Salt and freshly ground black pepper to taste
Vegetable oil for frying
Lemon wedges (optional)
Spicy Pepper Sauce for Fried Fish (page 42; optional)

Rinse and dry the fillets. Season the cornmeal with salt and pepper, then place it in a plastic bag. Heat at least 2 inches of oil to 350°F. A few at a time, shake the fillets in the cornmeal and fry in the oil, turning once, for a total of about 5 minutes. (The style at the festival is to overcook the fish slightly, making the crust super-crisp but the mullet a tad dry; if you want to try that, keep the fish in the oil until the crust is dark brown.) Drain on paper towels and serve immediately with lemon wedges or the hot sauce.

ALTERNATIVE FISH FOR THIS RECIPE:

Fillets of almost any fish at all. Adjust the cooking times accordingly.

MUSSELS

Latin name(s): *Mytilus edulis* (Atlantic), *M. californianis* (Pacific).
Other common names: Blue mussel, common mussel, New Zealand green-lipped mussel.
Common forms: Whole, in shell; cooked, shelled (infrequently).
General description: The familiar blue-black shell found on rocks, piers, pilings, and anywhere else they can gain an anchor in calm water.
For other recipes see: Clams, oysters.
Buying tips: Like all bivalve mollusks, mussels must be alive (or cooked or frozen) when sold (see page 8). This virtually guarantees relative freshness, but not necessarily quality. If mussels are especially muddy or dirt-encrusted, they'll be hard to clean. And if the meat doesn't fill the shell, they may be disappointingly small when cooked.

Dollar for dollar, mussels are the best bivalve you can buy. A pot of steamed mussels is as heavenly as a good lobster. The down side is that mussels can be a pain to clean, especially since you need at least a pound per person (and many people can devour twice that without much trouble).

To minimize hassles, start with clean mussels rather than muddy ones. Then, if you have the time, let them sit in a pot under slowly running cold water for a couple of hours. Next wash them carefully, discarding any with broken shells, those whose shells remain open after tapping them lightly, or those which seem unusually heavy (these might be filled with mud instead of meat). As you clean them, pull or scrape off the "beard"—the weedy growth attached to the bottom of shell—from each one. Rinse thoroughly.

You can easily gather your own mussels, as long as it's legal and the water is clean; I'd check with local health authorities or a bait shop before going ahead. Mussels sold in stores are, like clams and oysters, subject to Federal regulations. In general, mussels are considered safer than clams and oysters, but only because they are almost never eaten raw (although raw mussels can be quite good). After you gather or buy mussels, you can store them for at least a couple of days before cooking; just keep them cool and make sure they can breathe, which means don't let them sit in water or sealed plastic.

When you do cook mussels, think of them as you do spinach, and remember that they generate so much liquid that it's pointless to add any more liquid than you need to protect your pot for the first couple of minutes or for seasoning.

Some mussels contain pea crabs, pea-sized animals which live in a symbiotic relationship with the mussel. These crunchy little devils are not only harmless, they are edible. Although no one seems to like them, there doesn't seem to be much that can be done about ridding mussels of them.

STEAMED MUSSELS, VERSION I

Makes 4 servings
Time: About 15 minutes, plus cleaning time
These are basic steamed mussels. Note that they can readily be made more elaborate.

3 tablespoons olive oil
4 cloves garlic, smashed and peeled
1 medium-size onion, sliced
½ cup dry white wine
Juice of ½ lemon
½ cup roughly chopped fresh parsley
4 pounds or more large mussels, cleaned as described on page 183

In a large pot over medium heat, heat the oil, then add the garlic and onion and cook, stirring, just until the onion softens. Add the wine, lemon juice, parsley, and mussels, cover the pot, and turn the heat to high. Steam, shaking the pot frequently, until the mussels open, about 8 to 10 minutes. Spoon the mussels into a serving bowl, strain the liquid over them—I use a strainer lined with cheesecloth to be sure of removing any errant sand—and serve with plenty of crusty bread.

ALTERNATIVE FISH FOR THIS RECIPE:

Hard- or soft-shell clams, well-scrubbed oysters, or scallops in their shells.

MUSSELS WITH CREAM:

Bring the oil, onion, garlic, white wine, lemon juice, and parsley to a boil and add ½ teaspoon dried or 1 teaspoon minced fresh tarragon. Reduce to about ½ cup, turn the heat to low, then add 2 tablespoons butter, cut into bits. When it has melted, add 2 cups heavy cream. Do not boil. Taste the sauce for seasoning (feel free to add a little more tarragon) and pour it over the mussels.

MUSSELS WITH RICE:

Remove the mussels after they open and strain the liquid—using a strainer lined with cheesecloth—into a saucepan; keep it warm. Take the mussels from their shells (you might keep some in for garnish). Heat ¼ cup olive oil in a 12-inch skillet over medium heat and cook 1 cup chopped onion, stirring occasionally, until soft. Add 1 cup long-grain white rice and stir to coat. Pour 2 cups of the reserved liquid over the rice and cook, uncovered, stirring occasionally, until the liquid evaporates and the rice is cooked (in the unlikely event that there was not enough liquid from the mussels, finish the cooking with water or stock). Season to taste, then stir in the mussels and ½ cup minced fresh parsley. Check the seasoning and serve.

STEAMED MUSSELS, VERSION II

Makes 4 to 8 appetizer servings
Time: About 30 minutes, plus time for cleaning
This is slightly more elegant, and is fit for a cocktail party or other stand-up gathering.

30 to 40 good-size mussels, cleaned as described on page 183
½ cup dry white wine
1 tablespoon olive oil
1 clove garlic, minced
1 tablespoon fresh lemon juice

Place the mussels in a large pot with the wine and olive oil. Steam over medium-high heat, shaking occasionally, just until the mussels are open, about 10 minutes. Remove from the heat and take the mussels from the pot. While they cool slightly, strain the liquid—using a strainer lined with cheesecloth—and return it to the pot; add the garlic and cook, stirring, over medium-high heat, until there are only 2 tablespoons of liquid left. Remove the mussels from their shells and add them to the sauce along with the lemon juice, reheating gently. Serve hot or at room temperature, with toothpicks.

ALTERNATIVE FISH FOR THIS RECIPE:

Hard- or soft-shell clams, well-scrubbed oysters, or scallops in their shells.

STEAMED MUSSELS, VERSION III

Makes 2 servings
Time: 30 minutes

If I had to choose one mussel recipe as my favorite, this might be it. But don't even try to serve this without plenty of good bread, and don't hope to duplicate the results with olive oil.

If you like, you can prepare the mussels, without the sauce, in advance. Refrigerate them, covered, on their shells. Thirty minutes before serving, preheat the oven to 400°F, make the sauce, place the mussels in a baking dish or casserole, drizzle the sauce over them, and bake until the mussels are piping hot, about 10 minutes.

3 pounds mussels, cleaned as described on page 183
½ cup dry white wine
3 tablespoons butter
2 cloves garlic, minced
¼ cup minced fresh parsley
Salt

In a covered pot over medium-high heat, steam the mussels in the wine, shaking occasionally, until open, about 10 minutes. Drain the mussels, capturing the steaming liquid in a bowl. Immediately strain the liquid—using a strainer lined with cheesecloth—into a small saucepan and begin reducing over high heat.

Meanwhile, discard one shell of each mussel, and arrange the remaining shells, with the mussel meat, on a platter. Keep warm in a low oven while the liquid reduces.

When the steaming liquid is reduced to about ¼ cup, add the butter and let it melt. Add the garlic and parsley and cook over medium heat for 1 to 2 minutes. Check for salt, then drizzle over the mussel meats and serve immediately.

ALTERNATIVE FISH FOR THIS RECIPE:

Hard- or soft-shell clams, well-scrubbed oysters, or scallops in their shells.

MUSSEL BISQUE

Makes 4 servings
Time: 30 minutes

This poor man's lobster bisque is better than the "real" thing, if you ask me; it has the essence of mussels in every spoonful. Make the mussels in advance and shell them, using all but a few for a mussel salad such as the one on page 189 or for Seafood Salad Adriatic Style, page 49. Reserve the broth and make this soup when you're ready (mussel broth freezes beautifully for several weeks).

1 recipe Steamed Mussels, Version III (preceding recipe), made with shallots instead of garlic and with several sprigs thyme added
2 cups heavy cream
2 large egg yolks, lightly beaten
Salt and freshly ground black pepper to taste

Strain the steaming broth, using a strainer lined with cheesecloth. Shell the mussels and reserve four of the nicest for garnish.

Bring the broth to a boil and add the cream. Over medium heat, stirring, return the mixture to a boil. Turn off the heat and stir in the egg yolks. Turn the heat to low and cook, stirring, until the mixture thickens (do not boil). Taste for seasoning, stir in the mussels, and serve hot, garnished with salt and pepper and the reserved mussels.

CURRIED MUSSELS

Makes 4 servings
Time: 30 minutes

5 to 6 pounds mussels, cleaned as described on
   page 183
½ cup dry white wine
1 medium-size onion, minced
Salt and freshly ground black pepper to taste
Few sprigs fresh parsley
1 tablespoon butter
1 tablespoon flour
1 tablespoon curry powder or to taste
½ cup heavy cream

Put the mussels in a big pot with the wine, onion, salt, pepper, and parsley. Cook, covered, over medium-high heat, shaking the pot occasionally, until they're all opened, about 10 minutes. Remove the mussels and let cool for a few minutes; strain the cooking liquid—using a strainer lined with cheesecloth—into a saucepan and begin reducing it, over high heat, to about ½ cup.

Remove the mussels from their shells. In a 3- or 4-cup saucepan, melt the butter over medium heat. Add the flour and curry powder, turn the heat to low, and stir constantly for a couple of minutes. Add the mussel liquid a little at a time, stirring or beating to prevent lumps from forming. When the mixture is smooth, add the cream, stirring all the while. Do not boil. At the last minute, add the cooked mussels. Serve over rice.

MUSSELS PORTUGUESE STYLE OVER PASTA

Makes 4 to 6 servings
Time: 45 minutes
You can make this dish with any hard, dry sausage, but I think linguiça, the spicy Portuguese sausage,

works best. Use fresh tomatoes if you can find them, and be sure to serve this with plenty of crusty bread. Finish with a light green salad.

½ to 1 pound linguiça, chorizo, kielbasa, or
   other hard sausage
1 tablespoon olive oil
2 cloves garlic, chopped
3 or 4 plum tomatoes, roughly chopped
10 leaves fresh basil or parsley
½ cup water, more or less
3 pounds mussels, cleaned as described on page
   183
1 ½ pounds linguine or spaghetti

Bring a large pot of water to a boil for the pasta. Remove the skin from the sausage and chop into ¼- to ½-inch dice. Heat the olive oil in a large pot over medium heat, add the sausage, and cook, stirring. When it begins to brown, add the garlic. Cook 1 to 2 minutes, stirring occasionally, then add the tomatoes and basil. Cook, stirring, until the tomatoes soften, for a few minutes. Add the water, stir, add the mussels, cover, and raise the heat to high. Begin cooking the pasta.

Cook the mussels, shaking the pot occasionally, until all of them are open, about 10 minutes. Drain the pasta, place it in a very large serving bowl, and pour the mussels, with their sauce, on top. Dish it out at the table with chunks of bread.

ALTERNATIVE FISH FOR THIS RECIPE:
Hard-shell clams.

BROILED MUSSELS
WITH PERNOD BUTTER

Makes 3 to 4 servings
Time: 30 minutes

3 pounds mussels, cleaned as described on page 183
½ cup dry white wine
½ cup (1 stick) butter
2 cloves garlic, peeled
1 shallot, peeled
2 tablespoons chopped fresh parsley
2 tablespoons Pernod or other anise-flavored liqueur
3 tablespoons plain bread crumbs
1 teaspoon minced fresh tarragon or ½ teaspoon dried
Salt and freshly ground black pepper to taste

In a covered pot over medium-high heat, steam the mussels in the wine, shaking occasionally, until open, about 10 minutes. Drain the mussels, capturing the steaming liquid in a bowl. Immediately strain the liquid—using a strainer lined with cheesecloth—into a small saucepan and begin reducing over high heat. Cool the mussels.

Combine all the remaining ingredients in a food processor and process until smooth. Add enough of the reduced mussel liquid to make a thin paste.

Discard the top shell of each of the mussels; place a mussel in each of the remaining shells. Put the mussels on a baking sheet and top each with a bit of the sauce. (You may refrigerate the mussels for several hours, until ready to cook.)

When ready to serve, run the mussels under a hot broiler until lightly browned, about 2 minutes.

ALTERNATIVE FISH FOR THIS RECIPE:
Hard-shell clams.

STIR-FRIED MUSSELS WITH
BLACK BEAN AND OYSTER SAUCE

Makes 2 main course or 4 appetizer servings
Time: 30 minutes

Most of the mussels we eat in the shell are steamed, with the flavors common to Western Europe. But Asian spices complement mussels equally well, as this and the next recipe demonstrate, and stir-frying is, if anything, a more efficient cooking style. Like all mussel-in-the-shell dishes, this is far from elegant. Serve it piping hot—with plenty of rice, not bread—dig in, and enjoy.

2 tablespoons fermented black beans (available in Asian markets)
2 tablespoons dry sherry
3 pounds mussels, more or less, cleaned as described on page 183
2 tablespoons peanut or vegetable oil
1 tablespoon minced garlic
1 tablespoon peeled and minced fresh ginger
3 scallions, 2 roughly chopped, 1 minced
¼ cup any fish or chicken stock (pages 40–41) or water, if necessary
2 tablespoons oyster sauce (available in Asian markets)
1 tablespoon high-quality soy sauce

Soak the black beans in the sherry. Drain the mussels in a colander. Heat a wok or large pot over high heat until it begins to smoke, 5 minutes or so. Put the oil in the wok and immediately add the garlic, ginger, and chopped scallions. Stir for 30 seconds or so, then add the mussels. Keep the heat high and stir frequently; the mussels will begin to open quickly. As they do, they will generate a fair amount of liquid. (If this does not happen within a minute or two, add a little stock or water to prevent the spices from burning.)

Keep cooking and stirring until most of the mussels are open, about 5 minutes; at this point there will be plenty of liquid. Add the black beans and sherry, oyster sauce, and soy sauce, and stir until all of the mussels are open. Serve immediately.

STIR-FRIED MUSSELS WITH BASIL AND CHILES:

Omit the black beans and sherry. When the wok is hot, stir-fry 2 tablespoons minced garlic for 10 seconds. Add the mussels, along with ½ cup chopped fresh basil, several dried or fresh chiles (to taste), 4 or 5 scallions, cut into 1-inch sections, and 1 teaspoon sugar. Cook as above, using water or stock for liquid; omit the oyster sauce. Finish with 1 tablespoon soy sauce or Thai or Vietnamese fish sauce (available in Asian markets).

MUSSELS WITH CHIVES AND BLACK MUSHROOMS

Makes 2 servings

Time: About 45 minutes

This is a slightly more elegant stir-fry than the preceding one. Steam the mussels and remove them from their shells ahead of time, if you like, then cover and refrigerate them; they'll keep well for a day or two.

3 pounds mussels, more or less, cleaned as described on page 183
½ cup dry sherry or white wine
One 1-inch piece fresh ginger, cut into 3 or 4 pieces
1 large clove garlic, crushed and peeled
1 teaspoon chopped fresh or dried lemon grass (available in Asian markets; optional)
3 dried black (shiitake) mushrooms
1 tablespoon peanut oil
1 teaspoon minced garlic
1 teaspoon peeled and minced fresh ginger
1 tablespoon oyster sauce (available in Asian markets)

1 tablespoon high-quality soy sauce
1 teaspoon sesame oil
⅓ cup minced fresh chives

If using dried lemon grass, soak it in warm water for 10 minutes, then drain. Drain the mussels briefly in a colander and place them in a large, covered pot with the sherry or wine, ginger, garlic, and lemon grass. Steam over high heat, shaking occasionally, just until all the mussels open, about 10 minutes. Meanwhile, soak the black mushrooms in several changes of hot water to cover until softened; remove them and chop coarsely, discarding any wooden, stemmy parts.

When they're cool enough to handle, remove the mussels from their shells. Reserve about 1 cup of the cooking liquid.

Heat the oil in a wok or 12-inch nonstick skillet over high heat. Add the minced garlic and ginger and stir-fry until golden, about 1 minute. Add the mussel meat and cook, still over high heat, for about 1 minute. Add some of the reserved liquid—about ½ cup at first—and let it bubble away for a few seconds. Add the remaining ingredients and stir; if mixture seems too dry, add a little more stock. If it's too wet, cook another minute. Serve immediately, over rice.

ALTERNATIVE FISH FOR THIS RECIPE: Hard-shell clams.

GRILLED MUSSELS

Makes 4 servings

Time: 15 minutes

Grilled mussels are less messy than steamed ones. But, since they don't make their own sauce, you must provide one. I like simply scented olive oil, but you could use almost anything, such as pesto (page 41), cilantro pesto (page 235), light tomato sauce (page 209), or any of the dipping sauces for squid (page 295). Grilled mussels have a nice, natural, smoky flavor. Although you can do this with hard-shell clams or oysters, it's a lot easier with mussels, which are still cheap enough so that buying six or eight dozen doesn't require a trip to the cash machine.

½ cup extra virgin olive oil
2 cloves garlic, minced, or 1 tablespoon sherried garlic (page 306)
4 to 6 pounds mussels, cleaned as described on page 183

Preheat a gas grill or start a large charcoal fire; the heat should be high, and you need a lot of surface area on which to cook. In a saucepan slowly heat the olive oil with the garlic, until the garlic turns light brown.

Dump the mussels unceremoniously onto the grill, getting them in one layer as best you can. Those near the hottest part of the fire will open first, in 1 to 2 minutes; remove them to a platter and shift other mussels into their place. When they have all opened—total grilling time will be less than 10 minutes—bring the platter to the table and drizzle the sauce over the mussels. Serve immediately.

ALTERNATIVE FISH FOR THIS RECIPE:
Hard-shell clams, oysters, or scallops in their shells.

MUSSEL AND POTATO SALAD WITH MUSTARD DRESSING

Makes 4 servings
Time: 1 hour

You can easily make this with leftover mussels, should you have any, but it's worth starting it from scratch. If you don't have both kinds of mustard in the house, use one or the other—the salad will still be delicious.

3 to 4 pounds mussels, prepared according to the recipe for Steamed Mussels, Version I (page 183)
1 ½ pounds waxy potatoes
¼ cup Dijon mustard
¼ cup grainy French-style mustard
½ cup olive oil
1 tablespoon balsamic or sherry wine vinegar
3 tablespoons chopped fresh basil
Salt and freshly ground black pepper to taste

Shell the mussels. Strain the broth—using a strainer lined with cheesecloth—into a medium-size saucepan; bring it to a boil. Peel the potatoes if you like (or wash them well), then cut them into bite-size pieces; cook them in the mussel broth, covered until tender but not mushy, about 15 minutes. Drain. (Reserve the broth for another use, such as Mussel Bisque, page 185.) Mix together the mustards, oil, vinegar, and basil, and toss with the mussels and potatoes. Season with salt and pepper. Serve with or without greens.

OCEAN PERCH

Latin name(s): *Sebastes marinus* (Atlantic), *S. alutus* (Pacific), and others.
Other common names: Redfish, rosefish, sea perch, red bream.
Common forms: By far the most common form is skin-on fillets, usually scaled.
General description: The all-purpose inexpensive fillet, with pinkish flesh, rosy skin, and mild flavor; widely available. Note that this is not the overfished redfish of the Gulf, which is rightly called red drum, but a variety of the West Coast rockfish.
For other recipes see: Blackfish, catfish, cod, dogfish, flatfish, grouper, haddock, mullet, pollock, porgy, rockfish, red snapper, tilefish, weakfish, whiting, wolffish.
Buying tips: As with any fillet, gaping should be minimal, and there should be no brown or gray areas; smell should be clean and salty.

This is another of those wonderful but underrated fish. Because it's cheap (often three dollars a pound for fillets), because people associate it with fresh-water fish, because it's widely available (there are ocean perches in both the Atlantic and the Pacific), and maybe because no one ever gets to see one whole (they're all filleted), ocean perch is never mentioned as a high-class fish. But it is not unlike the European mullet (or goatfish, or rouget), and can be used in those recipes you see in European cookbooks calling for mullet.

Generally, ocean perches are more tender than other rockfish and can also be used, with great success, in almost any recipe for white-fleshed fish. The only caveat is that if the fish has not been scaled, take a minute to do so (it's easy; see page 19).

SAUTÉED PERCH WITH GARLICKED RUTABAGA

Makes 4 servings
Time: 60 minutes
Close as it is to the red mullet of the Mediter-ranean, the perch takes well to this nouvelle-style recipe. If you substitute, make sure the fillet you use has its skin on.

1 small rutabaga, about 1 pound, peeled and cut into chunks
3 medium-size potatoes, about 1 pound total
¾ cup olive oil
1 small clove garlic, crushed and peeled
8 ocean perch fillets, skin on but scaled, about 1 pound
Salt and freshly ground black pepper to taste
1 teaspoon minced garlic
Minced fresh parsley for garnish

Set the rutabaga chunks in a pot of salted water to boil. Peel the potatoes, cut them up, and add them to the pot (the rutabaga will probably take about 10 minutes longer to cook). When the vegetables are tender, puree them in a food processor or blender with 2 tablespoons of the olive oil and the clove of garlic. Taste for seasoning and keep warm (or put in a microwaveable dish and reheat just before serving).

Heat ½ cup of the olive oil in a 12-inch nonstick skillet over medium-high until it shimmers. Dry the fillets and place them in the oil one at a time, skin side down. Cook over high heat until the top is almost opaque, about 5 minutes; season with salt and pepper. While the fish is cooking, simmer the minced garlic in the remaining oil over low heat until it is just golden; turn off the heat.

Turn the fish and cook the flesh side for just 1 minute. To serve, spoon some of the rutabaga puree onto a plate, top with 2 fillets, and drizzle with a bit of the garlic oil. Top with the parsley and serve.

ALTERNATIVE FISH FOR THIS RECIPE:

(All should have skin on) haddock, rockfish, red snapper, or tilefish. Adjust the cooking times accordingly.

HERB-MARINATED PERCH, COOKED FOUR WAYS

Makes 4 servings
Time: 15 minutes, plus marinating time
This is among the most important recipes in this entire book, but it takes some flexibility on your part. Be willing to vary the herbs, the marinating time, the kind of fish (I start with perch because it is similar to rouget, a Mediterranean fish, and this is a Mediterranean recipe), the cut of fish, and the cooking method. Master this recipe and you're well on your way to mastering fish cooking.

½ cup fruity olive oil
2 bay leaves, crumbled
1 tablespoon minced garlic
3 tablespoons mixed chopped fresh herbs, such as tarragon, rosemary, basil, chives, parsley, thyme, marjoram
Salt and freshly ground black pepper to taste
1 to 1 ½ pounds perch fillets, skin on but scaled

Mix together all the ingredients except the fish. Marinate the fish in this mixture for 15 minutes to several hours (use the refrigerator if it will be more than 30 minutes or the weather is warm).

To grill: Use an oiled fish basket. Preheat a gas grill or build a medium-hot charcoal fire. Remove the fish from the marinade and grill about 4 inches from the heat source, turning once. The cooking time will be 6 to 8 minutes; the fillet will be opaque and firm when it is done. Brush lightly with the marinade before serving.

To broil: Use a lightly oiled baking pan (nonstick is nice). Remove the fish from the marinade and broil, skin side down, about 6 inches from the heat source. Do not turn. Cooking time will be about 6 to 8 minutes; the fillet will be opaque and firm when it is done. Brush lightly with the marinade before serving.

To roast: Use an oiled baking pan; preheat the oven to 500°F. Roast in the marinade, skin side down. Do not turn. Cooking time will be about 8 minutes; the fillet will be opaque and firm when it is done. Brush lightly with the marinade before serving.

To pan-grill: Use a 12-inch nonstick skillet; heat for 5 minutes or more over medium-high heat. Add 1 tablespoon olive oil to the skillet. Remove the fish from the marinade and pan-grill, skin side down for 5 minutes, then turn and cook 1 or 2 minutes more; the fillet will be opaque and firm when it is done. Brush lightly with the marinade before serving.

ALTERNATIVE FISH FOR THIS RECIPE:

This is a basic and always useful recipe for fillets or steaks of blackfish, catfish, dogfish, grouper, mackerel, mako, monkfish, Atlantic pollock, red snapper, rockfish, striped bass, tilefish, or wolffish. Adjust the cooking time according to thickness of fillets or steaks (see general guidelines, page 25).

CRUNCHY CURRIED PERCH

Makes 2 servings
Time: 20 minutes

¾ pound perch fillets, skin on but scaled
1 tablespoon red or white wine vinegar
Salt to taste
½ teaspoon freshly ground black pepper
½ teaspoon turmeric
1 ½ teaspoons ground cumin
½ teaspoon ground coriander
¼ teaspoon cayenne pepper
Peanut or vegetable oil as needed
½ cup unbleached all-purpose flour
Warm water as needed
Minced fresh parsley for garnish

Heat a 12-inch nonstick skillet over medium-high heat for 3 to 4 minutes. Rinse the perch with the vinegar. Combine the salt, pepper, turmeric, cumin, coriander, and cayenne and rub this mixture into the fish.

Add enough oil to the pan to reach a depth of about ⅛ inch. In a medium-size bowl, mix the flour with enough warm water to make a paste the thickness of yogurt. When the oil is hot (a pinch of flour will sizzle), dip each fillet into the batter and cook, raising the heat to high, until golden and crisp on each side, about 6 minutes total. As each piece is done, keep it warm in a low oven while you fry the remaining pieces. Serve immediately, garnished with parsley.

ALTERNATIVE FISH FOR THIS RECIPE:
Blackfish, catfish, clams, dogfish, grouper, oysters, Atlantic pollock, rockfish, red snapper,

shrimp, tilefish, or wolffish. Adjust the cooking times accordingly.

PERCH WITH ANCHOVY SAUCE

Makes 4 servings
Time: 30 minutes
Another recipe made with rouget throughout the Mediterranean. Some people sauté the fish, others roast it, and still others broil it. I prefer the last, because the sauce itself is little more than anchovy-scented oil, and the skin becomes crisp.

4 salted anchovies or 8 anchovy fillets
½ cup olive oil, plus 1 tablespoon
1 teaspoon minced garlic
Salt and freshly ground black pepper to taste
8 perch fillets, skin on but scaled, about 1 ¼ to 1 ½ pounds
Minced fresh parsley for garnish
Lemon wedges

Preheat the broiler. If you use salted anchovies, rinse them, then split them in half lengthwise and remove the backbone. Rinse again, then mince. If you use fillets, mince them, adding their oil to the olive oil (which you can reduce proportionately). Mix together the tablespoon of olive oil and the garlic; brush the fillets lightly with this mixture and sprinkle them with a little salt and some pepper.

Warm the remaining olive oil over low heat and add the anchovies. Cook, stirring, always over low heat, until the anchovies fall apart and the mixture becomes "saucy," about five minutes. Keep warm. Place the perch fillets in a baking pan and broil, skin side up, about 4 to 6 inches from the heat source, until the skin is crisp and the fish cooked through, about 3 to 4 minutes. Spoon a little of the sauce over each one, garnish with parsley, and serve with lemon.

Fillets of blackfish, catfish, dogfish, grouper, pollock, rockfish, red snapper, tilefish, or wolffish. Adjust the cooking times accordingly

GRILLED PERCH WITH NOODLES AND TOMATO SAUCE

Makes 4 servings
Time: 30 minutes

8 perch fillets, skin on but scaled, about 1 ¼ to
    1 ½ pounds
¼ cup olive oil
Salt and freshly ground black pepper to taste
8 plum tomatoes, fresh or canned (drained if
    canned)
1 teaspoon minced garlic
8 ounces linguine or spaghetti
3 tablespoons chopped fresh basil or dill

Preheat the broiler; set a pot of salted water to boil for the pasta. Brush the fillets with a little of the olive oil, sprinkle them with salt and pepper, and place them in a baking pan, skin side up. Puree the tomatoes in a food processor or blender and strain through a sieve. Place them in a saucepan with the remaining olive oil and the garlic and cook over medium heat until the flavors blend, about 10 minutes.

Cook the pasta according to the package instructions; while it is cooking, broil the fillets about 4 to 6 inches from the heat source until the skin is crisp and the fish cooked through, about 3 to 4 minutes. When the pasta is done, drain it and place a portion on each of four plates. Add 2 tablespoons of the basil to the sauce and spoon a bit of the sauce over the pasta. Top with two fillets, and garnish with the remaining basil.

ALTERNATIVE FISH FOR THIS RECIPE:

Fillets of catfish, dogfish, flatfish, haddock, rockfish, weakfish, or wolffish. Adjust the cooking times accordingly.

OCTOPUS

Latin name(s): *Octopus vulgaris.*
Other common names: Pulpo, devilfish.
Common forms: Whole, fresh; whole (usually cleaned), frozen.
General description: The eight-legged "monster of the deep," which usually is marketed between two and five pounds, frozen (or frozen and thawed) more often than not.
For other recipes see: Clams, conch, monkfish, squid.
Buying tips: As with other fish that is usually frozen (including shrimp), I'd rather thaw this myself than let the retailer do it. When you look at octopus that is fresh or already thawed, make sure that the purplish skin is not starting to brown, and that the smell is clean.

One of the last remaining great "undiscovered" seafoods—in this country at least. Most of our octopus is imported frozen. Of course most of that was caught off our own shores, processed, and shipped to Europe (see Monkfish for a similar story). The Europeans then have the good grace to ship it back to us.

Not that I'm complaining. All of the cephalopods—the "head-footed" fish, including squid and cuttlefish (which we see even less often than octopus)—are delicious. "I'd rather eat octopus than lobster," one old-time fishmonger always said to me, until I became (nearly) convinced.

Most of the octopus we buy are frozen; defrost in the refrigerator, or in cold water. They are also already cleaned. If you buy one that isn't, here's what to do: Turn the head inside out—like a sock, or the sleeve of a jacket—and remove the insides. That's it. It may not be appealing, but it doesn't take more than two minutes. The skin and everything else is edible.

Now for the controversy: Every country that admires the octopus (and this includes most, just not ours) has a different method of tenderizing. The Spaniards dip it into boiling water three times. The Japanese knead it with grated daikon. The Greeks hurl it against rocks or, more likely these days, against the kitchen sink. As far as I can tell, none of these methods has more merit than the other (the late A. J. McClane, dean of fish writers, preferred the first). My experience seems to indicate that each method yields some tender octopi and some tough ones. My guess is that some of these critters are just tougher than others. But even the tough ones are worth eating, so don't be put off. And don't bother to resort to extreme measures to tenderize.

Note that all the recipes here require some pre-cooking of the octopus, as in the first recipe; this can be done a day or two in advance. Refrigerate the octopus in a marinade or the cooking liquid.

OCTOPUS PROVENÇAL STYLE

Makes 4 servings
Time: 2 to 3 hours, mostly unattended
This basic preparation—note the spin-offs below—makes a rich, dark sauce that rivals intense meat sauces for complexity. Serve it with lots of bread and a light salad.

1 octopus, 2 to 3 pounds, cleaned (page 194)
3 cloves garlic, peeled and lightly crushed
1 bay leaf
3 tablespoons olive oil
1 large onion, coarsely chopped
1 teaspoon minced fresh thyme or ½ teaspoon
    dried
1 sprig fresh tarragon or ½ teaspoon dried
1 teaspoon minced fresh basil (do not use dried;
    optional)
10 fennel seeds
3 medium-size ripe tomatoes, cut into chunks
    (canned are fine; drain them first)
2 cups sturdy red wine: cabernet sauvignon
    (Bordeaux), merlot (Bordeaux), petite sirah
    (Rhone), etc.
Salt and freshly ground black pepper to taste
1 tablespoon minced garlic
½ cup minced fresh parsley

Place the octopus, garlic cloves, and bay leaf in water to cover; turn heat to medium, cover, bring to a boil, lower the heat, and simmer until the octopus is nearly tender, 1 hour or more. (Poke it with a sharp, thin-bladed knife; when the knife enters fairly easily, the octopus is ready. To make sure, cut a piece off and taste it; it should be pleasantly chewy.) Drain the octopus in a colander, reserving the cooking liquid.

Reduce the cooking liquid over high heat until needed (you'll need 1 cup or so, so don't reduce it more than that). Cut the octopus into bite-size pieces. Heat the oil in a large skillet, then sear the octopus over high heat, browning it lightly. Add the onion and lower the heat to medium. Cook, stirring, until the onion softens a bit. Add the herbs and tomatoes and stir. Cook for 1 minute, then add the wine. Raise the heat to high and boil for 2 minutes. Add 1 cup of octopus stock; bring to a boil, then lower the heat so the mixture simmers. Season with salt and pepper.

Cook until the octopus is good and soft and the liquid has reduced to a sauce (you can raise the heat if the octopus becomes tender but too much liquid remains). Add the minced garlic, stir, and cook another 5 minutes. Add half the parsley and stir. Garnish with the remaining parsley and serve.

OCTOPUS WITH POTATOES:

When the octopus is most of the way through its first cooking, peel and dice 4 medium-size potatoes. Sauté them in 3 tablespoons olive oil over medium-high heat in a nonstick skillet until nice and crisp all over, about 30 minutes. Stir into the octopus along with the minced garlic.

OCTOPUS WITH RICE:

Reduce the octopus cooking liquid to 3 cups rather than 1 (add water in the unlikely event that you don't have 3 cups). Use 2 cups of the liquid to cook 1 cup rice. Proceed as in original recipe, and serve the octopus over the rice.

OCTOPUS IN TOMATO SAUCE

Makes 4 servings
Time: 30 minutes, using precooked octopus
This dish is wonderful over pasta.

1 octopus, 2 to 3 pounds, cleaned, simmered,
    and drained as in the first recipe
⅓ cup olive oil
1 onion, peeled and chopped
2 tablespoons capers
½ cup good pitted black olives
½ cup red wine
3 cups chopped tomatoes (drained if canned)
1 teaspoon minced garlic
2 tablespoons minced fresh parsley plus more
    for garnish
Salt and freshly ground pepper

Cut the octopus into chunks as in the first recipe. Heat the olive oil over medium heat in a large skillet, then add the onion and cook, stirring, until softened; add the capers, olives, wine, and tomatoes. Cook until the tomatoes break up, then add the garlic, 2 tablespoons of parsley, and the cut-up octopus. Simmer a few minutes, season to taste with salt and pepper, and serve, garnished with additional minced parsley.

OCTOPUS WITH SPINACH AND PERNOD

Makes 4 servings
Time: 30 minutes, using precooked octopus

1 octopus, 2 to 3 pounds, cleaned, simmered, and drained as in the first recipe
⅓ cup olive oil
1 onion, peeled and chopped
4 cups washed spinach, tough stems removed
½ cup Pernod *or* ½ cup dry white wine and 1 teaspoon fennel seeds
Salt and freshly ground black pepper

Cut the octopus into chunks as in the first recipe. Heat the olive oil over medium heat in a large skillet, then add the onion and cook, stirring, until softened; add the spinach and sauté until the spinach begins to wilt. Add the cut-up octopus and Pernod or wine and fennel. Simmer for about 5 minutes, season to taste with salt and pepper, and serve.

GRILLED OCTOPUS

Makes 4 servings
Time: 30 minutes, using precooked octopus
This is one of the great grilled fish delicacies. You can precook the octopus (even a day or two in advance), and then it becomes a very quick dish to prepare. Or you can precook the octopus and marinate it for extra flavor; see variation 2.

1 octopus, 2 to 3 pounds, cleaned, simmered, and drained as in the first recipe
½ cup olive oil
Juice of 1 lemon
1 tablespoon minced fresh oregano or 1 teaspoon dried
3 cloves garlic, lightly crushed and peeled
1 bay leaf

Prepare a charcoal fire or start a gas grill; the fire should be quite hot. Cut the octopus into large pieces. Whisk together the oil, lemon juice, and oregano, then add the garlic and bay leaf. Brush the octopus pieces with this mixture and grill them on all sides, quickly, until they become slightly crisp. As they come off the grill, brush them with a little more of the oil and lemon juice mixture. Serve immediately, passing the remaining mixture at the table.

VARIATION 1:
You can use almost any basting-dressing mixture you like. See, for example, the dipping sauces for squid (pages 295–296).

VARIATION 2:
Marinate the cooked octopus for 12 to 48 hours in the olive oil-lemon mixture, or in any thin sauce you like. Grill as instructed above, basting with the marinade.

COLD MARINATED OCTOPUS

Makes 8 appetizer servings
Time: 2 hours or more, plus marinating time
This is an easy recipe, but it takes some time. To make a similar but far grander dish, see Seafood Salad Adriatic Style, page 49.

8 cups Flavorful Fish and Vegetable Stock (page 40), Court Bouillon (page 41), or 8 cups water

Salt and freshly ground black pepper to taste (if using water rather than stock)

1 medium-size onion, cut in half but unpeeled (if using water rather than stock)

3 cloves garlic, peeled and lightly crushed (if using water rather than stock)

1 medium-size carrot, cut into chunks (if using water rather than stock)

½ bunch fresh parsley (if using water rather than stock)

2 bay leaves (if using water rather than stock)

1 tablespoon any vinegar (if using water rather than stock)

½ cup dry white wine (if using water rather than stock)

1 octopus, about 3 pounds, cleaned (page 194)

½ cup fruity olive oil

3 cloves garlic, cut into slices

1 tablespoon paprika

2 tablespoons sherry or balsamic vinegar

½ cup minced fresh parsley

Bring the stock to a boil or simmer together the water, salt, pepper, onion, garlic, carrot, parsley, bay leaves, vinegar, and wine for about 10 minutes. Add the octopus and simmer until tender, 1 hour or more. (Poke it with a sharp, thin-bladed knife; when the knife enters fairly easily, the octopus is ready. To make sure, cut a piece off and taste it; it should be pleasantly chewy.) Turn off the heat and let the octopus cool in the water for 10 minutes. Strain and reserve the stock for another use. Cut the octopus into bite-size pieces.

In a small saucepan over medium-low heat, heat the olive oil and garlic until the garlic sizzles and colors slightly. Turn off the heat and cool; mix in the paprika and sherry vinegar, along with some salt and pepper. Pour over the octopus and mix well. Refrigerate at least 1 hour, or overnight. Garnish with the minced parsley before serving.

OCTOPUS SALAD WITH ASIAN SEASONINGS:

Dress the octopus with a mixture of ½ cup peanut oil, 1 teaspoon sesame oil, 3 minced scallions, the juice of 2 limes, 1 deveined, seeded, and minced jalapeño, and ¼ cup minced cilantro (fresh coriander).

ORANGE ROUGHY

Latin name(s): *Hoplostethus atlanticus*.
Other common names: Roughy.
Common forms: Fillets, often frozen.
General description: Ocean perchlike fish from New Zealand.
For recipes see: Any white-fleshed fish (see list, pages 11–12), especially ocean perch.
Buying tips: As with any fillet, gaping should be minimal, and there should be no brown or gray areas; smell should be clean and salty.

In the late eighties, when cod prices were high and roughy prices were low, this fish was widely imported as a substitute for cod. It's a good fish, but no better than a dozen others that are more likely to be sold fresh. Not widely available as of this writing (1993).

OYSTERS

Latin name(s): *Crassostrea virginica* (Eastern); *C. gigas* (Pacific); *Ostrea edulis* (European flat); *O. lurida* (Olympia).

Other common names: Blue Point, Apalachicola, Chincoteague, Wellfleet, etc. (Eastern); Japanese, Westcott Bay, Penn Cove, Kumamoto, etc. (Pacific); Belon, Westcott (European flat).

Common forms: Whole, live; shucked, in containers.

General description: The familiar, irregular, rough-shelled bivalve, commonly eaten raw.

For other recipes see: Hard-shell clams, mussels.

Buying tips: Like all bivalve mollusks, oysters must be alive when purchased (or cooked or frozen, see page 8). Out of the water, oysters are quite long-lived as long as they are kept cool. See text below.

Nomenclature and safety are the two big issues with oysters. To deal with the first: There are four major species (noted above). Almost every oyster grown from the Canadian Maritimes to the Mexican border, from the North Atlantic to the Gulf, is an Eastern oyster; any other name given them, and there are dozens—Wellfleet, Blue Point Apalachicola, whatever—is based on their geographic origin. Similarly, most West Coast oysters are Pacifics. Olympia, the only oyster native to the West Coast, is a tiny oyster related to the European flat which, in turn, is often called a Belon, although "belon"—in France at least—is a name that can be given only to oysters grown in a certain part of Brittany.

The Bretons insist that Belons are the world's best oysters, and charge eighty dollars a dozen for them (the more reasonably priced oysters in France are "Portugaises," closely related to the Eastern and Pacific oysters). They are, indeed, damned good. But so are the tiny, metallic Olympias. And a big, fat North Atlantic oyster raised in cold water can be incomparably delicious. It's all a matter of the oyster's upbringing, its shipping and storage conditions (if any), and the day on and circumstances

under which you eat it. They can all be wonderful or quite mediocre. (That goes not only for oysters but for days and circumstances, too.)

Now, safety: Oyster production, like that of mussels and clams, is monitored by local authorities under the auspices of the Federal Shellfish Sanitation Program. This means that tagged oysters—gathered by licensed shellfishermen from certified waters—are as safe as any other food. But oysters gathered by amateurs and unscrupulous sorts may be contaminated. Whatever the reason, there are those who feel that eating raw oysters (or clams) is like playing Russian roulette: eventually you will lose. And statistics do show that almost all reported illnesses related to seafood are the result of eating raw shellfish.

Even so, such illnesses are rare. Eating raw oysters is probably about as risky as eating an underdone egg yolk. It's unlikely to make you ill and, if it does, it's even more unlikely to cause permanent harm. (For a general discussion of seafood safety, see pages 14–17.)

In any case, I'm not here to tell you whether you should indulge in this simple pleasure. Suffice

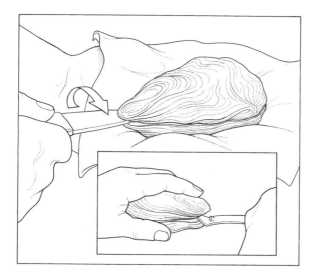

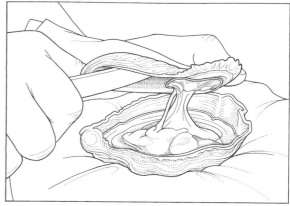

There are several ways to open oysters. As with clams, you can use a strong paring knife and insert it anywhere between the shells. Alternatively, you can use a can opener or specially designed oyster knife (bent at the end) to pry open the shell at the hinge—this is the best method for novices. In any case, always start with the rounded shell down to preserve the oyster liquid.

Once the oyster is opened, use the point of a knife to scrape the meat attached to the top shell into the bottom shell, taking care to keep as much of the liquid as possible in the shell.

it to say that I do at every single opportunity, and I've never been sorry. Oysters are at their best when raw and not fussed over (which is not to say they shouldn't be cooked; I love the recipes that follow).

The other more-or-less ongoing question about eating oysters has to do with the "R" month rule, which states that you shouldn't eat oysters in months with no "R"—May, June, July, August. This is because most oysters spawn in the summer and, at one time anyway, growers preferred that you didn't eat their product while it was trying to reproduce. In addition, the spawn can be milky and unattractive (I've met a couple of New Haven oystermen who claim that during the summer of 1930 the profusion of oyster spawn in Long Island Sound turned the water white).

After spawning, oysters tend to be fairly watery and somewhat less tasty, and they don't ship as well because they are relatively weak. Having said all of that, it's worth noting that some connoisseurs prefer their oysters in a prespawning state (the fatter the better) and that some oysters don't spawn in the summer. So don't pass up an offer of good-looking oysters in July.

Like clams and mussels, oysters in their shell must be alive when sold; dead oysters have loose shells (live ones take some work to shuck; see illustrations, below) and should be discarded. Good oysters, stored in a bowl or paper or mesh bag in the refrigerator, will keep for at least a week, but are best eaten soon after purchase. (Some oysters remain alive for weeks; in the eighteenth century many shoreline families kept a barrelful in their cellar through the winter as a hedge against starvation.) Shucked oysters may be pasteurized, which

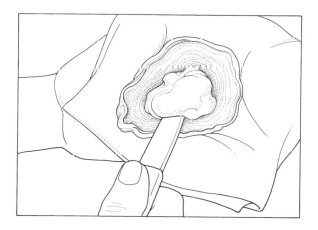

Cut the oyster from the bottom shell and remove or serve on the half-shell.

greatly extends their shelf life, but decreases their flavor; in any case they should be dated.

Shucking raw oysters is an art that requires practice. The first thing to do is scrub the shells well, removing any dirt that might contaminate the meat. Then prepare a plate with coarse salt, crushed ice, or seaweed—anything to hold the open shells steady. Finally, open oysters with the rounded shell down to keep as much liquid as possible in the shells (unless you're really good, you'll spill most of it anyway). Novices should try opening oysters with a common church key, or follow the directions accompanying the illustrations on page 200. I am of the school that the most you should put on a raw oyster is a squeeze of lemon; to me, adding horseradish, mignonette, vinegar, or Tabasco is the equivalent of putting ketchup on lobster.

If you have live oysters and want to use them in a recipe, you can steam or microwave them just until they open. Then cut the muscle that attaches them to the bottom shell. No matter what the cooking method—frying, poaching, baking, sautéing, steaming, or stewing—oysters must be cooked extremely gently and for a short period of time to avoid rubberizing the meat.

FRIED OYSTERS

Makes 4 snack or appetizer servings or 2 main course servings
Time: 30 minutes
Frying fish at home, as noted elsewhere, is not as much fun as, for example, having someone do it for you. But sometimes you have some nice oysters, and you get a hankering . . . No seafood is better fried than oysters. (They're good sautéed, also, and not as messy—see the variation.)

2 large eggs
¼ cup milk or light cream
Flour for dredging
Salt and freshly ground black pepper to taste
Vegetable oil for deep-frying
24 shucked oysters, drained and dried
Plain bread or cracker crumbs for dredging

Beat the eggs lightly with the milk. Season the flour with salt and pepper. Heat the oil to 350°F to 375°F. (If your fryer doesn't have a thermostat, or you don't have a frying thermometer, drop a small piece of bread in the oil; it should sink, then rise to the top and begin bubbling away.) Dredge the oysters, one by one, in the flour, then dip in the eggs, then roll in the bread crumbs. Let them stand on waxed paper until you are ready to start frying (you can refrigerate them for a few hours if you like). Fry a few at a time—do not crowd—for no more than 2 minutes. Serve immediately, with lemon wedges, Salsa Fresca (page 209), hot sauce, or Worcestershire sauce.

SAUTÉED OYSTERS:

Use a mixture of butter and good oil, enough to liberally coat the bottom of a large skillet. Heat the mixture over high heat until the butter foam subsides, then add the oysters prepared as instructed above. Do not crowd; you may have to cook in batches. Cook, turning once, until browned on both sides. You can, if you like, make a pan reduction of ½ cup dry white wine, 1 tablespoon minced shallots, and ½ cup minced fresh parsley to drizzle over the oysters. Or serve as suggested above.

GRILLED OYSTERS

Makes 4 appetizer servings
Time: 15 minutes
This is a great way to shuck your oysters, cook them, and flavor them lightly at the same time.

24 to 48 oysters in their shells
2 to 4 lemons, quartered

Start a charcoal or wood fire or preheat a gas grill; the fire should be moderately hot. Place the oysters rounded side down on the grill, 2 to 4 inches from the heat source. Grill until they begin to open, 5 minutes or so (it will depend on their size). As they open, remove them from the grill and move unopened ones to the hotter part of the grill. Shucking will be easy (just remember that the shells are hot); try to keep as much liquid as possible in the shell. If you like oysters fully cooked, return them to the grill and cook them until their edges curl (they may have done so already). Serve with the lemon wedges.

ALTERNATIVE FISH FOR THIS RECIPE:
Hard-shell clams or mussels.

OYSTER STEW
NEW ENGLAND STYLE

Makes 2 to 4 servings
Time: 15 minutes
The classic. Serve with hard crackers.

1 ½ dozen oysters, shucked (page 201), with their liquor
½ cup (½ stick) butter
¼ cup dry sherry
1 ½ cups milk
½ cup heavy cream (or any combination of cream and milk, half-and-half, or just milk to make 2 cups)

Combine all the ingredients except the cream and a little of the butter in a saucepan over very low heat. Cook and stir until the oysters begin to curl, just a couple of minutes. Add the cream and continue to stir; don't allow the stew to boil, but heat thoroughly. Top with the remaining butter.

ALTERNATIVE FISH FOR THIS RECIPE:
Hard-shell clams or mussels.

OYSTER STEW ASIAN STYLE

Makes 2 to 4 servings
Time: 30 minutes

4 cups any chicken stock (page 40)
1 stalk lemon grass, cut into 1-inch lengths, or 1 tablespoon dried (available in Asian markets)
Zest of 1 lime
1 fresh jalapeño, seeded, deveined, and roughly chopped, or 1 dried hot pepper
18 to 24 oysters, shucked (page 201), with their liquor
Juice of 3 limes
2 tablespoons minced cilantro (fresh coriander)

Salt and freshly ground black pepper to taste
Lime wedges
Minced deveined and seeded jalapeño (optional)

In a saucepan over medium heat, simmer together the stock, lemon grass, lime zest, and jalapeño for 15 minutes. Strain and return to the pan. Add the oysters and lime juice and cook over low heat until the edges of the oysters begin to curl, just a couple of minutes. Add the cilantro, season with salt and pepper, and serve. Pass the lime wedges and jalapeño at the table.

ALTERNATIVE FISH FOR THIS RECIPE: Hard-shell clams or mussels.

OYSTER STEW WITH POTATOES AND KALE

Makes 4 servings
Time: 45 to 60 minutes

2 pounds waxy potatoes
¼ pound bacon
1 pound kale, well washed, bottoms of thick stems trimmed
2 cloves garlic, minced
1 cup heavy cream, half-and-half, or milk
2 tablespoons balsamic vinegar
1 pint shucked oysters, preferably with their liquor
Salt and freshly ground black pepper to taste
¼ cup minced fresh chives

Peel the potatoes and place in just enough salted water to cover. Bring to a boil, lower the heat to a simmer, and cook until fork tender, 30 to 45 minutes. Remove the potatoes from the cooking liquid and cool slightly.

While the potatoes are cooking, cook the bacon until crisp in a 12-inch skillet. Remove the bacon with a slotted spoon to drain on paper towels;

crumble it when it's cool enough. Add the kale and garlic to the skillet, and cook over medium heat, stirring, until the kale wilts. Add the cream, cover, and simmer gently over low heat, until the kale is tender, 10 to 15 minutes. Turn off the heat.

Mash the potatoes slightly with a fork or potato masher. Combine them with about 6 cups of their cooking liquid, adding water (and strained oyster liquor, if you have any) as necessary. Stir in the kale-cream mixture and heat through; do not boil. Add the vinegar and oysters and cook for about 3 minutes. Season with salt and pepper. Top with the chives and reserved bacon and serve.

ALTERNATIVE FISH FOR THIS RECIPE: Hard-shell clams, mussels, scallops, or shrimp. Adjust the cooking times accordingly.

OYSTER PAN ROAST

Makes 4 appetizer servings
Time: 20 minutes
Another variation on classic oyster stew; you can use sage instead of thyme if you prefer. In either case, the seasoning should be subtle.

2 tablespoons butter
1 tablespoon minced shallot
½ cup dry white wine
1 cup heavy cream
½ teaspoon minced fresh thyme or 1 large pinch dried
Salt and freshly ground black pepper to taste
24 oysters, shucked (page 201), with their liquor if possible
4 to 8 pieces French or Italian bread, lightly toasted

In a 2-quart saucepan over medium heat, melt the butter. When the foam subsides, add the shallot and cook, stirring, until softened. Add the wine, raise the heat to high, and let it bubble away for a minute or so. With the heat on medium, add the cream, thyme, salt, and pepper, and stir. Bring to a simmer, add the oysters, and cook until their edges begin to curl, 2 minutes or so. Check the seasonings and serve immediately, over the toasted bread.

ALTERNATIVE FISH FOR THIS RECIPE: Hard-shell clams or mussels.

BROILED OYSTERS IN CHAMPAGNE SAUCE

Makes 4 to 6 appetizer servings
Time: 30 minutes

24 shucked oysters on the half shell (page 201), with their liquor
2 tablespoons butter
1 ½ tablespoons all-purpose flour
½ cup Champagne or dry white wine
Pinch cayenne pepper
Salt to taste
Coarse salt or seaweed

Using a strainer lined with cheesecloth, strain the oyster liquor and reserve ½ cup; discard the remainder. In a small saucepan, melt the butter over medium heat; add the flour, stir, and cook, stirring occasionally, for 2 or 3 minutes. Slowly add the oyster liquor, stirring to remove lumps (you can use a wire whisk if you prefer). Add the Champagne and stir. Add the cayenne and salt and stir until nicely thickened and blended. Cool slightly.

Preheat the broiler; nestle the opened oysters on a bed of seaweed or salt on a cookie sheet or baking pan. Top each oyster with a spoonful of the sauce. Broil about 4 to 6 inches from the heat source just until sauce begins to color, about 2 minutes. Serve immediately.

ALTERNATIVE FISH FOR THIS RECIPE: Hard-shell clams or mussels

OYSTERS WITH BREAD CRUMBS:

Nestle the oysters in seaweed or salt as directed above. In a food processor, mince 1 cup unseasoned bread crumbs, 1 clove garlic, and ½ cup fresh parsley. Sprinkle some of this mixture over each oyster and drizzle with olive oil. Broil as directed above.

OYSTERS WITH HORSERADISH:

Nestle the oysters in seaweed or salt as directed above. Top with a mixture of 1 cup heavy cream, 2 tablespoons prepared horseradish (or to taste), 2 tablespoons minced fresh chives, and salt and freshly ground black pepper. Broil as directed above.

OYSTERS BAKED WITH BUTTERED SPINACH

Makes 4 servings
Time: 30 minutes

5 tablespoons butter
1 cup minced onion
8 to 12 ounces fresh spinach, well washed, large stems removed, and roughly chopped
Salt and freshly ground black pepper to taste
Freshly grated nutmeg to taste
1 cup heavy or light cream or half-and-half
1 teaspoon minced garlic
24 oysters, shucked (page 201)
½ cup fresh toasted bread crumbs

Preheat the oven to 450°F. Melt 2 tablespoons of the butter in a large skillet over medium heat, add the onion, and cook, stirring, until wilted. Add the spinach to the skillet; turn the heat to high and cook, stirring, until it wilts. Season with salt, pepper, and nutmeg. Turn the heat to low and add the cream. Cook, stirring, for 2 minutes. Add the garlic and stir in 1 more tablespoon of butter.

Transfer the spinach to a buttered baking dish.

Nestle the oysters in the spinach and top with the bread crumbs. Dot with the remaining butter. Bake until the oysters cook through—their ends will curl, about 15 minutes.

ALTERNATIVE FISH FOR THIS RECIPE: Hard-shell clams or scallops.

ANGELS ON HORSEBACK

Makes 4 tiny servings
Time: 30 minutes

When I'm at a wedding with halfway decent food, and they start passing these things around, I eat as many as I can get my hands on, because I know the main course will never measure up. One of the world's easiest cocktail appetizers, they're even better if you throw them on the grill.

1 dozen oysters, shucked (page 201)
½ cup dry white wine (real Chablis if you have it)
1 clove garlic, peeled and crushed
Salt and freshly ground black pepper to taste
6 slices good bacon, halved

Marinate the oysters in the wine, garlic, salt, and pepper for about 15 minutes, while you preheat the broiler or grill, moderately hot. Wrap each oyster with a piece of bacon, secure with a toothpick, and broil or grill about 6 inches from the heat source. Turn once and cook just until the bacon is crisp.

POLLOCK

Latin name(s): *Nachius virens* (Atlantic); *Theragra chalcogramma* (Pacific).
Other common names: Atlantic: Saithe, coalfish, coley (especially in England), Boston bluefish; Pacific: Whiting, Pacific tomcod, Alaska (or Pacific) pollock.
Common forms: Fillets (almost exclusively), steaks and small whole fish (rarely); usually skin off but sometimes on (the skin is edible).
General description: Atlantic: a tannish gray, rather than white, codlike fillet; Pacific: white, soft, and quite codlike.
For other recipes see: Blackfish (very close to Atlantic), carp, catfish, cod (very close to Pacific), dogfish, flatfish, grouper, haddock, halibut, monkfish, ocean perch, rockfish, sablefish, sea bass, red snapper, striped bass, tilefish, weakfish, whiting, wolffish.
Buying tips: Atlantic and Pacific pollock are differnt. The fillets of East Coast fish are gray (giving it the name "Boston blue"); there should be no evidence of browning or dryness, gaping should be minimal, and the smell fresh. Pacific pollock is truly white and more codlike in appearance; it, too, should have no hint of dryness, browning, or off odors.

As you can tell from the above, we are really talking about two different fish here. Unlike kingfish, however (page 150), the name pollock at least applies to two fish that can be used interchangeably.

They are, however, different. Atlantic pollock is a wonderful fish, beloved in France (where it is called *lieu*) and England, where it has dozens of names. Here, it has suffered from its unfortunate alternative name—Boston bluefish—which reminds people, understandably, of the much stronger-tasting bluefish. The pollock fillet has the same shape as that of cod, is slightly blue, and it is somewhat oilier than cod. It's also firmer in texture, and the combination of oiliness and toughness makes it, along with blackfish, grouper, and a couple of other fish, one of the few fillets you can grill (see Blackfish and Grouper for recipes). It's usually inexpensive, to boot. All in all, Atlantic pollock is a worthy fish and, arguably, more useful than cod for which it theoretically substitutes.

Pacific pollock—of which there has been, until recently at least, an enormous resource—is now widely used in processing: It's the fish of millions of fish sandwiches, and it's the base for surimi, the highly processed fish food used in supermarket "seafood salads" and as a crabmeat substitute. But, since cod is becoming more difficult to find, more Pacific pollock fillets are making their way into retail stores. Use it interchangeably with cod although, like whiting, it is somewhat softer and lacks the distinctively large flake of that better-known fillet.

The recipes here can be used for either fish, but were developed to take advantage of the firmer, oilier nature of Atlantic pollock.

ROAST POLLOCK WITH SAUTÉED AND ROASTED CABBAGE

Makes 4 servings
Time: 40 minutes

Few inexpensive dishes are as elegant as this one, which combines an underappreciated fish with an underappreciated vegetable with wonderful results. The cabbage, half of which is sautéed and half roasted with the fish, lends a lovely sweetness to the mild pollock.

1 small head green or Savoy cabbage, about 2 pounds
2 tablespoons plus 1 teaspoon olive or peanut oil
1 teaspoon peeled and minced fresh ginger
1 teaspoon minced garlic
Salt and freshly ground black pepper to taste
One 1-inch-thick pollock fillet, 1 to 1 ½ pounds
1 tablespoon sesame oil
Chopped scallions, white and green parts, for garnish

Preheat the oven to 450°F. Shred the cabbage, then chop it coarsely. Divide it in half, and chop one half a little more finely. In a 12-inch skillet heat 2 tablespoons of the oil over medium-high heat, add the coarsely chopped cabbage, and cook, stirring occasionally, until softened. Add the ginger and garlic and continue to cook, stirring occasionally, until the cabbage is slightly browned. Season with salt and pepper; cover and keep warm.

Use the remaining oil to lightly grease the bottom of a baking dish slightly larger than the fillet. Cover the bottom of the dish with the finely chopped cabbage. Sprinkle with salt, then lay the fillet on top; salt the fish lightly. Roast until the fish is almost done (use a thin knife to peek inside; it should be opaque, and the knife should encounter little resistance), 6 to 8 minutes. Scatter the sautéed cabbage around the fish and roast another 2 min-

utes. Sprinkle with the sesame oil and chopped scallions and serve immediately.

ALTERNATIVE FISH FOR THIS RECIPE:
Blackfish, cod, dogfish, grouper, haddock, rockfish, sea bass, sablefish, red snapper, tilefish, or wolffish. Adjust cooking times accordingly.

POLLOCK BEIGNETS

Makes 4 servings
Time: 60 minutes or a bit more

Atlantic pollock is somewhat firmer than cod, so it lends a pleasant chewiness to these crisp, batter-dipped fritters. Make them walnut-size for appetizers, larger for an entrée. And, if you can, make the batter a couple of hours in advance for extra lightness.

1 cup lukewarm water
1 teaspoon dry yeast
1 ¼ pounds starchy potatoes, such as Idaho or Russet
1 large egg
1 ¼ cups unbleached all-purpose flour, more or less
1 large or 2 medium-size pollock fillets, about 1 ¼ pounds total
½ cup minced shallots, scallions (both green and white parts), or onions
2 tablespoons minced fresh parsley
1 tablespoon minced fresh chives
1 teaspoon minced fresh tarragon or ¼ teaspoon dried
Salt and freshly ground black pepper to taste
Milk as needed
Vegetable oil for deep-frying
Lemon wedges, Green Sauce (page 144), Light Tomato Sauce (page 209), any mayonnaise (such as the one on page 43), or Sesame Dipping Sauce (page 295)

Mix the water and yeast together in a medium-size bowl and let sit. Meanwhile, set a pot of water to boil for the potatoes; wash the potatoes if you haven't already done so. Beat the egg into the water-yeast mixture and add the flour, about ⅓ cup at a time, stirring to blend after each addition, until you have a batter slightly thicker than that for pancakes. Cover with plastic wrap and set aside in a warm place.

Salt the boiling water and add the potatoes (if you're in a hurry, quarter them first). Cook until they are quite tender—up to 45 minutes if they're large and whole. Lift them out gently and cool. Place the pollock fillet in the same water and simmer until it is done, about 10 minutes (a thin-bladed knife will easily pass through the fillet). Make sure the pollock is completely free of bones, then peel the potatoes and mash them with the pollock, shallots, herbs, salt, and pepper. The mixture should be pasty and thick; try rolling a piece between your hands, and add a little milk if it seems dry. (It's okay if the mixture is a bit sticky; if it is too moist to hold its shape, add flour 1 tablespoon at a time.)

Heat at least 3 inches of oil to about 375°F. (If your fryer doesn't have a thermostat, or you don't have a frying thermometer, drop a small piece of bread in the oil; it should sink, then rise to the top and begin bubbling away.) Salt the batter and stir it up. Roll the pollock-potato mixture into balls of any size, dip each ball into the batter, let the excess batter run off, and fry until golden on all sides, about 3 to 5 minutes, depending on their size (don't try to fry too many at once). As they finish cooking, drain the beignets on paper towels and keep warm in a low oven. Serve with lemon wedges or any sauce.

ALTERNATIVE FISH FOR THIS RECIPE:

Cod, dogfish, haddock, tilefish, weakfish, or whiting. Adjust the cooking times accordingly.

BROILED POLLOCK WITH PARSLEY PESTO

Makes 4 servings
Time: 20 minutes
An easy, flavorful recipe that translates well to steaks and fillets of many other fish.

2 cups loosely packed parsley leaves
1 large clove garlic, peeled
Zest and juice of 1 lemon
¾ cup olive oil
Salt and freshly ground black pepper to taste
1 large or 2 medium-size pollock fillets, about 1 ½ pounds total

Preheat the broiler. In a blender or food processor, mix together everything but the fish and blend until smooth. Spread 1 tablespoon or so of this mixture on a nonstick broiling or baking pan; place the fillets on top and sprinkle with salt and pepper. Spread a little more of the pesto on the fish.

Broil the fish about 6 inches from the heat source until cooked through (figure about 8 minutes per inch of thickness; use a thin knife to peek inside; the fillet should be opaque, and the knife should encounter little resistance). Serve, passing additional sauce at the table.

ALTERNATIVE FISH FOR THIS RECIPE:

Blackfish, carp, catfish, cod, dogfish, flatfish, grouper, haddock, halibut, ocean perch, rockfish, sea bass, red snapper, striped bass, tilefish, weakfish, or wolffish. Adjust the cooking times accordingly.

SAUTÉED POLLOCK WITH
SALSA FRESCA

Makes 4 servings
Time: 20 minutes
Another easily varied, easily adapted recipe.

2 cups chopped luscious fresh ripe tomatoes
1 small onion, minced
1 small clove garlic, minced
1 jalapeño or to taste, deveined, seeded, and
  minced
¼ cup minced cilantro (fresh coriander) leaves
1 teaspoon sherry, red, or white wine vinegar
Salt and freshly ground black pepper to taste
1 large or 2 medium-size pollock fillets, about
  1 ½ pounds total
¼ cup peanut oil
Flour for dredging

Combine the first seven ingredients; taste for seasoning (you may want more jalapeño, vinegar, salt, and/or pepper) and set aside.

Heat a 12-inch nonstick skillet over medium-high heat for 4 to 5 minutes. Cut the fillets into serving pieces if they are large. Add the oil to the skillet and, when it is hot (a pinch of flour will sizzle), dredge the fillets in the flour, shaking off any excess, and add them to the pan. Cook over high heat, turning once, until nicely browned, about 3 or 4 minutes per side. Serve immediately, with the salsa fresca.

Alternative fish for this recipe:

Blackfish, catfish, cod, dogfish, flatfish, grouper, haddock, halibut, monkfish (medallions are best), ocean perch, rockfish, sea bass, red snapper, tilefish, weakfish, or wolffish. Adjust the cooking times accordingly.

Variation:

Serve the pollock with Green Tomato Salsa (page 219) instead of salsa fresca.

POLLOCK SIMMERED
IN TOMATO SAUCE

Makes 4 servings
Time: 40 minutes
A basic recipe, easily varied, and useful for any thick white fillet.

4 slices good bacon, minced, or ¼ cup olive oil
1 medium-size onion, roughly chopped
½ cup dry white or red wine
2 cups chopped tomatoes (drained if canned)
Salt and freshly ground black pepper to taste
½ cup minced fresh parsley
1 ½ pounds pollock fillets, in 4 pieces

In a 10- or 12-inch skillet, cook the bacon over medium heat, stirring occasionally, until crisp (alternatively, heat the olive oil). Remove the bacon with a slotted spoon and drain on paper towels. Add the onion and cook, stirring, in the fat until softened. Add the wine and let it bubble away for a minute or so. Add the tomatoes, stir, and cook for about 10 minutes, stirring occasionally, until the tomatoes break down. Season with salt and pepper and add half the parsley.

Lay the fillets in the sauce and spoon some of the sauce over them. Cook until a thin-bladed knife will pass through the thickest part with little resistance, about 8 to 12 minutes depending on thickness. Serve each piece of fish with some sauce on it, sprinkled with parsley and bits of bacon.

Alternative fish for this recipe:

Fillets or steaks of blackfish, carp, cod, dogfish, grouper, haddock, halibut, monkfish, ocean perch, rockfish, sea bass, red snapper, striped bass, tilefish, weakfish, whiting, or wolffish. Adjust the cooking times accordingly.

Pollock Simmered in Spicy Tomato
Sauce:

Rub the fillets with a mixture of 1 teaspoon paprika and ½ teaspoon cayenne pepper. Add 2 teaspoons ground cumin or chili powder and 1 teaspoon minced garlic to the simmering tomato sauce. Substitute cilantro (fresh coriander) for the parsley if you like.

Pollock Simmered in Neapolitan Tomato Sauce:

Omit the bacon. Heat ¼ cup olive oil over medium heat. Add 2 cloves garlic, cut in half, and 2 dried hot peppers and cook, stirring, until browned. Discard the garlic and peppers and let the oil cool for 1 to 2 minutes. Add the tomatoes, along with 1 tablespoon capers and ½ cup roughly chopped pitted black olives (use a flavorful imported variety if possible). Proceed as directed above.

Pollock Simmered in Tomato-horseradish Sauce:

Add 2 tablespoons prepared horseradish (or to taste; or substitute freshly grated horseradish to taste) to the simmering tomato sauce just before it is done. Proceed as directed above.

POMPANO

Latin name(s): *Trachinotus carolinus*.
Other common names: Permit, butterfish, sunfish.
Common forms: Whole fish, skin-on fillets.
General description: Panfish size (usually under two pounds), but superior to most panfish in flavor and texture. Among the easiest to eat of all whole fish.
For other recipes see: Bluefish, butterfish, croaker, flatfish, mackerel, mahi-mahi, sardine, sea bass, red snapper, striped bass, tuna.
Buying tips: A similar fish, permit, which is sometimes sold as pompano, is larger and not as good. Stick to smaller fish. Skin should be shiny and bright, gills red, smell fresh. Buy it scaled, with skin left on.

This slim, silvery fish glistens in the sun as it rides the waves toward shore on the southeastern and Gulf coasts. The commercial catch is far from enormous, but pompano are shipped everywhere (although not in the kind of quantities its admirers would prefer). This is an esteemed fish that can be quite expensive (six dollars and more for uncleaned fish), but—assuming, of course, that it is fresh—its white, somewhat oily flesh is meaty and sweet, especially when broiled, grilled, or cooked in pouches.

Pompano have small scales which must be removed; have it done by your fishmonger, or do it yourself (page 19). Fillets almost always retain the skin; taking the skin off raw fish is tricky.

WHOLE POMPANO BAKED
EN PAPILLOTE

Makes 4 servings
Time: 45 minutes
Pompano baked in pouches is a classic, and not surprisingly; this method is great at preserving this fish's rich, incomparable flavor. As with all wrapped preparations (see Red Snapper, page 288, for several more), simplicity is the key.

¼ cup pine nuts
4 whole pompano, gutted and scaled, heads on or off, about 1 pound each (you can also use fillets; adjust cooking time accordingly)
2 tablespoons minced shallots
2 tablespoons minced fresh parsley
2 tablespoons dry white wine or any fish or chicken stock (pages 40–41)
1 tablespoon fresh lemon juice
Salt and freshly ground black pepper to taste

Preheat the oven to 450°F. Toast the pine nuts by heating them in a small dry skillet over medium heat, shaking occasionally, until lightly browned, about 5 minutes or less.

Tear off a piece of aluminum foil about 18 inches long (the more traditional parchment paper is, of course, acceptable). Place a pompano on it, and top the fish with a quarter of each of the remaining ingredients, including the pine nuts. Seal the package and repeat the process.

Place all the packages in a large baking dish and bake for about 30 minutes. Open one of the packages and check the fish for doneness (peer along the central bone with a thin-bladed knife; the fish should be white and flaky). Return to the oven if necessary. Serve the closed packages, allowing each diner to open his or her own at the table.

ALTERNATIVE FISH FOR THIS RECIPE:

Whole butterfish, croaker, mackerel, porgy; fillets of blackfish, bluefish, dogfish, grouper, haddock, mackerel, ocean perch, Atlantic pollock, rockfish, salmon, red snapper, trout, or wolffish. Adjust the cooking times accordingly.

POMPANO EN PAPILLOTE WITH MUSHROOMS:

Reconstitute 1 ounce dried cèpes (porcini) in warm water or stock, then drain and chop. Heat 2 tablespoons olive oil over medium heat, add the cèpes along with ½ pound chopped domestic mushrooms and 1 minced shallot, and cook, stirring, until softened, then season with salt and pepper. Top the pompano with this mixture, along with the parsley, wine, lemon juice, salt, and pepper, in the quantities described in the main recipe. Proceed as directed above.

POMPANO EN PAPILLOTE PROVENÇAL STYLE:

Mix together 1 shredded medium-size zucchini, 1 minced medium-size onion, 1 seeded and minced small to medium-size red bell pepper, 1 tablespoon minced garlic, salt and pepper to taste, and 1 teaspoon minced thyme (preferably fresh). Place half this mixture underneath the fish and half on top. Add the parsley (or basil), wine, lemon juice, and salt and pepper, in the quantities described in the main recipe. Proceed as directed above.

GRILLED POMPANO

Makes 2 servings
Time: 30 minutes
Pompano is among the best fish to grill.

Juice of 1 lemon
¼ cup dry (Fino) sherry or white wine
¼ cup olive oil
Salt and freshly ground black pepper to taste
2 whole pompano, about 1 pound or slightly larger, scaled and gutted
Several sprigs fresh rosemary or 1 tablespoon dried
Lemon wedges

Mix together the first four ingredients and marinate the fish in this while you start a charcoal or wood fire or preheat a gas grill or broiler; the fire should be medium-hot. If you have plenty of rosemary, throw some directly on the coals; in any case, sprinkle some on the fish, then place it directly on the rack or use a fish grilling basket (page 26). Grill or broil about 5 minutes per side, basting occasionally with the marinade, then check for doneness (peer along the central bone with a thin-bladed knife; the fish should be white and flaky). Garnish with rosemary sprigs and serve with lemon wedges.

ALTERNATIVE FISH FOR THIS RECIPE:

Whole bluefish (small ones), butterfish, mackerel, red snapper, or striped bass. Adjust the cooking times accordingly.

POMPANO GRILLED WITH MINT AND BALSAMIC VINEGAR:

Omit the marinade. Rub the fish with a little olive oil. As the fish grills, warm ¼ cup olive oil with ¼ cup balsamic vinegar, 1 teaspoon minced garlic, and ¼ cup chopped fresh mint. Season with salt and pepper. Serve the grilled fish with the sauce.

BROILED AND MARINATED POMPANO

Makes 6 appetizer servings
Time: 1 to 6 hours, mostly unattended

This is a fast escabèche with nontraditional seasonings.

6 pompano fillets
1 tablespoon peanut or vegetable oil
1 clove garlic, cut in half
Salt and freshly ground black pepper to taste
½ cup red or white wine vinegar
¼ teaspoon cayenne pepper
1 teaspoon minced garlic
1 tablespoon peeled and minced fresh ginger
1 tablespoon minced scallion, both green and white parts
2 tablespoons minced cilantro (fresh coriander), plus extra for garnish

Preheat the broiler. Rub the fillets with the oil, then with the cut sides of the garlic. Season with salt and pepper. Place in a nonstick pan or on a nonstick cookie sheet and broil, skin side up, about 4 inches from the heat source until the skin is crisp and the flesh white, about 4 to 6 minutes.

Remove the fish and place it on a serving platter, skin side down. Simmer together the remaining ingredients (except the garnish) for about 2 minutes. Pour, hot, over the pompano. Refrigerate for as little as 1 or as many as 6 hours, depending on your schedule and the intensity of flavor you desire, garnish, and serve.

ALTERNATIVE FISH FOR THIS RECIPE:

Fillets of bluefish, mackerel, mahi-mahi, or striped bass, or tuna steaks. Adjust the cooking times accordingly.

MARINATED POMPANO WITH JAPANESE SEASONINGS:

Season and broil the fish as directed above. Simmer together ½ cup rice vinegar, 2 tablespoons mirin (sweet cooking wine, available in Asian markets), 2 tablespoons soy sauce, 1 tablespoon peeled and minced fresh ginger, ½ to 1 teaspoon wasabe powder (Japanese horseradish, available in Asian markets; you can substitute 1 tablespoon prepared horseradish), and ¼ cup minced scallions, both green and white parts. Pour hot over the pompano and garnish with minced scallions.

PORGY

Latin name(s): *Stenotomus chrysops*.
Other common names: Scup, pogy, paugy.
Common forms: Whole, almost exclusively.
General description: Average one- to two-pound panfish with good flavor.
For other recipes see: Bluefish, croaker, flatfish, grouper, mackerel, mullet, pompano, rockfish, sea bass, red snapper, spot, tilefish, weakfish, whiting.
Buying tips: Porgy should be shiny and bright when you buy it, and look and smell like it just came out of the water. Get the fishmonger to scale (and gut) them for you.

There are a dozen or more fish known as porgy, most of them found in the warmer waters of the Atlantic and the Mediterranean. In addition to porgy, and the names above, they are called bream, jolthead, pink, white, or silver snapper, sheepshead, fair maid, and whitebone. Whether porgy or some related species, all are mild, sweet, white-fleshed fish with firm texture. But all are difficult to fillet and contain many small bones, which has limited their popularity in the United States.

There's no question that eating a porgy takes some work. Of course eating lobster takes some work, too, and few people complain about that. So think twice before you reject the inexpensive and quite versatile porgy.

Eating larger porgy is somewhat easier than eating pan-size fish, but, in my experience, small porgies taste better. For best flavor, try to find perfectly fresh porgy; although the shelf life of this fish is unusually long, the deterioration in flavor and texture is noticeable from day to day.

Make sure that porgy is scaled before you buy it (the lone exception is Porgy Baked in Salt, where it doesn't matter); scaling it at home is an exceptionally messy task.

ROAST PORGY WITH GARLIC AND VINEGAR

Makes 2 servings
Time: 45 minutes

Bony fish like porgy are good when they are roasted, not only because the bones soften somewhat, but because the flesh falls off of them fairly easily, especially if the fish is spanking fresh.

1 whole porgy, about 2 pounds, scaled and gutted, head on
Salt and freshly ground black pepper to taste
2 tablespoons minced fresh basil or 1 teaspoon dried
10 to 20 cloves garlic (do not peel)
½ cup dry white wine or any fish or chicken stock (pages 40–41)
½ cup (1 stick) butter
⅓ cup balsamic, sherry, or top-quality red or white wine vinegar
Minced fresh basil or parsley for garnish

Preheat the oven to 400°F. Season the fish with salt and pepper, then rub it with the basil. Place it in a baking dish with the garlic and wine. Dot it with about half the butter. Put the dish in the oven.

About every 5 minutes, put another dot of butter on the fish, along with 1 or 2 spoonsful of the vinegar. Baste with the pan juices. Repeat the process until all the butter and vinegar are used up and the porgy is cooked (use a thin-bladed knife to peek at the central bone; the flesh should be opaque and tender). Total cooking time will be 30 to 40 minutes. Garnish with the basil and serve with the remaining basting liquid and the garlic cloves (squeeze the garlic from its peel to spread on bread; it will be buttery and mild).

ALTERNATIVE FISH FOR THIS RECIPE:

Whole butterfish (you will need more than one), croaker, flatfish, mackerel, pompano, tilefish, or weakfish. Adjust the cooking times accordingly.

ROAST PORGY WITH OLIVE OIL AND ROSEMARY:

Cut two or three slits on each side of the fish, then stuff the slit and the body cavity with a mixture of minced fresh or dried rosemary, sage, or mint, coarse salt, 1 teaspoon minced garlic, 3 tablespoons plain bread crumbs, 3 tablespoons olive oil, and black pepper to taste. Roast on a rack in a baking pan with no added liquid. Garnish with minced fresh parsley and serve with lemon wedges.

ROAST PORGY WITH TARRAGON SAUCE:

Substitute 1 teaspoon fresh tarragon or ½ teaspoon dried for the basil in the original recipe; garnish with fresh tarragon sprigs.

COTRIADE
(Fish and Potato Stew)

Makes 4 servings
Time: 60 minutes

This is one version of the simple, classic Breton fish stew, often made with bream, one of the porgylike fishes of the eastern Atlantic.

3 slices bacon (the best you can find), minced
2 large onions, roughly chopped
1 pound potatoes, peeled and cut into eighths or sixteenths
Salt and freshly ground black pepper to taste
1 teaspoon fresh thyme or ½ teaspoon dried
8 cups Flavorful Fish and Vegetable Stock (page 40)
2 pounds porgy (1 or 2 fish), scaled, gutted, heads removed, and cut into chunks
Juice of 1 lemon
Minced fresh parsley for garnish

Cook the bacon in a 4- or 6-quart casserole over medium heat until it is crisp. Remove with a slotted spoon to a paper towel to drain. Cook the onions in the fat, stirring occasionally, until softened. Add the potatoes and cook, stirring occasionally, until they are well mixed with the onions and covered with fat. Season with salt, pepper, and thyme; stir, then add the stock. Simmer until the potatoes are almost tender, about 15 minutes. Add the fish and cook another 10 minutes or so, until the flesh pulls easily from the bone. Add the lemon juice, ladle into bowls, and garnish with the parsley.

ALTERNATIVE FISH FOR THIS RECIPE:

Whole croaker, rockfish, red snapper, tilefish, weakfish, or whiting. Adjust the cooking times accordingly.

PORGY BAKED IN SALT

Makes 2 to 3 servings
Time: 45 minutes

The most difficult thing about this impressive Mediterranean dish is the timing, since it's impossible to test the fish for doneness. What I do—and it's never failed me—is overcook the fish by a few minutes. The salt crust is such a good insulator that the flesh remains moist despite the extra heat.

After baking fish in salt using the method below for years, I learned another way in Seville: Make a 3-inch-deep bed of salt in a large baking pan, nestle the fish in it, and cover with another thick layer of salt. Bake as directed below; the crust is not as attractive, but the results are identical.

1 whole porgy, 2 pounds or so, gutted (scales can be left on or taken off), head on
2 pounds kosher or coarse sea salt
1 cup all-purpose flour
1 cup warm water

Preheat the oven to 450°F. Rinse and dry the fish. Mix together the salt and flour, then add enough water to make a paste about the consistency of thick cake batter. Spread this thickly all over the fish, completely covering it. You can decorate the crust if you like, or draw designs in the batter with a spoon or fork.

Lay the fish in a baking pan and cook, undisturbed, for 30 minutes. Remove the pan from the oven and take it directly to the table (where you can let it rest for a few minutes if you like, while everyone admires your genius). Crack the crust, peel off the fish's skin if it didn't come off with the crust, spoon the fish off the bone, and serve.

ALTERNATIVE FISH FOR THIS RECIPE:

Almost any whole fish under 3 pounds, including croaker, grouper, rockfish, sea bass (excellent), red snapper, tilefish, or weakfish. Increase cooking time by 10 minutes for 3-pound fish.

POUT

Latin name(s): *Macrozoarces americanus*.
Other common names: Eel pout, ocean pout.
Common forms: Fillets, almost exclusively.
General description: A tough, dry fish being marketed as a substitute for cod.
For recipes see: Any white-fleshed fillet.
Buying tips: My recommendation: Pass it by, except as an addition to chowder or stew, even if the price is irresistible.

This slender fish hails from the North Atlantic and vaguely resembles an eel. Because the stocks remain in good shape, it is being sold widely as a substitute for cod, and the fillet is a nice-looking one. But I have yet to find a way to make this fish stand by itself: the flavor is bland—which, in itself is not so bad—and the texture is tough and chewy.

ROCKFISH

Latin name(s): *Sebastes alutus* and many others in *Sebastes* genus.
Other common names: Ocean perch, Pacific red snapper, red, copper, brown, pink, blue, etc. rockfish, rock cod.
Common forms: Fillets (skin may be on or off), whole (less common).
General description: The West Coast equivalent of red snapper and ocean perch, shipped throughout the country. The flesh is firm, white, big-flaked, and tasty. Not quite red snapper, but excellent.
For other recipes see: Blackfish, carp, catfish, cod, dogfish, flatfish, grouper, haddock, halibut, ocean perch (especially), pollock, salmon, red snapper, striped bass, tilefish, weakfish, whiting, wolffish.
Buying tips: It's tough to generalize about rockfish (see below); just make sure fillets show no evidence of browning or graying, and that the smell is fresh.

There are more North American fish called "rock-fish" than anything else (forty are caught in the Gulf of Alaska alone). All have in common the virtue of firm, white, sweet fillets, which—although not quite sturdy enough to grill—can be considered all-purpose. (Whole fish can be grilled, but are not widely available.) Useful, wonderful fish, usually priced reasonably.

SAUTÉED ROCKFISH FILLETS WITH SAUTÉED APPLES

Makes 4 servings
Time: 30 minutes
I had a dish similar to this one in Brittany, made with cod. But rockfish, with its firmer texture, holds up better to sautéing.

4 crisp, not-too-sweet apples, such as Granny Smiths
6 tablespoons (¾ stick) butter
Flour for dredging
Salt and freshly ground black pepper to taste

1 large egg
Unseasoned bread crumbs for dredging
1 to 1 ½ pounds rockfish fillets (about 4), skin on or off
Juice of ½ lemon
1 tablespoon calvados or brandy (optional)

Peel and core the apples, then cut them into rings or thin wedges. Melt half the butter in a skillet over medium heat. Add the apples, raise the heat to medium-high, and cook, tossing and stirring occasionally, until nicely browned on all sides.

Once you've started cooking the apples, preheat a 12-inch nonstick skillet over medium-high heat. Season the flour with salt and pepper and beat the egg in a bowl. Add the remaining butter to the skillet and, when the foam subsides, dredge each fillet in the flour, then dip it in the egg, dredge it in the bread crumbs, and place in the pan. Cook until nicely browned on both sides, about 6 to 8 minutes total (when they're done, a thin-bladed knife will pass through the fillets with little resistance). Drizzle the apples with the lemon juice and calvados and spoon a portion onto each fillet. Serve immediately.

ALTERNATIVE FISH FOR THIS RECIPE:

Blackfish, grouper, ocean perch, Atlantic pollock, red snapper, or wolffish. Adjust the cooking times accordingly.

SAUTÉED ROCKFISH WITH GREEN TOMATO SALSA:

Dredge the fillets in 1 cup flour mixed with 2 tablespoons ground cumin. Cook in 4 tablespoons peanut or olive oil as directed above. Serve with a salsa made with ½ cup chopped green tomatoes or tomatillos, ½ cup chopped ripe red tomatoes, 2 tablespoons minced cilantro (fresh coriander), salt, freshly ground black pepper, and a pinch of cayenne pepper.

CRISP ROCKFISH FILLETS ON MASHED POTATOES

Makes 4 servings
Time: 45 minutes
This is a super dish, crisp, creamy, and—thanks to the quick reduction sauce—moist. Note the sautéing technique, which can be used with any fillet under ½ inch thick.

2 pounds starchy potatoes, such as Idaho or Russet, peeled
6 tablespoons (¾ stick) butter
1 cup milk
Salt and freshly ground black pepper to taste
2 tablespoons olive oil
1 cup unbleaded all-purpose flour, seasoned with salt and pepper
4 rockfish fillets, about 1 to 1 ½ pounds, skin on
2 tablespoons minced shallot
1 cup dry white wine or any stock (pages 39–41)
1 teaspoon Dijon mustard
3 tablespoons minced fresh parsley

Put the potatoes in a pot and cover with cold water; bring to a boil, lower the heat to medium, and simmer until tender, 20 to 40 minutes. Drain and mash with 3 tablespoons of the butter, ¼ cup of the milk, salt, and pepper. Cover and keep warm in a low oven (or set aside and microwave before serving).

Heat 2 tablespoons of the butter and the oil over medium heat in a 12-inch nonstick skillet that can later be covered. When the butter melts, dip each fillet in the milk, then dredge the skin side in the flour (the top should not be floured). When the butter foam subsides, place the fillets, skin side down, in the skillet. Cover and cook for about 5 minutes, undisturbed. At this point, the fillets should be white on top and crisp on the bottom; if not, cook another 2 minutes. Remove the fillets to a warm oven.

Raise the heat to high and cook the shallot, stirring occasionally, in the fat remaining in the pan until softened, 1 minute or so. Add the wine and stir, letting it bubble away for 1 minute or so. Stir in the mustard and parsley and cook for 30 seconds. Add the remaining butter and stir until the sauce is smooth.

To serve, spoon some mashed potatoes onto a plate, top with a rockfish fillet, and spoon some of the sauce over all.

ALTERNATIVE FISH FOR THIS RECIPE:

Haddock, ocean perch, salmon, red snapper, tilefish, or weakfish. Fillets should be under ½ inch thick and have their skin on. Adjust the cooking times accordingly.

CURRIED ROCKFISH FILLETS

Makes 4 servings
Time: 30 minutes

1 to 1 ½ pounds rockfish fillets (about 4), skin on or off
1 tablespoon minced garlic
2 tablespoons fresh lemon juice
1 teaspoon turmeric
2 cups plain yogurt
Salt and freshly ground black pepper to taste
2 tablespoons peanut oil
1 small onion, chopped
1 tablespoon peeled and minced fresh ginger
1 teaspoon ground cumin
1 teaspoon ground fenugreek
1 teaspoon ground coriander

Marinate the fish in a bowl with the garlic, 1 tablespoon of the lemon juice, the turmeric, yogurt, salt, and pepper while you cook the other ingredients. In a large, deep skillet, heat the oil over medium heat; add the onion and cook, stirring, until limp. Add the ginger and cook another minute. Add the cumin, fenugreek, and coriander and stir for 30 seconds. Carefully pour the fish and its marinade into the skillet, bring to a simmer, and cook until the fillets are white and firm, and a thin-bladed knife will pass through them with little resistance, about 10 minutes. Serve immediately, with rice (basmati is great with this).

ALTERNATIVE FISH FOR THIS RECIPE:
Blackfish, catfish, dogfish, grouper, Atlantic pollock, red snapper, tilefish, or wolffish. Adjust the cooking times accordingly.

BRAISED ROCKFISH FILLETS WITH SAUCE "HACHÉ"

Makes 4 servings
Time: 30 minutes

Some older recipes never finished a dish with sauce, but just minced (*haché*) the ingredients so finely that the sauce was made by chewing.

2 tablespoons olive oil
2 tablespoons butter
1 tablespoon minced garlic
1 tablespoon minced fresh rosemary
2 tablespoons minced onion
2 tablespoons minced celery
2 tablespoons minced carrot
Pinch minced fresh or dried thyme
1 cup chopped tomato, fresh or canned (drained if canned)
Salt and freshly ground black pepper to taste
4 rockfish fillets, 1 to 1 ½ pounds total, preferably with skin on
¼ cup dry white wine or water, if needed
Minced fresh parsley for garnish

Heat the olive oil and butter over medium heat in a skillet that can later be covered. When the butter foam subsides, add the garlic, rosemary, onion, celery, carrot, and thyme. Cook, stirring occasionally, over medium-low heat until the vegetables soften. Add the tomato and season with salt and pepper. Cook for about 3 minutes, then lay the fillets on top of the sauce. Cover and cook until the fillets are white and firm (a thin-bladed knife will pass through them with little resistance), about 5 to 8 minutes. Remove the fillets to a warm plate. (If the sauce is dry, add the wine and simmer for 1 minute.) Pour the sauce over the fillets, garnish with minced parsley, and serve.

ALTERNATIVE FISH FOR THIS RECIPE:
Blackfish, carp, catfish, cod, dogfish, flatfish, grouper, haddock, halibut, ocean perch, pollock,

salmon, red snapper, striped bass, tilefish, weakfish, whiting, or wolffish. Adjust the cooking times accordingly.

ROCKFISH SOUP WITH CITRUS

Makes 4 servings
Time: 45 minutes

3 tablespoons olive oil
½ cup shallots, quartered
2 medium-size waxy potatoes, peeled and cut into small pieces
2 medium-size carrots, sliced
1 medium to large parsnip, peeled and sliced
1 medium-size purple-top turnip, peeled and cut into small pieces
1 medium-size onion, thinly sliced
1 small bulb fennel, cut into small pieces (reserve a few of the feathery sprigs for garnish)
4 cups any fish stock (pages 40–41), warmed
1 bay leaf
Salt and freshly ground black pepper to taste
Juice of 1 lemon
Juice of 1 lime
Juice of 1 orange
1 pound skinless rockfish fillets, cut into chunks

Heat the olive oil over medium heat in a casserole. Add the shallots, potatoes, carrots, parsnip, turnip, onion, and fennel; cook, stirring occasionally, until the onion begins to wilt. Add the stock and bay leaf, bring to a boil, and turn the heat to medium. Simmer, uncovered, until the vegetables are tender, 20 to 30 minutes. Season with salt and pepper. Add the citrus juices, then nestle the fillets among the vegetables and cook just until the fish is white and firm (a thin-bladed knife will pass through them with little resistance), about 5 to 8

minutes. Serve immediately, garnished with fennel sprigs.

ALTERNATIVE FISH FOR THIS RECIPE:
Blackfish, catfish, dogfish, grouper, Atlantic pollock, scallops, shrimp, red snapper, or wolffish. Adjust cooking times accordingly.

ROCKFISH FILLETS IN SWEET SOY MARINADE

Makes 4 servings
Time: 1 hour or less
You can marinate the fillets for an hour or so before cooking, but it really isn't necessary; this is an assertive sauce.

½ cup sesame seeds
1 teaspoon sesame oil
¼ cup high-quality soy sauce
1 tablespoon peeled and finely minced or grated fresh ginger
½ cup minced scallion, both green and white parts
1 teaspoon minced garlic
1 tablespoon dry sherry
1 tablespoon honey or sugar
1 to 1 ½ pounds rockfish fillets (about 4), skin on or off

Toast the sesame seeds over medium heat in a dry skillet, shaking occasionally, until they brown and become fragrant, 3 to 5 minutes. Cool, then put them in a plastic bag and crush them with a rolling pin. Place in a large bowl with all the marinade ingredients (reserve half the scallions) and the fish. Marinate for as little as 5 minutes and as long as 1 hour.

Preheat the broiler, then place the fish on a rack on a baking sheet. Pour the remaining marinade over the fish and broil until lightly browned on top, 5 to 8 minutes. The fillets will be white and firm, and a thin-bladed knife will pass through them with little resistance. Garnish with the reserved scallions and serve immediately, with white rice.

ALTERNATIVE FISH FOR THIS RECIPE:

Blackfish, catfish, cod, dogfish, grouper, haddock, halibut, ocean perch, pollock, red snapper, striped bass, tilefish, or wolffish. Adjust the cooking times accordingly.

BROILED ROCKFISH FILLETS WITH JALAPEÑO BUTTER

Makes 4 servings
Time: 20 minutes

1 recipe Jalapeño Butter (page 45)
4 rockfish fillets, 1 to 1 ½ pounds total, preferably with skin on
Salt to taste
Lemon wedges

Preheat the broiler. Smear both sides of the fish with about half the jalapeño butter. Lay the fillets, skin side up, on a rack in a broiling pan. Broil about 4 inches from the heat source until the skin is nicely browned, about 3 minutes. Turn and brown the top lightly, about 2 minutes (the fillets will be white and firm, and a thin-bladed knife will pass through them with little resistance). Sprinkle with a little salt, top each fillet with a bit more of the butter, and serve with lemon wedges.

ALTERNATIVE FISH FOR THIS RECIPE:

Blackfish, catfish, dogfish, grouper, ocean perch, pollock, salmon, red snapper, striped bass, tilefish, or wolffish. Adjust the cooking times accordingly.

SABLEFISH

Latin name(s): *Anoplopoma fimbria*.
Other common names: Black cod, butterfish, coalfish, sable, skilfish.
Common forms: Whole (usually under ten pounds), fillets, steaks.
General description: Long, slender West Coast fish with black, furry (yes!) skin; meat is oily, pearly white, firm, and delicious.
For other recipes see: Blackfish, grouper, mackerel, monkfish, salmon (especially), sturgeon.
Buying tips: Fillets should glisten; sablefish does freeze well, and is often shipped, frozen and in good shape, from Alaska to the Lower 48.

If sablefish were more readily available, we'd eat it all the time. Its flesh is supremely oily, with deep, rich flavor and a meaty texture. Like salmon and swordfish, it is wonderfully juicy when cooked properly, and responds well to any basic cooking method.

But most sablefish is frozen at sea for shipment to Japan or for smoking for domestic use; smoked sable has been sold in Jewish delis since the turn of the century. That which remains may be sold fresh or frozen, usually as rather large (two-pound) fillets and somewhat smaller steaks. It freezes well, surprising given its high oil content. I buy sablefish whenever I see it, which isn't often enough.

MARINATED AND GRILLED SABLEFISH

Makes 4 servings
Time: 12 to 24 hours
This recipe showcases the supreme moistness of sablefish.

2 tablespoons cracked or freshly ground black pepper

2 tablespoons cracked or ground coriander seeds
2 tablespoons minced garlic
1 teaspoon coarse salt
One 2-pound sablefish fillet, skin on
Lemon wedges

Mix together the first four ingredients and smear on the flesh side of the sablefish. Refrigerate for several hours or overnight, pouring off any accumulated liquid from time to time.

When ready to cook, start a charcoal fire or preheat a gas grill or broiler. Wipe off the marinade but do not rinse the fillet. To grill, use a fish basket (page 26) if you have one, or rub the fish lightly with peanut or olive oil. Grill 4 to 6 inches from the heat source, turning once or twice and cooking until the fish is just lightly browned and begins to flake, about 10 minutes. To broil, keep the fish 6 to 8 inches from the heat, skin side down; do not turn. Broil until the fillet browns lightly and begins to flake, about 10 minutes. Serve with lemon wedges.

BASIC GRILLED OR BROILED SABLEFISH:
Omit the marinade entirely. Sprinkle with salt and pepper and grill or broil as directed above. Serve with lemon wedges.

SOY-GRILLED SABLEFISH:

Marinate for 15 minutes in a mixture of 1 tablespoon dry (Fino) sherry, 2 tablespoons soy sauce, 1 teaspoon sesame oil, 1 tablespoon fresh orange or lime juice, 1 teaspoon minced garlic, and 1 teaspoon peeled and minced fresh ginger. Grill or broil as directed above, basting frequently with the marinade. Garnish with minced cilantro (fresh coriander).

SABLEFISH POACHED ON A BED OF LEEKS

Makes 4 servings
Time: 30 minutes

2 pounds leeks
3 carrots, shredded on the large blade of a grater
2 cloves garlic, sliced
1 cup Full-flavored Chicken Stock (page 40) or Flavorful Fish and Vegetable Stock (page 40)
One 1- to 1 ½-pound sablefish fillet, skin off
Salt and freshly ground black pepper to taste
2 tablespoons butter

Trim the leeks of all tough green leaves, then cut in half. Wash thoroughly, fanning the leaves to get all the sand out. Shake dry, then dice.

Place the leeks, carrots, garlic, and stock in a broad skillet or casserole and bring to a boil. Lower the heat to medium, lay the sablefish on top, sprinkle with salt and pepper, and cover. Simmer until the sablefish is white, opaque, and just beginning to flake, about 10 minutes.

Remove the fish gently to a platter and place it in a low oven or cover with aluminum foil. Raise the heat to high and reduce the liquid in the skillet by about half, then lower the heat to medium and add the butter, stirring until it melts. If the sauce seems too wet, reduce some more, then pour over the fish and serve.

ALTERNATIVE FISH FOR THIS RECIPE:
Blackfish, grouper, halibut, Atlantic pollock, rockfish, salmon, red snapper, or striped bass. Adjust cooking times accordingly.

POACHED SABLEFISH SALAD WITH LEMON-OREGANO VINAIGRETTE

Makes 4 to 6 servings
Time: 1 hour

One 1-pound or slightly larger sablefish fillet, skin off
8 cups Court Bouillon (page 41), any fish stock (pages 40–41), or 7 ½ cups water mixed with ½ cup white or wine vinegar, 1 chopped onion, and several sprigs fresh parsley
Salt and freshly ground black pepper to taste
2 large ripe tomatoes, cut into chunks
8 cups washed, dried, and torn mixed greens
Lemon-oregano Vinaigrette (page 254)

Put the sablefish in a large skillet with the cold liquid and salt the liquid if it was not salted previously. Bring the liquid to a boil, then turn it off. Let the fillet rest for 20 minutes or so; it will be cooked. Drain the sablefish and dry it with paper towels (reserve the stock for another use). Season with salt and pepper, then flake it into a bowl. Toss with the tomatoes, greens, and about ½ cup vinaigrette. Taste for seasoning, add more dressing if you like, and serve immediately.

ALTERNATIVE FISH FOR THIS RECIPE:
Salmon or sturgeon. Adjust cooking times accordingly.

SMOKED SABLEFISH

Makes 8 appetizer servings
Time: 3 days, mostly unattended

Sake kasu, the lees of sake making, is available in one-pound packages in many Asian grocery stores. You need about half a package for this recipe, but the remainder can be frozen indefinitely. Alternatively, see the simpler variation.

One 2-pound sablefish fillet, skin on
2 tablespoons salt
2 tablespoons sugar
3 sheets sake kasu
1 cup dry white or rice wine
¼ cup mirin (Japanese sweet wine) or honey

Place the fillet on a baking dish or platter skin side down. Sprinkle with the salt and sugar, cover with plastic wrap, and refrigerate for about 24 hours. From time to time, pour off any liquid that accumulates. Rinse the fish and the platter briefly and dry them both.

Puree the sake kasu along with the wine and mirin in a food processor or blender. Smear this mixture all over the fish and return it to the platter. Cover and refrigerate 2 more days.

Rinse the fish again and smoke according to either of the methods on page 30. It will flake but still be quite moist when done. Serve cold over greens, flaked into a salad, or on sandwiches with cream cheese.

ALTERNATIVE FISH FOR THIS RECIPE:
Bluefish, mackerel (if you can get large fillets), salmon, or sturgeon. Adjust cooking times accordingly.

TEA-SMOKED SABLEFISH:
Omit the sake-kasu marinade entirely and smoke the fish indoors, using the recipe on page 31, after the salt-and-sugar cure. Add 1 cup tea leaves (preferably Lapsang souchong) and 1 cup white rice to the bottom of the smoking vessel. The results will be excellent.

SALMON

Latin name(s): *Salmo salar* (Atlantic), *Oncorhynchus* species (Pacific).
Common names: Atlantic salmon; five species of Pacific: Chinook (also called king), chum (dog), coho (silver), pink (humpback), and sockeye (red, or blueback).
Common forms: Whole fish (usually three to five pounds), fillets (up to two pounds), and (commonly) steaks.
General description: Pale pink to orange to red flesh that stays moist as long as it is not overcooked; one of the truly great fish. Skin is exceptionally delicious; smokes and freezes well.
For other recipes see: Char and trout, both of which are in the salmon family. Salmon is an unusual fish and not easily substituted for.
Buying tips: See text below. Note, too, that not all salmon is scaled before sale; if you intend to eat the skin (and, usually, you will), ask the fishmonger to scale the fish, or do it yourself (see page 19).

Like most fish, salmon was once strictly seasonal; if you wanted to eat it in the winter months, you bought a can. Now, however, farm-raised fish is available year-round, and new freezing techniques have reduced the amount of Pacific salmon destined for cans and given us top-grade frozen salmon in months when the fresh product is unavailable. You should be able to find good salmon any day of the year, at a reasonable price. The harvest period for Alaskan salmon, which comprises about 95 percent of the Pacific salmon sold in this country, peaks in midsummer. But since the catch numbers in the hundreds of millions of fish, much of it is frozen and sold throughout the year. Farm-raised production has no peak, but it does slack off a bit in the summer months.

Despite the abundance of relatively inexpensive salmon, it's not always easy to make a sound decision about what you're buying. This is due, in large part, to perplexing retail practices. Many fish markets and restaurants sell "Norwegian" salmon as if it were a distinct species. That is not the case: Farm-raised salmon from Norway, like most farm-raised salmon, is Atlantic salmon, the only species of salmon living in the Atlantic ocean. Because it is an endangered species, there is no wild Atlantic salmon for sale; it's all farm-raised, from the Pacific Northwest, Maine and the Atlantic Maritimes, Norway, Chile, and elsewhere.

What confuses the issue is that there are also five species of wild Pacific salmon. Most East Coast chefs, and probably consumers, prefer the flavor, fat content, and pinkish orange color of Atlantic salmon, though this may be more the result of habit than culinary logic. Farm-raised Atlantic salmon is rich and fatty; it actually looks marbled. But the best Pacific salmon, especially king and sockeye, can sport the same richness along with a pronounced, wilder flavor. At a tasting I ran comparing the five species of wild salmon to two types of Atlantic, West Coast people preferred the lean wild sockeye; Easterners liked the fatty Atlantic.

Buying Pacific salmon is a challenge, especially in supermarkets. The same purveyors who insist that their farm-raised salmon is Norwegian will tell you that their Alaskan salmon is "king." But king salmon (also called chinook) accounts for a mere 1 percent of the total Alaskan catch. This large (up to forty pounds), prized, fatty fish winds up in many prestigious West Coast restaurants when the season begins in late winter. But precious little makes its way East. West Coast salmon lovers refer to kings by the rivers in which they spawn. As salmon leave the ocean they are laden with fat; since they stop feeding when they enter their rivers, those with the longest trips to make are the fattest. A Yukon River king, then, with more than two thousand miles to travel before spawning, is considered a real prize, one which few East Coast dwellers will ever see.

The sockeye, sometimes called red salmon, has the darkest flesh of all species, and its flavor rivals that of king (many, including me, prefer it). Once almost exclusively canned, much of the sockeye catch is now shipped, frozen, to Japan, where it is in great demand. The balance is sold fresh, in season, and frozen for shipment throughout the country; even frozen, sockeye is worth looking for.

Coho is a Pacific species which is farm-raised in Chile and elsewhere. It may be grown to just under ten pounds, as is much Atlantic salmon. Wild coho is available fresh in the fall.

Chum salmon has a reputation far below that of sockeye and king, but chum, with bright silver skin and deep orange flesh, can be delicious. It freezes well, and is in supermarkets year-round, fresh or frozen, often at rock-bottom prices—as little as three dollars a pound for steaks.

Finally, there is pink salmon, the least valuable species, most of which is canned or frozen. Although it is occasionally sold fresh or frozen in supermarkets (sometimes for a dollar a pound in the West), its dry, sometimes bitter flesh makes it best suited for salmon croquettes and similar preparations.

Given all these choices, what is the best salmon for any given recipe? Usually, there are several. The first choice to make, as always, is the one of quality. If fresh or thawed salmon looks suspect—the flesh dry, the skin lacking sheen, the smell slightly off—consider choosing still-frozen product.

Next, give the pairing some thought. For simple preparations, such as Salmon Roasted in Butter (page 235), you should start with the most beautiful fillet you can find, preferably one of sockeye, king, or farm-raised Atlantic. (Not finding a farm-raised fish to my liking recently, I made this dish with a frozen sockeye fillet and was delighted by the results.) With dishes of more complexity, such as Salmon Fillets in Red Wine (page 233), chum or coho can be added to the list. If you're grilling or broiling, farm-raised fish is the best choice because its high fat content makes it difficult to overcook. And, for smoking (page 31), choose king or farm-raised salmon.

As with many dark-fleshed fish, the cooking time for salmon varies according to your taste. (Of course raw salmon, when perfectly fresh, is delicious.) I prefer my salmon cooked to what might be called medium-rare to medium, with a well-cooked exterior and a nearly raw center. Cold poached salmon is especially delicious when under-done. Remember that fish steaks and whole fish retain enough heat to continue cooking after they're removed from the heat source, so stop cooking just before the fish reaches the desired state of doneness.

MARINATED GRILLED SALMON

Makes 4 to 6 servings
Time: 90 minutes
Make sure the salmon used for these cubes has its skin on (make equally sure that it has been scaled; see page 19). The skin not only protects the fish, it helps it to retain its shape and integrity; further-more, salmon skin is delicious. The marriage of fla-

vors here is ideal; you can substitute other fish for salmon, but the taste will not be the same.

⅓ cup high-quality soy sauce
1 teaspoon grated lemon rind
¼ cup fresh lemon juice
2 tablespoons olive oil
2 cloves garlic, minced
2 teaspoons Dijon mustard
2 teaspoons sesame oil
1 tablespoon minced fresh herbs: parsley, basil, rosemary, thyme
2 pounds salmon fillets, preferably from the middle of the fish, skin on
Assorted vegetables for grilling, such as red bell pepper, red onion, zucchini or summer squash, and/or mushrooms

Whisk together all the ingredients except the fish and vegetables; taste and correct the seasoning (it should be pungent, salty, rich, and delicious).

Cut the salmon into 1 ½- to 2-inch cubes (the center cuts should be about that thick; if there are thinner portions of the fillet, cut them into large rectangles). Skewer the fish if desired. Marinate for about 1 hour, refrigerated if the weather is warm. Cut up the vegetables and skewer if desired; marinate with the fish for as long as possible.

The fish and vegetables can be grilled on skewers, in a basket, or—the most convenient method—on skewers in a basket. The salmon will take about 8 to 10 minutes to cook over high heat (its interior should be rare); some vegetables, especially raw onions, can take a little longer, so you may want to cook them first (I usually grill the vegetables and put them on the table before beginning the salmon).

ALTERNATIVE FISH FOR THIS RECIPE:

Any very firm-fleshed fish—mako shark, monkfish, swordfish, or tuna—large enough to cut into chunks and skewer.

CRISPY SKIN SALMON WITH GINGERY GREENS

Makes 4 servings
Time: 40 minutes

The skin of most fish is neutral, the skin of some inedible. The skin of salmon, however, is a delicacy. (You can even sauté it, without the fish, and enjoy it by itself.) For the best chance of keeping the salmon skin whole, oil it liberally, make the grill grate very hot, and don't move the fish until it's done. Incidentally, gardeners beset by collards and kale will love this dish, but so will everyone who appreciates the rich flavor of salmon, cut by sharp greens sparked with ginger. Steam the greens well in advance if it's more convenient for you.

One 2-pound salmon fillet, skin on
1 pound kale, collards, or other dark greens (can be a combination)
5 tablespoons olive oil
1 teaspoon minced garlic
1 teaspoon peeled and grated fresh ginger
1 tablespoon high-quality soy sauce
1 teaspoon sesame oil

Rinse the fish well, remove any of the large "pin bones" that run down the center of the fillet (use a needlenose pliers as illustrated on page 229), and let it rest between paper towels, refrigerated, while you prepare the greens.

Wash the greens in several changes of water, and steam them in an inch of water brought to a boil until good and soft, 20 minutes or more. Drain, rinse in cool water, squeeze dry, and chop.

Preheat a covered gas grill or start a charcoal fire in a grill that can be covered. Heat 2 tablespoons of the olive oil in a 10-inch nonstick sauté pan. Add the garlic and cook, stirring occasionally, 1 minute; do not brown. Add the greens and cook, stirring occasionally, for about 3 minutes; add the ginger and cook another minute, then add the soy sauce

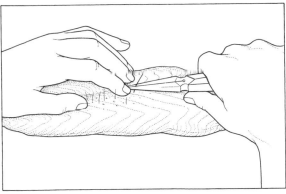

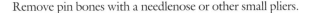

Remove pin bones with a needlenose or other small pliers.

and sesame oil and turn off the heat. Remove to a platter and keep warm.

With a sharp knife, score the skin of the salmon in a crosshatch pattern. Oil the fish well with the remaining olive oil. Put the fillet on the preheated grill, skin side down, and cover. Cook, undisturbed, until done (use a thin-bladed knife to check the salmon's interior; it is done before it becomes completely opaque), 5 to 8 minutes. Remove carefully with a large spatula, and place atop the greens. Serve immediately, making sure everyone gets a piece of skin.

SALMON STEAKS WITH CHIVE-TARRAGON SAUCE

Makes 4 servings
Time: 20 minutes
Butter sauces need not contain a lot of butter, nor need they be especially complicated. Here's a dazzling salmon recipe that is almost as easy as throwing a couple of steaks on the grill.

1 tablespoon olive oil
4 salmon steaks, ½ pound each
Salt and freshly ground black pepper to taste

½ cup dry white wine
⅓ cup minced fresh chives
3 sprigs fresh tarragon
2 tablespoons butter
2 fresh meaty plum tomatoes, seeded and minced
½ lemon
Several whole fresh chives for garnish

Preheat a 10- or 12-inch nonstick pan over medium-high heat until it is quite hot, about 5 minutes. Preheat the oven to about 200°F. Add the oil, turn the heat to high, and cook the steaks 3 to 4 minutes per side, depending on their thickness; season them as they cook. They should be nicely browned, but not cooked through. Remove the steaks to a platter and place the platter in the oven.

Add the wine, reduce the heat slightly, and let it bubble away for 1 minute or so. Add the herbs and butter and stir. When the butter has melted, add the tomatoes and cook another 30 seconds. Taste for seasoning; if the sauce is flat after you've added salt and pepper, add a few drops of lemon juice. Spoon the sauce over the salmon steaks and garnish with chives.

ALTERNATIVE FISH FOR THIS RECIPE: Swordfish.

PAN-GRILLED SALMON FILLETS
WITH LENTILS

Makes 4 servings
Time: 45 minutes

If you ever doubted the value of nonstick pans, try this recipe. The salmon cooks perfectly without the benefit of any fat (if you're on a strict low-fat diet, eliminate the olive oil from the lentils).

2 to 3 cups dried whole green lentils
2 medium-size carrots, diced into ¼-inch cubes
1 small potato, peeled and diced into ¼-inch cubes
1 medium-size onion, diced
2 cloves garlic, minced
A bouquet garni of fresh parsley, thyme, bay leaf, and chives, wrapped in cheesecloth for easy removal
Salt and freshly ground black pepper to taste
2 tablespoons extra virgin olive oil
Coarse salt
4 center-cut salmon fillets, about ½ pound each, skin on (but scaled) or off
Minced fresh parsley or chives for garnish

Rinse and pick over the lentils, then place in a large saucepan with water to cover. Simmer over medium heat until they begin to soften, 15 to 20 minutes, then add the carrots, potato, onion, garlic, and bouquet garni. Continue to cook, adding water if necessary (keep this to a minimum), until the lentils and vegetables are tender, 45 to 60 minutes total. Remove the herbs, season with salt and pepper, add the olive oil, and keep warm.

Heat a 12-inch nonstick skillet over high heat for about 5 minutes. Sprinkle the bottom of the skillet with coarse salt, then add the salmon, skin side down. Cook over high heat until well browned on the bottom, about 5 minutes. Flip the salmon and cook 1 additional minute (more if you

like your salmon well done). Place about a cup of lentils in the center of each of four serving plates and top with a salmon fillet. Garnish and serve immediately.

SMOKY SALMON WITH LIME
MAYONNAISE

Makes 4 to 6 servings
Time: About 60 minutes

Smoking fish can be done on top of the stove or in a covered grill. Since the fish cooks fairly quickly in either case, I prefer the grill method, which yields a subtler flavor, but you could certainly use the stove (in either case, see the general guidelines for smoking fish, page 30). Since this dish is best cold or at room temperature, it can be prepared as much as a day in advance. Crispy Skin Salmon (page 228) is also good with this mayonnaise.

2 salmon fillets, about 1 pound each, skin on
2 tablespoons olive oil
1 teaspoon Dijon mustard
1 small shallot
1 teaspoon minced fresh tarragon, dill, chervil, or parsley, or a combination
Juice of 1 lime
Salt and freshly ground black pepper
1 large egg
1 cup oil—olive, peanut, vegetable, or a combination
⅓ cup sour cream

Prepare a grill or stovetop pan for smoking according to the directions on page 30.

Scale the salmon if necessary (page 19). Rinse and dry the fillets, then rub the skin side with the olive oil. When the wood is smoldering, place the fillets on the grill, skin side down, away from the source of heat. Cover the grill and cook until the salmon is done, 15 to 30 minutes (use a thin-bladed knife to peek into the thickest part of the fillet; salmon should not be completely opaque when fully cooked).

Using a wide spatula, remove the fillets to a serving platter (some of the skin will undoubtedly stay behind, but in this instance it is no great loss) and let cool. Refrigerate if you will not be eating the fish within an hour or two.

To make the mayonnaise, put the mustard, shallot, herbs, lime juice, salt, pepper, egg, and 1 tablespoon of the oil in a food processor or blender. Process for about 10 seconds, then slowly add the remainder of the oil in a very thin stream. The mayonnaise is done when all the oil is added and it is creamy thick. Taste for seasoning and mix in the sour cream; you will have about 1 ⅓ cups. (Mayonnaise keeps, refrigerated, for 1 week or longer.) Refrigerate until ready to serve, then pass along with the salmon.

SALMON SCALLOPS WITH GARLIC CONFIT

Makes 4 servings
Time: 60 minutes
This is the kind of dish you'd pay a small fortune for in a restaurant, yet it's quite simple and very impressive. If you can't get fresh basil because it's January and the herbs are more expensive than the fish, don't worry about it—the dish is almost as good without it.

2 whole heads garlic
1 cup extra virgin olive oil
1 teaspoon salt plus salt to taste
½ teaspoon freshly ground black pepper plus pepper to taste
8 to 10 sprigs fresh thyme or 1 teaspoon dried

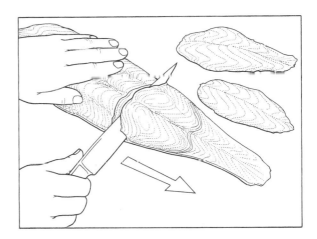

Cut salmon into scallops by cutting thin slices almost parallel to the surface of the fillet.

2 salmon fillets, about 1 pound each, or one 2-pound fillet, skin on
10 leaves fresh basil (omit rather than substitute dried)
1 teaspoon fresh lemon juice

Peel the garlic (this is the most difficult part of the recipe), lightly crushing the cloves to make it easier to remove the skin. Combine them with the olive oil in a small saucepan over very low heat, and add the teaspoon of salt, the ½ teaspoon of black pepper, and the thyme. Simmer as slowly as possible until the garlic is soft and lightly browned, about 30 minutes.

Meanwhile, cut 8 to 10 scallops from the salmon fillets (see illustration above). (You may be left with a fair amount of meat on the skin; use it for Galette of Salmon and Potatoes, page 232.) Sprinkle them with salt and pepper.

When the garlic is done, pour off most of the oil (reserve it; you'll use a little in the next step, and find ways to use the rest within days). Puree the garlic with 5 of the basil leaves.

Place a 12-inch nonstick skillet over high heat

and add 1 to 2 teaspoons of the garlic oil. Cook the scallops for 1 minute per side—no more—keeping them warm in a low oven until they're all done. Cut the remaining basil leaves into strips—not quite minced. Divide the scallops among four plates, and spread each with 1 teaspoon or so of the garlic puree and a few drops of lemon juice. Garnish with the basil strips and serve.

ALTERNATIVE FISH FOR THIS RECIPE:

Sturgeon, swordfish, or tuna (use steaks and increase the cooking time).

GALETTE OF SALMON AND POTATOES

Makes 4 servings
Time: 40 minutes

Although you can make this hashlike dish from salmon leftovers, I always do it when I have accumulated a number salmon skeletons from making gravlax (page 237) or from cutting my own scallops (page 244). In that case, simmer or microwave the skeletons until they are barely cooked, just enough to release the meat from the bone. When you cook the galette, you can add an egg for a more cakelike consistency; I prefer the pure crunch of this flaky pie.

2 cups grated peeled potatoes
1 tablespoon salt plus salt to taste
2 cups flaked cooked salmon
2 tablespoons minced fresh basil or 1 teaspoon minced fresh thyme or rosemary
Freshly ground black pepper to taste
2 tablespoons butter
2 tablespoons olive oil

Put the grated potatoes in a colander and sprinkle them with the tablespoon of salt. Let them sit for about 15 minutes, tossing and squeezing occasionally. Meanwhile, combine the salmon, basil, pep-per, and a little more salt. Heat a 12-inch nonstick skillet over medium heat for 5 minutes or so.

Put the potatoes in a kitchen towel and squeeze out as much remaining moisture as possible. Combine them with the salmon. Melt 1 tablespoon of the butter along with 1 tablespoon of the olive oil in the skillet. Keeping the heat on medium, add the salmon-potato mixture and flatten out into a cake.

Cook for 10 minutes, then slide the galette onto a large plate and cover with another plate of equal size. Add the remaining olive oil and all but a bit of the remaining butter to the skillet; when the butter melts, invert the plates and slide the galette back into the skillet. Cook another 10 minutes, then slide onto a serving plate. Gild with the remaining bit of butter. Serve immediately, keep warm in a 200°F oven for up to 1 hour, or serve at room temperature.

ALTERNATIVE FISH FOR THIS RECIPE:

The galette will work with almost anything, but nothing will give it as much flavor as salmon. My second choice is cod or another mild, white-fleshed fish.

SALMON CROQUETTES

Makes 4 servings
Time: 20 minutes, using leftovers

Cooking whole salmon often results in leftovers; this is the ideal use for them. If you don't want to pan-fry these croquettes, you can broil or even grill them. Keep them 6 to 8 inches away from the heat source to avoid burning. If you've only made croquettes from canned salmon, you're in for a treat when you make these.

1 to 2 cups leftover salmon meat
1 to 2 cups leftover mashed potatoes
½ to 1 cup minced onion or scallion, both green and white parts

¼ cup minced fresh parsley
1 teaspoon peeled and minced fresh ginger or
  garlic (optional)
1 or 2 large eggs
1 teaspoon Dijon mustard
Salt and freshly ground black pepper to taste
Unseasoned bread crumbs for dredging
½ cup olive oil
Lemon wedges

Combine the first eight ingredients; add enough
bread crumbs to make the mixture stiff and not too
wet. Shape into small cakes; dredge in bread
crumbs, then dry on a rack for 15 to 30 minutes.
Heat the oil in a large skillet over medium-high
heat. When the oil begins to shimmer, raise the
heat to high and add as many croquettes as will
comfortably fit in the pan. Cook until browned on
both sides, adjusting the heat so the patties brown
but do not burn. You may need to do this in several batches. Serve with lemon wedges.

ALTERNATIVE FISH FOR THIS RECIPE:
Char or trout.

SALMON FILLETS IN RED WINE

Makes 4 servings
Time: 30 minutes
This is a great recipe in which to use leaner, less
expensive chum salmon, since the fish retains its
moisture. Serve it with crusty bread or crisp potatoes.

2 tablespoons butter
1 tablespoon olive or vegetable oil
4 skinned salmon fillets, about 6 ounces each,
  of roughly the same thickness
Flour for dredging
Salt and freshly ground black pepper to taste
1 medium-size onion, diced

2 cloves garlic, minced
1 medium-size carrot, cut into ¼-inch dice
½ cup minced fresh parsley
¼ cup any fish or chicken stock (pages 40–41)
  or water
1 cup dry, full-bodied red wine, such as Bor-
  deaux or Cabernet, Barolo, or Rioja

Heat a 12-inch nonstick skillet over medium-high
heat. Add the butter and oil, turn the heat to high,
and wait for the butter foam to subside. Quickly
dredge each of the fillets in the flour, shaking off
the excess, and place them, flesh side down (not the
side that originally had skin) in the skillet. Season
with salt and pepper, brown them quickly, remove
them from the pan to a plate (flesh side up now),
and keep warm in a low oven.

With the heat on medium, add the onion, garlic,
and carrot to the pan and cook, stirring, until the
onions soften slightly. Add half the parsley and
some salt and pepper and stir. Add the stock, raise
the heat to high, and reduce until it is almost evaporated. Add the wine and reduce by about half.
Return the fillets to the pan, skinned side down,
and cook over medium heat until the fillets reach
the desired degree of doneness (peek inside with a
thin-bladed knife), about 3 to 5 minutes. Sprinkle
with the remaining parsley and serve immediately.

ALTERNATIVE FISH FOR THIS RECIPE:
Bluefish, mackerel, or pompano.

STIR-FRIED SALMON WITH ASPARAGUS AND BLACK BEANS

Makes 4 servings
Time: 20 minutes

1 ½ pounds not-too-thin asparagus (½-inch diameter or more at bottom)
1 tablespoon fermented black beans (available in Asian food stores)
2 tablespoons dry sherry
2 tablespoons peanut oil
1 tablespoon peeled and minced fresh ginger
2 cloves garlic, peeled and crushed
¼ cup minced scallions, both green and white parts
One 1- to 1 ½-pound salmon fillet, skin removed and cut into 1-inch cubes
⅓ cup scallions, both green and white parts, cut into 2-inch lengths
1 tablespoon high-quality soy sauce
Salt to taste

Peel the asparagus. Microwave or parboil it for about 3 minutes, until it is no longer crisp. Cut off the tips and cut the stems into 1-inch lengths. Soak the black beans in the sherry.

Heat 1 tablespoon of the oil over high heat in a wok or 12-inch nonstick skillet (I prefer the latter). Brown the asparagus stems stirring, frequently. Remove them with a slotted spoon.

Add the remaining oil, then the ginger, garlic, and minced scallions. Cook 1 minute, stirring. Add the salmon and cook it, turning and shaking the skillet or wok until the salmon browns a bit, 3 to 5 minutes. Add the black beans and sherry, the cut-up scallions, the soy sauce, and the asparagus tips. Cook to blend the flavors; taste for seasoning and add salt if necessary. Serve immediately over rice.

ALTERNATIVE FISH FOR THIS RECIPE:
Chunks of mako shark, monkfish, sturgeon, or swordfish.

BAKED SALMON FILLET WITH BUTTERED ALMONDS

Makes 4 to 6 servings
Time: 30 minutes

It's fine to leave the scales on the fillet for this preparation; you'll just be scooping the meat off the skin to serve the fish anyway.

1 tablespoon vegetable oil
3 tablespoons butter
1 cup blanched slivered almonds
Salt and freshly ground black pepper to taste
One 1 ½- to 2-pound salmon fillet (one whole side), skin on

Preheat the oven to 450°F. When the oven is hot, add the oil to a baking dish large enough to hold the salmon (you can cut the fillet in half if you need to). Heat the baking dish for 5 minutes or so. Meanwhile, melt the butter over medium heat in a small saucepan, add the almonds, and season with salt. Cook, stirring, until some of the almonds brown.

Remove the baking dish from the oven and put the salmon in it, skin side down. Season with salt and pepper; spoon the browned almonds on top. Place the fish in the oven and set the timer for 10 minutes. Check for doneness—this dish is best on the rare side—and serve immediately.

ALTERNATIVE FISH FOR THIS RECIPE:
Char or trout.

SALMON ROASTED IN BUTTER

Makes 4 to 6 servings
Time: 15 minutes

If you make this with the most flavorful, beautiful fillet you can find—such as Alaskan sockeye in season, or a lovely side of farm-raised salmon—you will be stunned at the richness of flavor. There is nothing simpler, and few things better.

One 2- to 3-pound salmon fillet, skin on (but scaled) or off
¼ cup (½ stick) butter
Salt and freshly ground black pepper to taste
Minced fresh parsley for garnish

Preheat the oven to 475°F. Melt the butter in a roasting pan—either on top of the stove or in the oven as it preheats—until the foam subsides. Place the salmon in the butter, flesh side down, and put the pan in the oven. Roast about 5 minutes, then turn and roast 3 to 6 minutes longer, until the salmon is done (peek between the flakes with a thin-bladed knife). Sprinkle with salt, pepper, and parsley and serve immediately.

SALMON ROASTED WITH CILANTRO "PESTO"

Makes 4 servings
Time: 30 minutes

1 clove garlic
1 cup loosely packed cilantro (fresh coriander) leaves
3 tablespoons olive oil
Juice of 1 lime
Salt and freshly ground black pepper to taste
One 2- to 3-pound salmon fillet, skin on
1 large ripe tomato, seeded and coarsely chopped

Preheat the oven to 400°F. Place the garlic, cilantro, 2 tablespoons of the olive oil, the lime juice, salt, and pepper in a blender or food processor. Process until creamy. Brush a baking pan or sheet with the remaining oil and place the salmon in it. Spread the cilantro mixture on the salmon, scatter the tomato over it, and sprinkle with a little more salt and pepper. Bake, uncovered, until the salmon is done (peek in between the layers of flesh with a thin-bladed knife), 12 to 15 minutes. Serve immediately.

ALTERNATIVE FISH FOR THIS RECIPE:
Because the pesto is strong-flavored, I'd prepare this only with strong-flavored fish, such as bluefish, bonito, mackerel, or pompano.

SALMON FILLETS EN PAPILLOTE

Makes 4 servings
Time: 30 to 40 minutes

This is a master recipe than can be used with any fillet you like. For more suggestions about cooking en papillote, see page 211; for variations, see Red Snapper Fillets en Papillote, page 288.

2 medium-size ripe tomatoes, each cut into 4 slices
½ cup minced fresh basil
1 cup cooked chick-peas (canned are fine)
4 skinless salmon fillets, ⅓ to ½ pound each, all roughly the same shape
2 tablespoons fruity olive oil
2 teaspoons balsamic vinegar
Salt and freshly ground black pepper to taste

Preheat the oven to 400°F. Tear four sheets of aluminum foil, each slightly longer than a foot. On one sheet, place a thick slice of tomato, a sprinkling of basil, a few chick-peas, a piece of salmon, some more basil and chick-peas, and another slice of tomato. Drizzle with a quarter of the olive oil and vinegar and season with salt and pepper. Close up the package, leaving as much air inside as possible. Repeat this for each of the fillets.

Place the packages on a cookie sheet or baking pan and bake until the tomatoes are slightly lique-fied and the salmon is done (you will have to open one of the packages to check doneness), 15 to 20 minutes. Serve immediately, letting the diners open the packages on their plates.

ALTERNATIVE FISH FOR THIS RECIPE:

Fillets of any fish at all; adjust cooking times according to thickness and density of flesh (flatfish fillets will be done in less than 10 minutes; striped bass may take 30 to 40).

COLD POACHED SALMON WITH GARLICKY GREEN MAYONNAISE

Makes 4 to 6 servings
Time: 30 minutes, plus time to cool
Much fish poaching is done in court bouillon—too much, in my view. For although court bouillon adds a wonderful flavor to milder fish, a meaty cut of salmon needs no such help. Poached in salty water using a foolproof, easy technique, it is deli-cious on its own. Serve this dish on a hot summer day when Alaska salmon is cheap and plentiful (try to get sockeye or king) with boiled new potatoes and barely blanched green beans.

One 2- to 3-pound cut of salmon, preferably tail end, skin on
5 heaping tablespoons salt
1 teaspoon any good vinegar
Salt and freshly ground black pepper to taste
1 large egg
¼ cup chopped fresh chives
2 sprigs fresh tarragon
½ cup chopped fresh parsley

1 medium-size clove fresh peeled garlic or to taste
1 cup olive oil
1 tablespoon sour cream

Place the salmon in a pot large enough to hold it, then cover with cold water. Add the salt and bring to a boil. Turn off the heat immediately and let the salmon sit in the hot water for about 30 minutes. This results in a moist fish that is not overdone. Remove the fish from the water and chill.

To make the mayonnaise, put the vinegar, salt, pepper, egg, chives, tarragon, parsley, garlic, and 1 tablespoon of the oil in a food processor or blender. Process for about 10 seconds, then slowly add the remainder of the oil in a very thin stream. The mayonnaise is done when all the oil is added and it is creamy thick; there will be about 1 cup. Taste for seasoning and mix in the sour cream. Refrigerate until ready to serve. (Mayonnaise keeps, refrigerated, for 1 week or longer.)

To serve the salmon, insert the tine of a fork under the skin at the midline of each side of the fish, then run it lengthwise, splitting the skin. The skin will then peel off easily. Take the salmon off the bone in the kitchen or at the table, using a spoon and following the natural contours of the fish.

ALTERNATIVE FISH FOR THIS RECIPE:

If you can get a large cut of cod, red snapper, striped bass, or tilefish, you can follow the same directions as those given here. The taste, of course, will be different.

SALT-AND-SUGAR CURED SALMON
(Gravlax)
....

Makes 12 or more appetizer servings
Time: 20 minutes, plus 3 days to cure
Lovely, impressive, and superbly fragrant, gravlax is also among the simplest cured dishes. Use king or sockeye salmon when they're in season, Atlantic farm-raised salmon from a good source otherwise. In either case, the fish must be spanking fresh.

One 3- to 4-pound salmon, weighed after cleaning and beheading, skin on
3 tablespoons salt
2 tablespoons sugar
1 teaspoon freshly ground black pepper
1 good-size bunch dill, roughly chopped, stems and all
1 tablespoon spirits: brandy, gin, aquavit, lemon vodka, etc.

Fillet the salmon (page 23) or have the fishmonger fillet it for you; the fish need not be scaled. Lay both halves, skin side down, on a plate. Sprinkle with the salt, sugar, and pepper, spread the dill over them, and splash on the spirits. Sandwich the fillets together, tail to tail, then wrap tightly in plastic wrap. Cover the sandwich with another plate and something that weighs about a pound—an unopened can of coffee or beans, for example. Refrigerate.

Open the package every 12 to 24 hours and baste, inside and out, with the accumulated juices. On the second or third day, when the flesh has lost its translucence, slice thinly as you would smoked salmon—on the bias and without the skin—and serve with rye bread or pumpernickel, lemon wedges and, if you like, the Garlicky Green Mayonnaise on page 236.

ALTERNATIVE FISH FOR THIS RECIPE:
Gravlax is a curing method than can be applied to almost any fish. I like it most with highly flavored fish, such as bluefish or mackerel.

SAUTÉED AND MARINATED SALMON
(Escabèche)
....

Makes 12 appetizer servings
Time: 30 minutes, plus marinating time
You can find recipes for preparing almost any fish imaginable this way. To me, however, it's absurd to smother a subtle white fish in such a flavorful marinade. Salmon, I believe, is ideal; bluefish, mackerel, pompano, and other dark-fleshed fish are also wonderful prepared in this traditional Spanish manner.

½ cup olive oil
2 medium-size carrots, diced
2 large onions, sliced
1 jalapeño, stems and seeds removed and minced (or cayenne pepper to taste)
5 cloves garlic, sliced (not minced)
3 bay leaves
3 sprigs fresh thyme or ½ teaspoon dried
Salt and lots of freshly ground black pepper
½ cup red wine
½ cup water
½ cup red wine vinegar
One 3- to 4-pound skinned salmon fillet or 2 or 3 smaller ones
1 tablespoon chili powder or more, according to its strength and your taste
Flour for dredging
Minced cilantro (fresh coriander) for garnish
1 orange, sliced
1 lime, sliced
1 lemon, sliced

Heat ¼ cup of the oil in a 12-inch skillet over medium heat, then add the carrots and onions. Cook, stirring to prevent browning, until the onions soften, 5 to 10 minutes. Add the jalapeño, garlic, bay leaves, and thyme, and cook 5 minutes more, stirring frequently. Add the salt and pepper, wine, water, and vinegar. Simmer over medium heat about 2 minutes; cover and keep warm over the lowest flame possible.

If you have a large piece of salmon, cut it into two or three pieces so it is more convenient to sauté. Heat a large nonstick skillet over medium-high heat while you prepare the fish. Rinse and dry it, then rub it all over with the chili powder. Add the remaining oil to the pan. When it is hot (a pinch of flour will sizzle) dredge the salmon in the flour and cook it over high heat (in batches if necessary) until lightly browned, about 3 minutes per side.

Remove the salmon to a deep platter and pour the warm marinade over it. Let cool to room temperature, cover, and refrigerate for 12 to 24 hours, or longer (the fish will retain its flavor and quality for 3 days, no more). To serve, remove the fish from the marinade and garnish it with the cilantro and citrus slices.

ALTERNATIVE FISH FOR THIS RECIPE:
See headnote.

SARDINE

Latin name(s): *Sardinella anchovia*.
Other common names: Sprat, Spanish sardine, pilchard.
Common forms: Whole (also, of course, canned).
General description: Small, silvery fish with rich, delicious dark flesh.
For other recipes see: Anchovy, bluefish, mackerel, pompano, smelt.
Buying tips: Like anchovies, fresh sardines become rancid pretty quickly, and begin to smell as they deteriorate. Look for relatively firm, unbruised fish with shiny skin and bright eyes.

"For most people," writes Alan Davidson, "sardines are canned sardines." True enough, and most unfortunate, since fresh sardines are a great pleasure. Canned sardines from the United States and Canada are actually Atlantic herring (*Clupea herengus herengus*); from Norway they are the sprat (*C. strattus*). The classic American canning sardine, which is the Pacific or California sardine (*Sardinops sagax*), seems to be nearly extinct, perhaps not surprising since it was canned at the rate of about a billion pounds a year through the 1930s.

None of these is the fresh sardine that shows up in our markets from time to time. Which is good, because the fish that is most commonly sold fresh—the Atlantic or Spanish sardine—is the best for cooking fresh, and especially for broiling (or "grilling," as the Europeans say; see recipes, page 240).

Like all oily fish, sardines should be iced immediately after catch and eaten as soon as possible.

MARINATED SARDINES WITH ENDIVE

Makes 4 to 6 appetizer servings
Time: 30 minutes, plus a few hours to marinate

24 small sardines, each about 4 inches long
2 tablespoons olive oil
Salt to taste
Fresh lemon juice or sherry vinegar as needed
1 tablespoon minced garlic (optional)
Endive leaves, rinsed and dried

To bone the sardines, snap off the heads by grasping the body just behind the head and pulling down on the head. Most of the innards will come out with the head. Run your thumb along the belly flap, tearing the fish open all the way to the tail and removing any remaining innards. Then grab the backbone between your thumb and forefinger and gently pull it out. This is easier than it sounds; stay with it and after five fish you'll be an expert; see the illustrations. As you finish each fish, drop it into a bowl of ice water.

Rinse the fish and dry them with paper towels. Place them in a shallow bowl, sprinkle with the olive oil and salt, then add enough lemon juice to

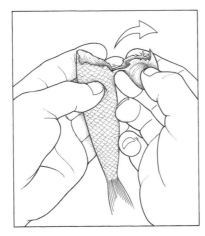 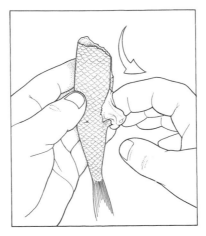 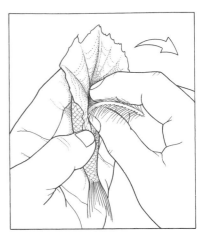

Beheading and boning anchovies (or sardines): Snap off the fish's head and pull straight down. Most of the entrails will come along with it.

Use your fingers to remove any remaining innards.

Grasp the backbone between your thumb and forefinger and gently pull it out of the fish.

barely cover them; add the garlic if you like. Refrigerate for a day or so, gently stirring occasionally. The fish are done when they have turned white, and will keep for several days after that. When ready to serve, lay a fillet on an endive leaf and sprinkle a little of the marinade on each.

ALTERNATIVE FISH FOR THIS RECIPE: Fresh anchovies.

"GRILLED" SARDINES

Makes 2 servings
Time: 15 minutes

These are not grilled, but broiled, as they are throughout Europe, where they are enormously popular as an appetizer, and always referred to as grilled. If you have a grilling basket, you can cook these over hot coals, but the broiler does a wonderful job.

6 to 12 large fresh sardines, a total of about 1 pound, gutted (they may be sold gutted, if not see above), with heads on

Melted butter or olive oil
Salt and freshly ground black pepper to taste
Minced fresh parsley for garnish
Lemon wedges

Preheat the broiler. Brush the fish inside and out with a little butter; sprinkle with salt and pepper. Lay them in a baking dish, side by side. Broil, turning once, about 4 inches from the heat source, until browned on both sides, about 6 minutes total. (Sometimes these fish are too delicate to turn; just finish the cooking on the top side, moving them a little farther from the heat if necessary to prevent burning.) Sprinkle with parsley and serve with lemon wedges.

GRILLED SARDINES WITH HERB OR MUSTARD BUTTER:

Brush very lightly with butter before grilling. Before garnishing, spread with about ½ tablespoon (per fish) of Herb or Mustard Butter (page 44).

GRILLED SARDINES WITH GARLIC SAUCE:

Brush very lightly with butter or oil before grilling. Over low heat cook 1 tablespoon minced garlic in 2 tablespoons melted butter or olive oil, just until softened. Add 2 tablespoons minced fresh parsley, 1 tablespoon fresh lemon juice, and salt and pepper to this mixture. Spoon over the sardines when they are finished.

GRILLED SARDINES WITH TOMATO PESTO:

Mix ½ cup pesto (page 41) with 1 cup minced fresh tomatoes. Brush the sardines very lightly with oil before grilling. Spoon the room-temperature pesto mixture over the hot sardines just before serving.

PAN-STEAMED SARDINES
WITH CILANTRO

Makes 4 servings
Time: 20 minutes
Two cooking techniques and contemporary spicing combine to make a splendid sardine dish.

12 to 24 medium to large sardines, about 2
    pounds, gutted (page 240), with heads on
2 tablespoons olive oil
1 tablespoon minced garlic
Several thin slices peeled fresh ginger
¼ cup fresh lemon juice
¼ cup high-quality soy sauce
½ cup minced cilantro (fresh coriander)
Freshly ground black pepper to taste

Rinse the sardines and dry them well. Heat a 12-inch nonstick skillet (that can later be covered) over medium-high heat for 3 to 4 minutes. Add the olive oil, garlic, and ginger and cook, stirring, until the garlic begins to color. Add the lemon juice, soy sauce, half the cilantro, some pepper, and the sardines. Cover and steam, still over medium-high heat, until the sardines are tender (a fork will meet no resistance), about 5 minutes. Remove the sardines to a platter, reduce the sauce slightly, taste it for seasoning (it may need salt), and spoon it over the fish. Garnish with the remaining cilantro and serve.

ALTERNATIVE FISH FOR THIS RECIPE:

Bluefish, butterfish, eel, mackerel, mullet, or pompano. Adjust the cooking times accordingly.

SPICY PAN-STEAMED SARDINES
WITH THYME:

Follow the recipe above, substituting 2 dried hot red peppers for the ginger, red wine vinegar for the lemon juice, dry red wine for the soy sauce, and 2 teaspoons minced fresh thyme for the cilantro.

STUFFED SARDINES
SICILIAN STYLE

Makes 4 servings
Time: 45 minutes
Between cleaning and stuffing, the preparation for this dish takes some time. But the dish is as good cold or at room temperature as it is hot, so you can prepare it in advance. Besides, it's delicious.

12 to 24 medium to large sardines, about 2
    pounds
½ cup unseasoned bread crumbs
3 tablespoons freshly grated Parmesan or
    pecorino Romano cheese
1 tablespoon chopped fresh herbs in combina-
    tion: parsley, dill, chives, basil, sage
1 teaspoon minced fresh rosemary or ½ tea-
    spoon dried
1 tablespoon minced garlic
Salt and freshly ground black pepper to taste
¼ cup pine nuts
2 tablespoons raisins (optional)
Olive oil as needed, about ½ cup
2 tablespoons fresh lemon juice
Minced fresh parsley for garnish
Lemon wedges

Clean the fish as in Marinated Sardines with Endive (page 239), making certain that the fillets remain attached by the "hinge" of flesh on their back. Mix together the bread crumbs, cheese, herbs, garlic, salt, pepper, pine nuts, and raisins. Moisten with olive oil until the mixture is fairly smooth. Taste the mixture and adjust the seasonings as necessary.

Preheat the oven to 400°F and brush the bottom of a baking pan with a little olive oil. Put a bit of the stuffing into the body cavity of each sardine and fold them along their backs to enclose the stuffing; lay them, side by side, in the baking pan. Sprinkle with a little salt and pepper and drizzle with a little more olive oil and the lemon juice.

Bake until cooked through and tender, about 15 minutes. Garnish with parsley and serve with lemon wedges.

ALTERNATIVE FISH FOR THIS RECIPE: Fresh anchovies or smelts.

ROASTED AND MARINATED SARDINES

Makes 8 to 12 appetizer servings
Time: 30 minutes, plus several hours to marinate
Another escabèchelike dish (see other recipes in the entries for Pompano and Salmon), in which the fish is marinated after cooking, then served cold or at room temperature. These are great with almost any mayonnaise (see Index), or straight from the refrigerator.

12 to 24 medium to large sardines, about 2 pounds, gutted
¼ cup olive oil
2 teaspoons minced fresh thyme
2 bay leaves, crumbled
Salt and freshly ground black pepper to taste
2 cups sliced onions
3 tablespoons minced garlic
1 fresh jalapeño, deveined, seeded, and minced, or dried hot pepper, seeded
¾ cup red or white wine or cider vinegar
Minced fresh mint or parsley for garnish

Preheat the oven to 450°F. Clean the fish as described for Marinated Sardines with Endive (page 239). Spread about 1 tablespoon of the olive oil in a baking pan (preferably nonstick) and lay the sardines on top. Sprinkle them with thyme, bay leaves, salt, and pepper, then drizzle with another tablespoon of olive oil. Roast until the sardines are fork-tender, about 10 minutes.

Meanwhile, heat the remaining oil in a 12-inch skillet. Cook the onions, stirring, over medium heat until soft, then stir in the garlic and jalapeño and cook 1 minute more. Add the vinegar, raise the heat to high, and reduce until syrupy, about 5 minutes. Season with salt and pepper and cool for about 10 minutes.

When the sardines are done, place them on a platter and top them with the onion-vinegar mixture. Marinate in the refrigerator for several hours (or, if you like, several days). Garnish with mint just before serving.

ALTERNATIVE FISH FOR THIS RECIPE: Fresh anchovies, bluefish, mackerel, or pompano. Adjust the cooking times accordingly.

SCALLOPS

Latin name(s): *Placopecten megellanicus* (sea); *Argopecten irradians* (bay); *Aequipecten gibbus* (calico); *Chylmis hericius* (pink).
Other common names: Giant, smooth (sea); cape (bay); southern bay (calico); singing, spiny (pink).
Common forms: Shucked, muscle only (almost exclusively); shucked with roe (rarely); live, in shell (rarely).
General description: The familiar muscle of the fan-shaped scallop shell.
For other recipes see: Clams, cod, crab, dogfish, halibut, lobster, monkfish, mussels, oysters, shrimp, red snapper.
Buying tips: Scallops should not be sitting in liquid, they should show no browning, and they should smell sweet. See below for more.

Many people believe that the creamy and almost translucent scallop offers the most complex flavors and enjoyable texture of any mollusk. In any case, scallops certainly are cooked in more ways than any of their cousins.

Scallops differ in an important way from clams, mussels, and other bivalve mollusks: Because their shells never close completely, whole scallops are especially prone to spoilage, and are therefore almost always shucked immediately after harvest (the relatively rare West Coast pink scallops are the exception; they're often steamed like mussels). To further safeguard against spoilage, the scallop's guts are removed and discarded. What remains is the massive muscle. (It is that muscle, powerful enough to slam the scallop's shells together and expel a jet of water, which the scallop uses for locomotion.) Sometimes the muscle is sold together with the reddish orange roe or pale, creamy milt, both of which are delicious.

Once shucked, scallops are almost never eaten raw. (Having said that, I'll report that the best scallops I've ever had were whole and raw; I caught them myself off Nantucket and ate them immedi-

ately.) They are, however, extremely popular as seviche, in which the cooking is done not by heat but by acidity.

Beyond that, it is not that easy to make generalizations about scallops. The best, depending on your wealth and geographic orientation, are either bay scallops, sea scallops, or pink scallops. The least desirable (and, predictably, the least expensive), are the tiny calicos, not much bigger than pencil erasers and just as rubbery when overcooked.

Here's how the different types of scallops break down:

Sea scallop: Harvested year-round in the North Atlantic, sea scallops range from mild to quite briny. They are best cooked so that their interior remains creamy. Some shells are as big as salad plates, with muscles the size of small dinner rolls; others are the size of a small stack of quarters. Market weight is from a half ounce (thirty per pound) to several ounces.

Bay scallop: Caught between Massachusetts and Long Island in an ever-shrinking area (the only remaining commercial catch is centered around the island of Nantucket), these are the most expensive scallops and, it's generally agreed, the best. Winter is their season. Cork-shaped and about the size of pretzel nuggets, they are slightly darker in color than other scallops, and are very expensive. If you're not paying at least eight dollars a pound—and more likely twelve dollars—you're not buying bay scallops but large calicos, no matter what the sign says. Market weight ranges from fifty to a hundred per pound.

Calico scallop: These are the little scallops that sell for four dollars a pound in supermarkets, referred to above as pencil erasers (they're actually a bit bigger than that). They can be good if they're cooked very quickly, but they're never terrific. Found in warmer waters, off the Atlantic and Gulf coasts, and also in Central and South America, these are shucked by blasting the shells with a hit of steam. Of course this semicooks them as well, further contributing to their already high propensity to become overcooked. Calicos run to two or even three hundred per pound, although larger ones are also harvested (and frequently passed off as bays).

Pink scallop: Calico-size specimens taken in small quantities from the Puget Sound, off the coasts of Washington and British Columbia. Never shucked, they are sold in their pearly pink shells and steamed like mussels. Rarely seen outside of the Northwest.

Many scallops are soaked in phosphates, which—in addition to the obvious objection we have to additives in seafoods—cause them to absorb water, which, needless to say, is less expensive than scallop meat. This is another of those objectionable practices that will only be halted by consumer resistance; as always, buy from someone you trust, and let him or her know that you want unsoaked (sometimes called "dry") scallops.

SCALLOP SEVICHE, VERSION I

Makes 6 to 8 appetizer servings
Time: About 2 hours, mostly unattended

As in all seviches, the acid in the citrus juice "cooks" the scallops, resulting in chemical changes similar to those produced by heat.

1 pound bay or sea scallops
Juice of ½ lime, ½ lemon, and ½ orange
4 scallions, minced, both green and white parts
2 tablespoons chopped cilantro (fresh coriander) or parsley
⅛ teaspoon cayenne pepper
Romaine lettuce leaves, washed

Cut cork-shaped bay scallops in half; cut large sea scallops into chunks or slices. As an optional refinement, you may choose to remove the stark white hinge that attaches the scallop to the shell; it is tougher than the muscle itself.

Combine the scallops with the remaining ingredients (except the lettuce), cover, and refrigerate, stirring now and then. Scallops are "cooked" when they are white throughout, about 2 hours. Serve seviche on a bed of lettuce, which may be used to roll up portions of the fish, fajita style. Or serve with bread or crackers.

ALTERNATIVE FISH FOR THIS RECIPE:
Spanking-fresh fillets of flatfish, mackerel, or sea bass.

SCALLOP SEVICHE, VERSION II

Makes 4 appetizer servings
Time: 15 minutes

This is a fast seviche, similar to one created by Eberhard Mueller when he was at New York's Le Bernardin. Use super-fresh scallops.

½ pound large sea scallops
Juice of 1 large lemon
¼ cup extra virgin olive oil
Salt and freshly ground black pepper to taste
3 tablespoons minced fresh basil

Cut the scallops horizontally into ⅛-inch-thick slices; divide among four plates. Drizzle a quarter of the lemon juice and olive oil over the scallops on each plate, then sprinkle with a little salt and pepper. Top with the basil, let rest 5 minutes, then serve.

ALTERNATIVE FISH FOR THIS RECIPE:

Spanking-fresh fillets of flatfish, mackerel, or sea bass.

GRILLED OR BROILED SCALLOPS AND SHRIMP

Makes 4 to 6 servings
Time: 30 minutes

Nothing fancy is needed here, just a quick brush with five elemental ingredients and a less-than-five-minute grilling time. Peeling the shrimp is an optional step; the peels offer good protection, but removing them at the table is messy work.

Juice of 1 lemon
2 tablespoons olive oil
2 cloves garlic, minced
1 teaspoon coarse salt
½ teaspoon freshly ground black pepper
1 pound large or extra-large (not jumbo) shrimp, peeled and deveined if desired
1 pound large sea scallops

Start a charcoal or wood fire or preheat a gas grill or broiler; the fire should be quite hot. Combine the lemon juice, oil, garlic, salt, and pepper, and toss with the shrimp and scallops (do not marinate—the lemon juice will begin to cook these delicate fish within minutes). Skewer the fish (the scallops should be skewered through their equator rather than their axis, or they may break), or put it in a basket. Grill 2 to 4 inches from the heat source, until just brown. Turn and brown again. Total cooking time should be just about 5 minutes—stop cooking before the scallops' interior becomes opaque.

ALTERNATIVE FISH FOR THIS RECIPE:

Chunks of grouper, lobster, mahi-mahi, monkfish, octopus, squid, or swordfish; whole clams, mussels, oysters, singly or in any combination. Adjust the cooking times accordingly.

GRILLED SCALLOPS WITH BASIL STUFFING

Makes 6 appetizer or 3 main course servings
Time: 1 hour

These are among the most impressive appetizers I know, yet the hardest part is finding good sea scallops and fresh basil. Don't be put off by the time estimate, either; the actual work takes less than 10 minutes.

15 to 20 fresh basil leaves
1 clove garlic, peeled
1 teaspoon salt
¼ teaspoon freshly ground black pepper
2 tablespoons extra virgin olive oil
6 large sea scallops, about 1 pound
½ lemon, cut into 6 pieces

Mince the basil, garlic, salt, and pepper together until very fine, almost a puree (you can do this in a food processor, but it really won't save you time or effort). Mix in a small bowl or cup with 1 tablespoon of the olive oil and let sit 30 minutes or more.

Make a deep horizontal slit in each of the scallops, but don't cut all the way through. Fill each scallop with a bit of the basil mixture; close with a toothpick. Put the scallops on a plate and drizzle with the remaining oil. Preheat a gas grill or start a charcoal fire; it should be very hot before grilling.

Place the scallops on the grill (don't pour the remaining oil over them, as it will catch fire), and grill 2 to 3 minutes per side, no more. Serve immediately, with lemon wedges.

ALTERNATIVE FISH FOR THIS RECIPE: Thick steaks of swordfish or tuna. Cooking time will be considerably longer; see Semeon's Grilled Arugula-stuffed Tuna Steaks, page 330, for details.

ROASTED SEA SCALLOPS
GALICIAN STYLE

Makes 4 servings
Time: 30 minutes
Sea scallops are absolutely essential for this dish; even bay scallops are likely to overcook.

1 medium-size fresh ripe tomato, roughly chopped
1 medium-size onion, minced
2 tablespoons minced fresh parsley
1 teaspoon paprika
1 tablespoon olive oil
Salt and freshly ground black pepper to taste
1 ½ pounds sea scallops

Preheat the oven to 400°F. Mix together all the ingredients except the scallops in a baking dish just large enough to hold the scallops in one layer (alternatively, divide the mixture into four portions and place in large scallop shells). Bake until the juices begin to bubble, about 10 minutes. Mix in

the scallops, return to the oven, and bake just until the scallops are opaque about halfway through, about 10 minutes more, depending on their size. Serve with rice.

ALTERNATIVE FISH FOR THIS RECIPE: Shrimp.

BAKED SCALLOPS WITH
TOMATOES AND PISTOU SAUCE

Makes 4 servings
Time: 25 minutes
Pistou, the Provençal equivalent of pesto, is also basil based, but thinner than the now standard Genovese version. For me, this is a late-summer classic: sea scallops are large and relatively inexpensive, and real tomatoes and fresh herbs are widely available. The herbs in this recipe are interchangeable: Use whatever you can get your hands on, in combination with your judgment.

½ cup loosely packed fresh basil leaves
1 tablespoon minced cilantro (fresh coriander)
2 tablespoons minced fresh parsley
1 tablespoon minced fresh oregano
1 tablespoon minced fresh chives
2 cloves garlic, minced
Salt and freshly ground black pepper to taste
Juice of 1 lime
1 cup olive oil
1 ¼ pounds sea scallops
2 or 3 large, perfectly ripe tomatoes

Preheat the oven to 425°F. Combine the herbs, garlic, salt, pepper, lime juice, and 2 tablespoons of the olive oil in a blender or food processor. Turn on the machine, then add the remainder of the olive oil in a drizzle, as if you were making a mayonnaise (the sauce will remain thin). Taste for salt, lime juice, and garlic, and add more if you like.

Drizzle a few tablespoons of the sauce on the

bottom of a baking pan that will hold the scallops in one layer. Add the scallops and season with salt and pepper. Slice the tomatoes about ¼ inch thick and layer over the scallops; season again. Spoon most of the rest of the sauce over the tomatoes. Bake until the tomatoes begin to liquefy, 10 to 15 minutes. Serve immediately, with crusty bread; pass the remaining sauce at the table.

ALTERNATIVE FISH FOR THIS RECIPE:

Fillets or steaks of blackfish, bluefish, grouper, mackerel, mahi-mahi, mako shark, Atlantic pollock, pompano, striped bass, or swordfish; shrimp. Adjust the cooking times accordingly.

SAUTÉED SEA SCALLOPS
WITH ROE

Makes 4 appetizer servings
Time: Less than 10 minutes

These are very filling, and so rich that you won't want to eat more than one or two. Lemon is essential for cutting the richness; herbs help as well. Overcooking, as with all scallops, is death. When you buy them, the roe should be gleaming and bright, deep orange-red, and the muscle should be glistening.

1 tablespoon extra virgin olive oil
1 teaspoon minced fresh rosemary or ¼ teaspoon dried
4 to 8 sea scallops with roe, depending on size, about ½ pound
Lemon wedges

Heat a 10- or 12-inch nonstick skillet over high heat until quite hot, 3 to 5 minutes. Add the olive oil and, a minute or so later, the rosemary and, one at a time, the scallops. Cook until browned on one side, 2 to 3 minutes, then turn and cook another 2 minutes on the other side. The scallops should still be quite rare—you may prefer them cool—on the inside. Serve immediately, sprinkled with a few drops of lemon juice.

SAUTÉED SCALLOPS,
WITH VARIATIONS

Makes 4 servings
Time: 15 minutes, more or less

It's imperative not to overcook scallops. To avoid doing so in sautés, you must remove the scallops from the pan after an initial browning, then return them for a brief cooking period once you have built a sauce. The basic recipe remains the same; there are four variations here, but the possibilities are just about infinite.

Do not attempt this with the tiny calico scallops, which inevitably overcook and become rubbery.

2 tablespoons olive oil
1 teaspoon minced garlic
1 to 1 ½ pounds large sea scallops
Salt and freshly ground black pepper to taste
Juice of 1 lemon
1 tablespoon minced fresh chives

Heat a 12-inch nonstick skillet over high until almost smoking; add the olive oil, garlic, and, one or two at a time, the scallops. Turn them individually, as they brown, allowing about 2 minutes per side (less for scallops under an inch across, somewhat more for those well over an inch). Season them as they cook; remove them to a bowl as they finish.

Add the lemon juice to the liquid in the pan and cook over medium-high heat until the liquid is reduced to a glaze, 3 to 5 minutes. Return the scallops to the skillet, along with the chives, and stir to coat with the sauce and reheat, 1 to 2 minutes. Serve immediately.

SCALLOPS WITH PERNOD AND TARRAGON:

Use half butter, half olive oil. Begin by cooking the garlic and adding the scallops, as above. Add a sprig of tarragon and ⅓ cup Pernod (or other anise-flavored liqueur such as Raki) for the reduction instead of the lemon juice. Substitute parsley for the chives.

BALSAMIC-GLAZED SCALLOPS:

Use olive or vegetable oil. Begin by cooking the garlic and adding the scallops, as above. Sprinkle the scallops with ¼ teaspoon cayenne pepper as they brown. Use ¼ cup balsamic vinegar for the reduction instead of the lemon juice. Finish with ¼ cup chopped cilantro (fresh coriander) instead of the chives.

GINGER SCALLOPS:

Use peanut or vegetable oil. Cook 1 tablespoon peeled and minced fresh ginger with the garlic. Add 3 scallions, chopped (both green and white parts), to the skillet with the scallops. Use a mixture of 1 tablespoon soy sauce, 1 tablespoon dry sherry, and 2 tablespoons water or chicken or fish stock for the reduction instead of the lemon juice. Finish with the chives.

SCALLOPS WITH BREAD CRUMBS:

Cook as in original recipe (including the garlic). After removing the scallops from the skillet, lower the heat to medium and add 3 tablespoons butter. When the butter foam subsides, add ½ cup fresh bread crumbs. Toss until lightly browned, return the scallops to reheat, and serve, with lemon wedges.

"BLASTED" SCALLOPS WITH CREAMY TOMATO SAUCE

Makes 4 servings
Time: 30 minutes
You don't need fat to cook the scallops in this recipe, but the butter gives the tomato sauce a lovely creaminess; substitute olive oil if you like.

¼ cup (½ stick) butter
1 clove garlic, minced
1 shallot, minced
1 ½ cups chopped tomatoes, canned (drained} or fresh
1 teaspoon sherry or balsamic vinegar
Salt and freshly ground black pepper to taste
1 teaspoon minced fresh tarragon or ½ teaspoon dried
1 pound fairly large sea scallops
1 or 2 tablespoons olive oil
Minced fresh basil for garnish

Melt half the butter in a small saucepan; cook the garlic and shallot, stirring occasionally, over medium heat until softened. Add the tomatoes and cook until they release their juices, about 10 minutes, stirring occasionally. Stir in the vinegar, salt, pepper, tarragon, and the remaining butter. Cool slightly and puree in a blender or food processor; keep warm.

Heat a 12-inch nonstick skillet over high heat until smoking. While it heats, place the scallops on a plate and brush or drizzle them with a little olive oil. Add the scallops, one at a time; turn as they brown, allowing about 2 minutes per side (they should not cook through). Pour a little sauce onto each of four plates and top with the scallops and basil.

ALTERNATIVE FISH FOR THIS RECIPE:

Cod, grouper, haddock, ocean perch, pollock, rockfish, red snapper, tilefish, or wolffish. Adjust cooking times accordingly.

SCALLOP SOUP

Makes 4 servings
Time: 20 to 30 minutes
An adaptation of a subtle, ethereal dish created by my friend Jean-Louis Gerin of Greenwich, Connecticut. Use true bay scallops if at all possible.

3 cups any chicken or fish stock (pages 40–41)

1 medium-size carrot, minced into tiny cubes

1 medium-size zucchini, minced into tiny cubes

1 small leek, white part only, well washed and
  cut into julienne

1 small onion, thinly sliced

2 tablespoons butter

1 tablespoon fresh lemon juice

Salt and freshly ground black pepper to taste

1 ½ pounds bay scallops

Bring the stock to a boil in a large saucepan. Add the carrots and cook until barely tender, about 5 minutes. Add the zucchini and leek and cook about 3 minutes. Add the onion and cook 2 minutes more. Reduce the heat as low as possible and whisk in the butter bit by bit. Season with the lemon juice, salt, and pepper. Add the scallops and any juices from them. Cook 2 minutes, turn off the heat, and serve.

ALTERNATIVE FISH FOR THIS RECIPE:

Freshly shucked littleneck clams or oysters, alone or in combination. Adjust the cooking time accordingly.

SOUP OF BITTER GREENS
WITH SCALLOPS

Makes 4 servings

Time: 30 minutes

The heat of the soup is enough to cook the scallop slices in the bowl.

8 cups any chicken or fish stock (pages 40–41)

Salt to taste

1 teaspoon freshly ground black pepper or to
  taste

1 pound bitter greens: mustard, turnip, watercress, arugula, or whatever is available

1 large onion, chopped

1 tablespoon minced garlic

8 to 12 large sea scallops, cut in half horizontally to make 16 to 24 pieces

½ cup minced cilantro (fresh coriander) leaves

2 fresh jalapeños, deveined, seeded, and minced

2 limes, quartered

Bring the stock to a boil and add the salt and pepper. Wash the greens well and chop them roughly. Add them to the stock, along with the onion and garlic, and cook until the greens are tender, about 3 to 10 minutes depending on their toughness. Add the scallops and immediately ladle into bowls. Garnish with the cilantro; pass the jalapeños and limes at the table.

ALTERNATIVE FISH FOR THIS RECIPE:

Freshly shucked littleneck clams or oysters, alone or in combination. Adjust the cooking time accordingly.

KATE'S PASTA WITH SCALLOPS

Makes 3 to 4 servings

Time: 30 minutes

Here's a recipe designed especially for calico scallops. Take care to keep the cooking time brief, not only to avoid overcooking but to preserve the liquid exuded by the scallops.

¼ cup olive oil plus extra for sprinkling if
  desired

¼ cup (½ stick) butter

1 tablespoon minced garlic

¾ pound calico or other scallops

Salt and freshly ground black pepper to taste

½ cup minced fresh parsley

¼ cup toasted unseasoned bread crumbs

1 pound linguine or spaghetti

Set a large pot of salted water to boil. In a small saucepan, warm the olive oil, butter, and garlic over low heat until the garlic turns pale tan, gently shaking the pan occasionally. Add the scallops, salt, and pepper, and cook just until the surface of the scallops turns opaque. Add half the parsley and the bread crumbs and turn off the heat.

Cook the pasta according the package instructions. When it is just about done, reheat the scallops. Drain the pasta, toss with the sauce, and top with the remaining parsley. Add a sprinkling of olive oil if the dish seems dry.

SPICY SCALLOPS EN PAPILLOTE

Makes 4 servings
Time: 30 minutes
Scallops are great cooked in packages; see the Blackfish, Flatfish, Pompano, Salmon, and Red Snapper entries for other suggestions.

2 large shallots, minced
4 jalapeño or other small hot chiles or to taste, deveined, seeded, and minced
1 tablespoon high-quality soy sauce
1 tablespoon peanut oil
1 cup chopped tomato, fresh or canned (drained if canned)
16 large sea scallops

Preheat the oven to 450°F. Mix together the shallots, chiles, soy sauce, oil, and tomato. Tear four squares of aluminum foil and place four scallops in the center of each piece. Top with the sauce; fold and seal the packages. Bake until the scallops are opaque outside and barely warm in the center, 10 to 15 minutes. Serve the closed packages, allowing each diner to open his or her own at the table.

ALTERNATIVE FISH FOR THIS RECIPE:
Fillets of cod, dogfish, flatfish, haddock, mackerel, mahi-mahi, ocean perch, Pacific pollock, pompano, rockfish, sea bass, red snapper, tilefish, turbot, or weakfish; shrimp. Adjust the cooking times accordingly.

SCALLOP SALAD WITH MIRIN-SOY VINAIGRETTE

Makes 4 to 6 servings
Time: 20 minutes

2 tablespoons mirin (sweet rice wine; available in Asian markets)
2 tablespoons high-quality soy sauce
¼ cup sherry or cider vinegar
½ cup olive oil, plus 2 tablespoons
1 tablespoon minced shallot
4 cups fresh mixed salad greens: radicchio, chicory, lettuce, arugula, etc.
1 medium-size red bell pepper, seeded and cut into rings
1 pound sea scallops, the larger the better
Salt and freshly ground black pepper to taste

Preheat the broiler. Mix together the mirin, soy sauce, vinegar, ½ cup of the olive oil, and the shallot; bring just to a boil, then turn off the heat.

Wash and dry the greens. Heat a 12-inch nonstick ovenproof skillet over high heat until it begins to smoke. Add 1 tablespoon of the olive oil and the pepper rings and cook, stirring, until they wilt and brown slightly, about 2 to 3 minutes. Add the remaining tablespoon of olive oil and place the scallops in the pan, one at a time so as not to lower the heat too suddenly. Season with salt and pepper and cook them until brown on the bottom, then run under the broiler until they are brown on top.

Toss the greens with most of the dressing and place them on four to six plates; top with a portion of scallops and peppers, sprinkle with the remaining dressing, and serve.

STEAMED SCALLOPS WITH VEGETABLES AND LEMON-OREGANO VINAIGRETTE

Makes 4 servings
Time: 30 minutes

1 leek
Several sprigs fresh tarragon or 1 teaspoon
    dried
2 medium-size carrots, cut into rounds
2 medium-size turnips, peeled and diced
2 medium-size potatoes, peeled and diced
12 to 16 large sea scallops, 1 pound or more
½ cup Lemon-oregano Vinaigrette (page 254)

Cut the tough green parts from the leek, then cut the leek into quarters. Wash well, fanning out the leaves to remove all the sand. Cut it into 1-inch sections. Place half the tarragon in the bottom of a steamer in the steaming water and steam the vegetables until they are almost tender, 5 to 10 minutes. Slice the scallops in half (through their equator, not their axis) and place them on top of the vegetables. Steam until the scallops are just opaque, 3 to 5 minutes. Spike the vinaigrette with the remaining tarragon (minced if it is fresh). Serve the scallops and vegetables hot or warm, with a bit of the vinaigrette on top.

SCROD

Latin name(s): None.
Other common names: Schrod.
Common forms: Fillet.
General description: See below.
For recipes see: Cod, haddock, pollock, tilefish, etc.
Buying tips: As for cod.

Scrod is not a fish; in Massachusetts markets the word is used to distinguish among sizes of cod, haddock, cusk, and pollock. But in places where cod is more popular, it might be used to describe haddock; elsewhere, it might be used to describe cod. Or any other white fillet. Basically, the term is meaningless. If the price is right, and the fillet looks good, there's no reason not to buy scrod. Just don't pay a premium thinking you're getting something exceptional; it could be a white fillet of any species.

SEA BASS

Latin name(s): *Centropristis striata* and many others.
Other common names: Black sea bass, blackfish, rock bass, etc.
Common forms: Whole, usually in the one- to three-pound range but sometimes much larger (the giant sea bass of the West Coast can reach five hundred pounds); fillets (rarely precut).
General description: A firm-fleshed fish that is among the best of small fish to cook whole. Delicious skin.
For other recipes see: Butterfish, cod, dogfish, grouper, haddock, ocean perch, pollock, rockfish, red snapper, striped bass, tilefish.
Buying tips: Sea bass is an attractive fish; if it doesn't look lovely at the fish counter, pass it by. The flesh should be distinctively marked, the gills bright red, the fish alive-looking and sweet smelling. Avoid skinned, precut fillets; there's no way to tell if the fish is indeed bass. And, when buying whole sea bass, make sure the upper (dorsal) fin is removed; these are especially sharp and can cause infection.

The word *bass* is common in the fish kingdom. Freshwater bass—largemouth, smallmouth, shoal, redeye, spotted, and others—are the most pursued inland game fish of America (just tune into any fishing program until your eyes start to close). But they are almost never found on restaurant menus, and are even more scarce in fish markets.

Along with striped bass (page 305), sea bass is the most important commercial bass. Although there are many related species, the most commonly seen is the relatively small and quite attractive black sea bass of the North Atlantic. Its firm flesh makes it especially suitable for frying, steaming, broiling, or roasting whole. And its relatively simple bone structure—similar to that of grouper or red snapper—makes it easy to eat.

STEAMED SEA BASS

Makes 2 servings
Time: 20 minutes
The rendered fish juices turn this simple spice paste into a delicious sauce during the steaming process.

2 black sea bass, about 1 pound each, gutted and scaled, with heads on
1 clove garlic, peeled
1 hazelnut-size chunk peeled fresh ginger
1 small onion, peeled
1 tablespoon ground bean paste or hoisin sauce (available in Asian markets)
1 tablespoon fermented black beans (available in Asian markets)
1 tablespoon dry sherry
1 tablespoon high-quality soy sauce
2 scallions, thinly shredded

Score each side of the fish two or three times, from top to bottom, right down to the bone. Place all the remaining ingredients except the scallions into a blender or food processor and puree. Rub this paste into the fish; place the fish on a plate, cover, and refrigerate the fish until ready to cook, up to 4 hours.

Place the fish, still on the plate, in a bamboo or other steamer (see page 38 to learn how to improvise a steamer) and cover. Steam over boiling water, undisturbed, for 10 minutes. Check for doneness (since you scored the fish, you will be able to see clear to the bone and can easily tell if the fish is cooked through); cook an additional 3 to 4 minutes if necessary. Garnish with the scallions and serve immediately, with rice.

ALTERNATIVE FISH FOR THIS RECIPE:

Almost any small whole, firm fish: Butterfish, croaker, flatfish, porgy, red snapper, spot, or tilefish.

GRILLED OR BROILED SEA BASS WITH LEMON-OREGANO VINAIGRETTE

Makes 2 servings
Time: 30 minutes

Black sea bass looks so appealing when grilled or broiled that I find this a good dish to serve to people who think they don't like whole fish. It's quick and very satisfying, since the meat comes off the bones cleanly and with little effort. Use fresh rosemary, thyme, savory, mint, or basil to vary this recipe.

2 black sea bass, about 1 pound each, scaled and
    gutted, with heads on
¼ cup dry white wine or sherry
¼ cup extra virgin olive oil
1 clove garlic, minced
Several sprigs fresh oregano
½ cup olive oil
Juice of 1 lemon
1 tablespoon chopped fresh oregano
1 tablespoon chopped fresh parsley

2 tablespoons minced onion
Salt and freshly ground black pepper to taste

Preheat a gas grill or the broiler, or start a charcoal fire; heat should be medium-hot. Rinse the fish with the wine, and let it sit for a few minutes in a mixture of the wine, extra virgin olive oil, garlic, and sprigs of oregano. Make the vinaigrette by whisking or shaking together the olive oil, most of the lemon juice, the herbs, onion, salt, and pepper. Taste and adjust the seasoning, adding more lemon juice if necessary.

Grill or broil the fish until nicely charred on each side, about 8 to 10 minutes total. If you grill, use a fish basket or move the fish around on the grill to keep it from sticking. (See general grilling directions for whole fish, page 28.) If you broil, baste once or twice with the pan juices. Serve immediately, with the vinaigrette.

ALTERNATIVE FISH FOR THIS RECIPE:
Same as for Steamed Sea Bass, page 253.

GRILLED OR BROILED SEA BASS WITH CITRUS SAUCE

Makes 2 servings
Time: 30 minutes

1 lemon
1 orange
1 grapefruit
½ cup olive oil
1 teaspoon fresh thyme or ½ teaspoon dried
1 clove garlic, minced
1 small onion, minced
Salt and freshly ground black pepper to taste
2 black sea bass, about 1 pound each, scaled and
    gutted, with heads on

Preheat a gas grill or the broiler, or start a charcoal fire; heat should be medium-hot. Zest the lemon and mince the zest; section the lemon, orange, and grapefruit and place the zest and sections in a small saucepan. Stir in the olive oil, thyme, garlic, onion, salt, and a fair amount of pepper. Season the fish, too.

Grill or broil the fish until nicely charred on each side, about 8 to 10 minutes total. If you grill, use a fish basket or move the fish around on the grill to keep it from sticking. (See general grilling directions for whole fish, page 28.) While the fish is cooking, warm the citrus mixture gently; do not boil. When the fish is done, serve immediately with the citrus sauce.

ALTERNATIVE FISH FOR THIS RECIPE:
Same as for Steamed Sea Bass, page 253.

CRISPY SEA BASS WITH GARLIC-GINGER SAUCE

Makes 2 servings
Time: 30 minutes
You can serve these fish on a bed of plain white rice if you like.

¾ cup vegetable oil, more or less
2 black sea bass, each about 1 pound, gutted and scaled, with heads on
2 tablespoons peanut oil
1 tablespoon minced garlic
1 teaspoon peeled and minced fresh ginger
1 tablespoon high-quality soy sauce
1 teaspoon sesame oil
Minced cilantro (fresh coriander) for garnish (optional)

Heat a 12-inch nonstick skillet over medium-high heat for about 5 minutes. Add the vegetable oil to a depth of ¼ of an inch, more or less. When the oil shimmers, put the fish in it. Cook, undisturbed, for about 8 minutes. Turn carefully.

As the fish is cooking, in another pan heat the peanut oil over medium heat. Add the garlic and ginger and cook, stirring, until the garlic begins to color. Add the soy sauce and sesame oil and keep warm.

Cook the fish 8 to 10 minutes on the second side. Remove them carefully to two plates, drizzle with the sauce, and sprinkle with the chopped cilantro. Serve immediately.

ALTERNATIVE FISH FOR THIS RECIPE:
Same as for Steamed Sea Bass, page 253.

RAW SEA BASS SALAD

Makes 6 first course servings
Time: 20 minutes
Like the recipe for Raw Flatfish Salad on page 132, this variation on seviche can be made with almost any fish, as long as you are sure it's perfectly fresh. The fish does not quite cook through here, but does lose its rawness.

1 pound sea bass fillets
Juice of 2 lemons
1 small onion, minced
2 tablespoons flavorful olive oil
Salt and freshly ground black pepper to taste
Minced fresh parsley for garnish

Using a fillet knife, slice the fillets into scallops, as thin as possible (see page 231, cutting salmon fillets into scallops, for an illustration). Mix them in a bowl with about half the lemon juice, then arrange on a plate. Sprinkle the onion over the fish, then sprinkle the remaining lemon juice, the olive oil, salt, and pepper over all. Allow to sit about 10 minutes, garnish with the parsley, and serve.

ROASTED SEA BASS

Makes 4 servings
Time: 1 hour

A basic recipe that can be used for almost any small to medium-size whole fish.

One 3- to 4-pound sea bass, or 2 smaller ones, scaled and gutted, preferably with heads on
2 tablespoons olive oil
2 tablespoons fresh lemon juice
1 bay leaf
Several sprigs fresh thyme or 1 teaspoon dried
½ cup minced fresh parsley
1 teaspoon minced garlic
Salt and freshly ground black pepper to taste

Score each side of the fish two or three times, from top to bottom, right down to the bone. Mix together all the other ingredients and marinate the fish in it, refrigerated, for 30 to 60 minutes. Preheat the oven to 450°F.

Roast the fish, undisturbed, in a lightly greased baking dish until done, 20 to 30 minutes, depending on size. Check for doneness (since you scored the fish, you will be able to see clear to the bone and can easily tell if the fish is cooked through); cook an additional few minutes if necessary. Serve with the pan juices.

ALTERNATIVE FISH FOR THIS RECIPE:
Same as for Steamed Sea Bass, page 253.

ROASTED SEA BASS WITH FENNEL:
Add some fennel seeds to the marinade. Slice and blanch (for about 2 minutes) 1 fennel bulb. Layer the fennel with tomato slices before adding the fish to the roasting pan. Stuff the fish with a little minced parsley, any remaining marinade, and a few fennel tops. Roast the fish for 15 minutes, then add 1 cup fish stock (page 40) or dry white wine. Serve the fish with the vegetables and sauce spooned over it.

SHAD

Latin name(s): *Alosa sapidissima* and others.
Other common names: Ohio shad, Gulf shad, Atlantic shad, etc., poor man's salmon.
Common forms: Whole fish, with or without roe; roe only; fillets.
General description: A three- to five-pound fish (some run larger) that, like salmon, swims into our rivers each spring. The egg sac (roe) of the female is the foie gras of the fish world.
For other recipes see: Blackfish, bluefish, carp, cod, grouper, mackerel, ocean perch, pompano, rockfish, salmon, red snapper, striped bass, swordfish.
Buying tips: Whole fish are *very* bony; see below. Fillets should be true fillets—run your finger along the bone lines if the fishmonger will allow you to. Roe, usually a fairly bright orange, should be moist; ideally, you'll see the fishmonger take it from a fish for you; you may have to buy the whole fish for this to happen, but it's worth it. All parts of the fish should be sweet-smelling; a whiff of mud is not bad.

The Indian myth about shad has it that the fish began existence as an unhappy porcupine. When it complained, the great spirit turned it inside out and cast it into the water. This served to explain the curse of the shad, often considered the world's boniest good-eating fish. In some ways, its boniness has probably saved shad from the fate of the Atlantic salmon, which nearly became extinct from overfishing; because it is difficult to eat whole, shad was never as popular.

The meat of this five-pound fish, however—which is native to the Atlantic but was introduced on the West Coast in the nineteenth century—is nearly as delicious (that's what its species name, *sapidissima*, means) as that of salmon, and it can be filleted by a skilled knife-wielder. Note the word skilled, though; it takes me an hour to fillet a shad, and the result is not especially pleasant to look at. The best shad-boner I ever met told me I gave up too easily: "If you practiced on a few fish a day for six weeks, you could do it perfectly," he said. I suppose I did give up too easily. If you can buy shad fillets—real fillets, that is, with all of the bones removed, not just some, as seems to happen these days—do so. It's a delicious fish.

There is a traditional theory that maintains that long baking softens the shad's bones to the point of edibility. This theory also stresses the importance of sorrel in baked preparations; the acidic herb is said to further break down the bones. I have tried this many times, and it is nonsense. If you cook a shad for long enough, the meat becomes so dry that it sticks in your throat, along with the bones. As for the sorrel, its acidity does make a nice counterpoint to the richness of shad, but its effectiveness is questionable.

Now, to the roe. Once the roe (and milt, the male organs) of many fish—cod, herring, and salmon, for example—were eaten routinely. Many of these are delicious, but we no more savor them than we do calves' brains or pigs' feet. The exception is caviar, the salted roe of sturgeon (which I don't consider in this book because it is already prepared when you buy it, and because the real thing costs thirty dollars an ounce), and shad roe, which is sublime.

When cooked properly, that is. One fine spring day, I walked into a friend's house and he announced we were having shad roe for lunch, making me ecstatic. He then proceeded to cook it in butter for thirty minutes, making me depressed. If you want to eat sand, go to the beach; if you want to appreciate shad roe, please leave it pink in the center. All you need to know about enjoying shad roe is buy it fresh and keep the cooking time short; overcooking results in tough, individual eggs.

CLASSIC SHAD ROE

Makes 2 servings
Time: 10 minutes
There's nothing easier than this, and few things as satisfying. As with most fish, the key is freshness—if you can see the fishmonger take the roe from a nice-looking fish, so much the better. And, at all costs, avoid overcooking.

¼ cup (½ stick) butter (you can use half this amount if you want to), cut into chunks
1 pair shad roe, about 6 ounces
Salt and freshly ground black pepper to taste
Lemon wedges

Preheat a 10-inch skillet pan over medium heat for 3 to 4 minutes. Add the butter and let it melt. When the foam subsides, add the roe and cook until lightly browned, 3 to 4 minutes. Turn and brown the other side. Sprinkle with salt and pepper and serve immediately, with lemon wedges.

SHAD ROE WITH GARLIC BUTTER:
Dredge the roe lightly in flour, shaking to remove the excess, before cooking. When it's cooked, remove it from the pan and keep warm. Add 2 more tablespoons butter to the skillet, then 1 teaspoon minced garlic. Cook, stirring occasionally, over medium heat until the garlic softens, then add 2 tablespoons fresh lemon juice and 2 tablespoons minced fresh parsley. Spoon this mixture over the roe and serve.

SHAD ROE WITH CAPERS AND BALSAMIC VINEGAR

Makes 2 servings
Time: 10 minutes
A simple twist on the basic roe recipe; this is about as elaborate as I would ever want to get with shad roe, which needs little help in the flavor department.

2 tablespoons olive oil
1 pair shad roe, about 6 ounces
Salt and freshly ground black pepper to taste
½ cup red wine
1 tablespoon butter
1 tablespoon capers, drained
1 tablespoon balsamic vinegar

Preheat the oven to 300°F. Heat a small nonstick skillet over high heat until almost smoking. Add the olive oil and, a minute later, the roe. Sear over high heat for 2 minutes per side, seasoning with salt and pepper as it cooks. Remove to a plate; put the plate in the oven. Add the wine to the pan and reduce to 2 tablespoons, stirring to get up any browned bits. Lower the heat to a minimum and gently swirl or stir in the butter; stir and cook until the sauce is smooth. Add the capers and vinegar and cook to blend the flavors, about 1 minute. Check the seasoning (remember capers are salty), pour the sauce over the roe, and serve immediately.

BROILED SHAD FILLET

Makes 4 servings
Time: 15 minutes

Because shad is so fatty, simple treatment is best (although this never stopped anyone from serving it with bacon or butter; see the variations). I prefer it this way.

2 shad fillets, ¾ to 1 pound each
Salt and freshly ground black pepper to taste
1 tablespoon capers
½ lemon, cut in half

Preheat the broiler. Place the shad, skin side down, on a rack in a baking pan and sprinkle with salt and pepper. Broil without turning about 6 inches from the heat source, until the top is lightly browned and the fish is cooked through, about 6 minutes (peek between the flakes with a thin-bladed knife to check for doneness; there should be the barest trace of rawness in the center). Sprinkle with the capers and serve with lemon.

ALTERNATIVE FISH FOR THIS RECIPE:

Bluefish, mackerel, pompano, salmon, or sword-fish. Adjust the cooking times accordingly.

SHAD FILLETS WITH BACON:

Lay 3 or 4 strips of bacon on top of the shad and broil as directed above. (Traditionally, you would broil a pair of roe alongside the fillet; they will need less cooking time.) Sprinkle with minced fresh parsley rather than capers.

SHAD FILLETS WITH BUTTER:

Cook ¼ cup (½ stick) butter slowly over low heat until it turns nut brown. Drizzle some of this butter over the fillet before broiling, and the remainder after the fillet is done. Sprinkle with minced fresh parsley in addition to the capers; a few pieces of diced raw tomato is also nice.

SHAD FILLETS WITH VINAIGRETTE:

Brush the fillets with about ½ cup of Basic Vinaigrette (page 43) before and during broiling.

SHRIMP

Latin name(s): Several genuses (there are literally thousands of species worldwide), the most important of which is *Peneaus*.
Other common names: Prawns, rock, white, black tiger, red, etc. shrimp.
Common forms: Head-on, head-off, shell-on, shell-off, cooked. Almost always previously frozen.
General description: The single most important shellfish in the world.
For other recipes see: Cod, conch, crab, crayfish, lobster, mako shark, monkfish, octopus, rockfish, scallop, red snapper, squid, tilefish, wolffish.
Buying tips: See Buying Shrimp, page 261.

Americans eat more shrimp than any other fresh or frozen seafood; only canned tuna is a more popular fish. Yet although buying shrimp offers a myriad of choices, most of us give no more thought to buying ten-dollar-a-pound shrimp than to two-dollar-a-pound tuna.

This was understandable half a century ago, when the choices were limited: Almost all shrimp was local, or was iced and shipped by rail or truck, to be sold within days of the catch. But improved freezing technology made fresh shrimp rare, and now it is safe to say that any shrimp you buy has been frozen and thawed by the retailer or chef. There are certainly exceptions to that rule, but they're not nearly as common as many fishmongers and restaurateurs would have you believe.

That doesn't mean that all shrimp are the same; far from it. The South ships about as much shrimp to the rest of the country as it ever did—about 200 million pounds in 1992—but three times that amount is imported, mostly from Asia and Central and South America. And there are other important differences: About 80 percent of all imported shrimp is farm-raised, while virtually all of the domestic catch is wild. For my money, the best shrimp is Gulf white, especially when it's fresh. But I don't wait around for it, because it isn't easy to find.

Both farm-raised and wild shrimp can be rich, flavorful, and firm, or insipid, bitter, and mushy. Some farm-raised shrimp are raised on high-protein pellets not unlike those fed to aquacultured salmon, but others live in sealed bays, where they get their nutrients from seawater. And, since the population is high and the diet not as dense, there are times when these are downright watery.

Many chefs simply buy the best shrimp available, and that's what you should do, too. I think it makes sense to buy frozen shrimp rather than those that have been thawed. Since only 2 percent of the shrimp sold in this country are fresh, (and much of that is eaten within fifty miles of the water from which it was taken), and since the shelf life of previously frozen shrimp is not much more than a couple of days, buying thawed shrimp gives you neither the flavor of fresh nor the flexibility of frozen. Stored in the freezer, however, shrimp retain their quality for several weeks.

Most frozen shrimp are sold in blocks of five pounds (or two kilos, slightly less than that), and should be defrosted in the refrigerator or in cold water. Defrosting in a warm place or microwave robs shrimp—or anything else, for that matter—of moisture, nutrients, and even weight (in the industry, this is called "drip loss"). Partial defrosting to cut a block in half in order to freeze some for later use, while not ideal, is still preferable to buying thawed shrimp.

Another strategy, routinely practiced by chefs and retailers, is to return shrimp that are mushy or smack of iodine. Cook a couple as soon as you get home. If you buy shrimp in a frozen block, soak it in cold water until you can remove a shrimp or two from the edges for sampling; then return the block—either to the freezer, if it's good, or to the store, if it isn't.

Several other tactics can help you make the most of your shrimp: Avoid prepeeled and deveined shrimp; cleaning before freezing may deprive shrimp of some of their flavor and texture. Processors may compensate for this by using tripolyphosphate, an additive that aids in water retention.

If your palate is sensitive to iodine—not everyone's is—you might also want to steer clear of brown shrimp, especially large ones, which are most likely to taste of this naturally occurring mineral. The iodine is found in a type of plankton which makes up a large part of the diet of brown shrimp.

You can also improve the flavor and texture of almost any shrimp by brining them slightly: Stir 1 cup salt and ½ cup sugar into 2 cups boiling water until dissolved; pour the mixture into a large bowl filled with ice and water, and add up to 2 pounds shrimp. Let the shrimp sit in the brine, refrigerated (or adding ice occasionally) for 2 hours or so. Rinse the shrimp well. A 30-minute marinade in olive oil and garlic, an unceremonious dump on a hot grill, and you have yourself a feast. Remember shrimp cook in as little as three minutes; when they're pink, they're done.

Finally, there are the questions of peeling and deveining. To the first question—should the shell be removed before cooking?—I answer, "Sometimes." I remove the shell if I'm serving a dish where the shrimp will be served in hot liquid. I leave it on if I'm poaching the shrimp for later use, or if I'm grilling it, in which case I want the protection it gives the meat. Peeling at the table obviously demands a certain level of informality that is almost always part of dinners at my house but may not be at yours. It's really a judgment call, but the shell does have good flavor, and if you cook the shrimp with it on you gain from that. (Shrimp shells also make excellent stock, as in Stir-Fried Shrimp with Garlic and Green Beans, page 264.)

The next question: Deveining. I never bother to devein shrimp unless I'm butterflying it, in which case deveining is unavoidable. There's no harm in it, of course. But do you remove the intestine from a lobster before you eat it? Do you separate the viscera when you're chowing down on a quart of steamers or mussels? I doubt it.

BUYING SHRIMP

There are few rules governing the sale of shrimp. Small, medium, large, extra-large, jumbo, and other size classifications are subjective and relative. Small shrimp of seventy or so to the pound are frequently labeled "medium," as are those twice that size and even larger. So learn to judge shrimp size by the number it takes to make a pound, as retailers do. Shrimp labeled "16/20," for example, require sixteen to twenty (usually closer to twenty) individual specimens to make a pound. Those labeled "U-20" require fewer (under) twenty to make a pound. Shrimp of from fifteen or twenty to about thirty per pound usually give the best combination of flavor, ease (peeling tiny shrimp is a nuisance), and value (really big shrimp usually cost more than ten dollars a pound).

Shrimp should have no black spots, or

melanosis, on their shell, which indicates a breakdown of the meat has begun. Be equally suspicious of shrimp with yellowing shells, or those that feel gritty, either of which may indicate the use of sodium bisulfite, a bleaching agent sometimes used to remove melanosis. Shrimp should smell of saltwater and little else and, when thawed, should be firm and fill the shell fully.

There are three hundred species of shrimp worldwide, but six are most commonly found in our markets:

Gulf White (Panaeus setiferus): Certainly the most expensive shrimp, and frequently the best. Good flavor, firm texture. May be wild or farm-raised. Usually grayish white in color, these are similar in appearance to the less desirable Gulf brown shrimp, so be careful. Ask to see the box, which may be of some help.

Ecuadorean or Mexican White (P. vannamei): Similar to Gulf whites, these may be wild (as are most Mexicans) or farm-raised (more Ecuadorean shrimp, all of which is farm-raised, is imported to the United States than any other).

Black Tiger (P. monodon): Widely farmed shrimp from Asia. May be dark gray with black stripes and red feelers or bluish with yellow feelers; when cooked, they are pink. Inconsistent but frequently quite flavorful and firm.

Gulf Pink (P. duorarum): Another high-quality shrimp, wild or farm-raised. Shell is usually redder than that of whites, but may be light brown.

Gulf Brown (P. aztecus): The wild shrimp most likely to taste of iodine, these tend to be reddish brown, but can easily be confused with whites or pinks.

Chinese White (P. chinensis): Asian farm-raised shrimp with grayish white color, soft, sometimes watery texture, and mild flavor. Usually relatively inexpensive. Benefits greatly from brining treatment described above.

Rock shrimp (Sicyonia brevirostris): These are caught off the mid-Atlantic and southern states and in the Gulf of Mexico. Good-tasting, but very hard to peel, they are usually sold peeled and frequently cooked.

SPICY GRILLED SHRIMP

Makes 4 servings
Time: 20 minutes
Be forewarned: This is the kind of dish that makes people eat more than they should. Make extra; I always do.

2 pounds large shrimp
1 large clove garlic
1 tablespoon coarse salt
½ teaspoon cayenne pepper
1 teaspoon paprika
2 tablespoons olive oil
2 teaspoons fresh lemon juice
Lemon wedges

Peel the shrimp (you can butterfly them if you like; just cut along the line of the vein, a little deeper than usual). Mince the garlic with the salt; mix it with the cayenne and paprika, then make it into a paste with the olive oil and lemon juice. Smear the paste all over the shrimp. Start a charcoal or gas grill or preheat the broiler; the fire can be as hot as you like. Grill or broil the shrimp, 2 to 3 minutes per side. Serve immediately or at room temperature, with lemon wedges.

ALTERNATIVE FISH FOR THIS RECIPE:
Crayfish.

GRILLED SHRIMP WITH PASTA AND FRESH TOMATOES

Makes 4 servings
Time: 45 minutes

1 pound large to extra-large shrimp, about 20, peeled
¾ cup fruity olive oil, more or less
Salt and freshly ground black pepper to taste
2 to 3 tablespoons balsamic or sherry vinegar
1 shallot, minced
1 teaspoon Dijon mustard
4 large ripe tomatoes, cut into chunks
20 leaves fresh basil, roughly chopped
1 pound penne or other cut pasta

Set a large pot of salted water to boil for the pasta; start a charcoal fire or light a gas grill. Brush the shrimp with about ¼ cup of the olive oil; sprinkle them with salt and pepper. Mix together the remaining olive oil, 2 tablespoons of the vinegar, the shallot, and mustard, and season with salt and pepper. Taste and add more vinegar if needed. Set the tomatoes in a large bowl to marinate with the vinaigrette and basil. Grill the shrimp over high heat until they turn pink, about 3 to 4 minutes per side; meanwhile, cook the pasta according to the package instructions. Drain the pasta, toss with the tomatoes, top with the grilled shrimp, and serve.

ALTERNATIVE FISH FOR THIS RECIPE:
Crayfish.

GAMBAS À LA PLANCHA
(Blast-sautéed Shrimp)

Makes 2 to 4 servings
Time: 20 minutes

There are few things simpler or better than the Spanish method for "grilling" shrimp and other seafood.

16 to 20 medium to large shrimp, about 1 pound, peeled
Coarse or kosher salt
¼ lemon

Heat a large skillet, preferably nonstick, over high heat until very hot, about 5 minutes. Sprinkle the bottom of the pan liberally with salt. Place only as many shrimp in the pan as will fit without crowding (you probably will need to do this in two batches; salt the pan again before cooking the second batch). Turn the shrimp after about 2 minutes; cook other side for 1 minute. Sprinkle with a little lemon juice and serve.

ALTERNATIVE FISH FOR THIS RECIPE:
Crayfish or scallops. Adjust the cooking times accordingly.

SCAMPI

Makes 4 servings
Time: 20 minutes

There are more variations on this dish, which is made in every country in southern Europe and, indeed, all over the world, than you can count. I only give one here, but you can make some others by adding anchovies, cayenne, or slivered hot pepper (with the first batch of garlic), and/or wine or lemon juice at the end. All have this in common: lots of olive oil, lots of garlic, salt, pepper, and parsley. And lots of crusty bread.

1 pound or more large shrimp
¾ cup fruity olive oil
2 large cloves garlic, slivered
2 large cloves garlic, minced
¼ cup minced fresh parsley
1 teaspoon salt or to taste
Freshly ground black pepper to taste
1 tablespoon dry sherry (optional)

Peel the shrimp if you like. Warm the olive oil in a large skillet over medium-low heat. Add the slivered garlic and cook gently until it is golden brown, stirring occasionally. Put the shrimp in the pan in one layer, and add the minced garlic. Simmer, undisturbed, for 1 to 2 minutes. When the shrimp are pink on one side, turn them over. Add the parsley, salt, pepper, and sherry, raise the heat slightly, and cook until all the shrimp are pink, about 2 minutes more. Serve immediately.

ALTERNATIVE FISH FOR THIS RECIPE:
Crayfish or scallops. Adjust the cooking times accordingly.

SHRIMP WITH SPICY ORANGE FLAVOR:
Add 2 or more dried hot red peppers and the roughly chopped peel of 1 orange along with the slivered garlic. Add ½ teaspoon ground cumin and the juice of the orange along with the minced garlic. Substitute cilantro (fresh coriander) for the parsley; omit the sherry.

JOHNNY EARLES' "BARBECUED" SHRIMP

Makes 4 servings
Time: 10 minutes
As everyone must know by now, the term "barbecue" legitimately refers only to foods that are slow-cooked by wood heat. The Worcestershire sauce in this dish, however, lends the shrimp a smoky fla-vor. Serve this as an appetizer or main course, with bread or rice. And please don't substitute for the butter here; the dish will just not be the same.

1 pound large shrimp, peeled
Salt to taste
½ cup (1 stick) butter
1 tablespoon Worcestershire sauce
Juice of ½ lemon
Freshly ground black pepper to taste
1 tablespoon water

Sprinkle the shrimp with salt. Melt the butter over medium heat in a large skillet. Add the remaining ingredients and cook, shaking the pan continuously, until the shrimp are cooked, 3 to 5 minutes (they'll all be bright pink). Serve immediately.

ALTERNATIVE FISH FOR THIS RECIPE:
Crayfish.

STIR-FRIED SHRIMP WITH GARLIC AND GREEN BEANS

Makes 4 servings
Time: 30 minutes
This is one instance where you must buy shell-on shrimp; the shells are used to make a quick, wonderful-tasting stock.

1 pound large shrimp, shells on
1 cup water
1 ½ teaspoons sugar
2 tablespoons high-quality soy sauce
1 clove garlic, sliced
1 teaspoon salt
1 tablespoon dry sherry
2 teaspoons sesame oil
¾ pound green beans, trimmed
2 tablespoons peanut oil
2 tablespoons minced garlic

1 tablespoon peeled and minced fresh ginger
¼ teaspoon chili-garlic paste (available in Asian
  markets; optional)
¼ cup minced scallions, both green and white
  parts
Juice of ½ lime

Peel the shrimp and simmer the shells for 5 minutes or so in the water while you work on the rest of the recipe. Marinate the shrimp in a mixture of ½ teaspoon of the sugar, 1 tablespoon of the soy sauce, the sliced garlic, salt, sherry, and 1 teaspoon of the sesame oil while you assemble the other ingredients. Drain the shrimp shells, reserving ¾ cup of the stock.

If the green beans are tough, parboil them for 1 minute or so, then plunge them into ice water. If they are large, cut them into pieces.

When you are ready to cook, preheat a wok or 12-inch nonstick skillet over medium-high heat for 3 to 5 minutes. Add 1 tablespoon of the peanut oil and raise the heat to high. When it begins to smoke, add the minced garlic and, immediately thereafter, the shrimp and its marinade. Cook the shrimp about 1 minute per side. Spoon it out of the wok or skillet.

Put the remaining peanut oil in the wok, still over high heat, and, when it smokes, add the ginger, followed immediately by the green beans. Cook, stirring occasionally, until they are lightly browned, 3 to 5 minutes, then add the shrimp stock and let it bubble away for 1 or 2 minutes. Return the shrimp to the wok and stir; add the chili-garlic paste, the scallions, and the remaining sugar and soy sauce. Stir and cook for 1 minute. Turn off the heat, drizzle with the lime juice and the remaining sesame oil, and serve.

FRIED SHRIMP

Makes 4 servings
Time: 20 minutes

Shrimp are easier to fry at home than most other fish: They cook quickly, don't overcook too easily and, most important, don't spatter. If you prefer, however, you can use this same recipe and sauté the shrimp quickly; they'll be almost as crunchy, you'll use less oil, and cleanup will be easier.

1 ½ to 2 pounds large shrimp
Vegetable oil for deep-frying
Flour for dredging
2 large eggs, beaten
Unseasoned bread crumbs for dredging
Salt to taste
Lemon wedges

Peel the shrimp, leaving the tails on if you like. Butterfly them if you like (just cut halfway through the shrimp, following the vein). Heat the oil to 350°F to 375°F (if your fryer doesn't have a thermostat, or you don't have a frying thermometer, drop a small piece of bread in the oil; it should sink, then rise to the top and begin bubbling away).

Dredge the shrimp in the flour, then shake off the excess. Dip them in the eggs, then in the bread crumbs, patting the bread crumbs on to help them adhere. If there is time, refrigerate them, on a rack, for 30 to 60 minutes. Fry in batches, depending on the size of your fryer (I can do about a pound of shrimp per batch in mine). Drain on paper towels, sprinkle with salt, and serve with lemon wedges.

ALTERNATIVE FISH FOR THIS RECIPE:
Crayfish or scallops. Adjust the cooking times accordingly.

CURRIED SHRIMP, VERSION I

Makes 4 to 6 servings
Time: 45 minutes

This is a good dish for a party, since you can make the sauce hours in advance, then add the shrimp and lemon juice at the last minute. You can also use more potatoes to expand this dish to serve more people.

2 tablespoons peanut or vegetable oil
2 large onions, minced
1 tablespoon curry powder
¼ teaspoon cayenne pepper or to taste
2 tablespoons minced cilantro (fresh coriander)
1 pound small new (or other waxy) potatoes, peeled and halved
2 cups canned or fresh tomatoes, with their liquid
Salt to taste
1 pound medium to large shrimp, peeled and cut into halves or thirds
2 tablespoons fresh lemon juice

Heat the oil over medium heat in a 12-inch skillet. Add the onions and cook, stirring occasionally, until golden. Add the curry powder, cayenne, and half the cilantro and stir. Add the potatoes, tomatoes, and salt, stir, cover, and cook over low heat, stirring occasionally, until the potatoes are tender, about 30 minutes. Add the shrimp and lemon juice and cook, uncovered, until the shrimp turn pink, 3 to 5 minutes. Add the remaining cilantro and serve with white rice.

ALTERNATIVE FISH FOR THIS RECIPE:
    Chunks of monkfish; crayfish, scallops; cut-up squid. Adjust the cooking times accordingly.

CURRIED SHRIMP, VERSION II

Makes 4 servings
Time: 30 minutes

This is an unusual curry, spiked with mint.

2 tablespoons peanut or vegetable oil
1 large onion, chopped
1 medium-size red bell pepper, seeded and chopped
2 cloves garlic, peeled and smashed
Salt and freshly ground black pepper to taste
1 tablespoon fresh mint or 1 teaspoon dried
¼ teaspoon cayenne pepper
1 teaspoon ground cumin
½ cup dried unsweetened shredded coconut
Juice of 1 lemon
Any fish or chicken stock (pages 40–41) or water, as needed
1 pound large shrimp, peeled

In a large, fairly deep skillet, heat the oil over medium heat. Add the onion and red pepper and cook, stirring occasionally, until softened. Add the garlic and salt and pepper and cook, stirring occasionally, 2 to 3 minutes more. Turn off the heat and let cool for a few minutes. Place the mixture in a blender or food processor with the mint, cayenne, cumin, coconut, lemon juice, and enough stock to make a thick liquid when blended. Blend until smooth. Return to the pan, bring to a boil, and reduce the heat to a simmer. Taste and adjust the seasonings as necessary. Add the shrimp and cook until pink, 3 to 5 minutes. Serve immediately, with white rice.

ALTERNATIVE FISH FOR THIS RECIPE:
    Chunks of monkfish; crayfish, scallops; cut-up squid. Adjust the cooking times accordingly.

CURRIED SHRIMP, VERSION III

Makes 6 servings
Time: 30 minutes

This white-sauce-based curry is similar those once found in French restaurants throughout America. It has a classic appeal.

1 cup any fish or chicken stock (pages 40–41) or water
½ cup chopped onion
1 tablespoon turmeric
1 tablespoon peeled and minced fresh ginger
1 teaspoon salt
2 pounds medium to large shrimp, shells on
2 tablespoons peanut or vegetable oil
1 ½ tablespoons all-purpose flour
1 tablespoon curry powder
Salt and freshly ground black pepper to taste
Juice of ½ lemon

Mix the stock, onion, turmeric, ginger, and salt in a medium-size saucepan and bring to a boil. Add the shrimp, stir, cover, and simmer over medium heat until the shrimp turn pink, 3 to 4 minutes. Remove the shrimp with a slotted spoon. Strain and reserve the broth; peel the shrimp.

In a medium-size saucepan, heat the oil over medium heat. Add the flour and stir, cooking until it browns a bit, 3 to 4 minutes. Add the curry powder, stir, and cook an additional minute. Add the shrimp broth a little at a time, stirring after each addition to keep it smooth; the sauce will not become extremely thick, but creamy. Add the shrimp, salt and pepper, and lemon juice. Cook until the shrimp are hot, 2 minutes, and serve immediately, over white rice.

SHRIMP AND BEANS

Makes 4 servings
Time: 60 minutes plus soaking time

These are classic Tuscan beans with shrimp; but you can vary this dish easily by changing the spices or seafood and adding a vegetable or two. I offer two variations here.

2 cups dried white beans: cannelini, navy, pea, Great Northern, etc., picked over
20 fresh sage leaves or 1 tablespoon dried
Freshly ground black pepper to taste
2 teaspoons minced garlic
Salt to taste
1 pound shrimp, peeled and cut into bite-size pieces
2 tablespoons extra virgin olive oil

Cover the beans with 3 inches of water and soak overnight (alternatively, boil for 2 minutes and soak for 2 hours). Drain the beans, transfer them to a pot, and cover with water. Add the sage and pepper and bring to a boil. Reduce the heat to medium and simmer until the beans are tender but not mushy, about 1 hour. Drain the cooking liquid if necessary, then add the garlic, salt, and shrimp. Cook over low heat until the shrimp turn pink, about 5 minutes. Drizzle with the olive oil and serve.

SEAFOOD CASSOULET:

Keep the beans soupy when they are cooked or, if they are dry, add 2 cups fish, shrimp-shell (page 264, Stir-fried Shrimp with Garlic and Green Beans), or chicken stock. For the shrimp, substitute 2 pounds mixed seafood: shrimp, cut-up squid, shucked clams or oysters, cut-up cooked octopus, and/or any white-fleshed fillet. Top with minced fresh parsley.

PASTA AND BEANS WITH SHRIMP:

Add 2 cups chopped fresh or canned tomatoes, with their juice, to the cooked beans. Simmer 10 minutes. When the shrimp is cooked, add ½ pound cooked cut pasta, such as penne, and stir. Add more liquid if necessary—stock or reserved pasta cooking liquid—and serve garnished with the olive oil and minced fresh parsley.

RISOTTO WITH SHRIMP AND GREENS

Makes 4 servings
Time: 45 minutes
This is a basic risotto recipe; you can use it for almost any combination of fish and vegetables that appeals to you.

½ to ¾ pound medium to large shrimp
4 to 6 cups any fish or chicken stock (pages 40–41)
¼ cup olive oil
1 medium-size onion, minced
1 ½ cups arborio or other short-grain rice
Salt and freshly ground black pepper to taste
½ cup dry white wine
3 cups washed, roughly chopped fresh greens, such as arugula, spinach, mustard, collards, or a combination, large stems removed
2 fresh plum tomatoes, seeded and roughly chopped
3 tablespoons butter, softened

Shell the shrimp and simmer the shells in the stock for 10 minutes; strain the stock and keep it warm. Cut each shrimp into two or three pieces.

In a large saucepan or 12-inch skillet (preferably nonstick), heat 2 tablespoons of the oil. Add the onion and cook, stirring occasinally, until it softens. Add the rice and stir until it is coated with oil. Add a little salt and pepper, then the wine. Stir and let it bubble away. Begin to add the stock, a ½ cup or so at a time, stirring after each addition and every minute or so. When the stock is just about evaporated, add more. The mixture should be neither soupy nor dry.

Meanwhile, in another skillet, heat the remaining oil over medium heat. Add the greens and cook, stirring occasionally, until they are limp. When the rice is done—it will take 20 to 30 minutes, and should be slightly al dente—add 1 more ladleful of stock, then the greens, tomatoes, and shrimp. Continue to cook until the shrimp turn pink and the stock is just about evaporated; stir in the butter and serve immediately.

ALTERNATIVE FISH FOR THIS RECIPE:
Chunks of blackfish, catfish, precooked conch, dogfish, eel, grouper, lobster, mahi-mahi, mako shark, monkfish, precooked octopus, squid, swordfish, or tuna; clams, mussels, oysters, or snails. Adjust the cooking times accordingly.

PERLOW

Makes 4 servings
Time: 30 minutes
You might consider this relative of jambalaya to be our indigenous risotto (or pilaf, from which it undoubtedly got its name). When it was first made for me, in northern Florida, I was told that authentic perlow is "damned peppery."

½ pound bacon or fatty leftover ham, chopped
2 medium-size onions, chopped
1 tablespoon minced garlic
1 medium-size red bell pepper, peeled, seeded, and minced
2 cups chopped tomatoes (canned are fine; don't bother to drain)
Salt and freshly ground black pepper to taste
½ teaspoon dried thyme or 1 teaspoon minced fresh
Several drops Tabasco or other red pepper sauce or to taste

1 ½ cups long-grain white rice
2 cups water
1 pound shrimp, shelled and cut into pieces if they are large
Minced fresh parsley for garnish

In a medium-size saucepan, fry the bacon over medium heat until crisp. Remove it with a slotted spoon and drain on paper towels, leaving its fat behind. Cook the onions, stirring, in the fat until softened; add the garlic and red pepper and cook, stirring, until the red pepper begins to soften, 2 to 3 minutes. Add the tomatoes, salt, lots of black pepper, the thyme, and Tabasco. Cook, stirring occasionally, until the tomatoes begin to fall apart, 5 to 10 minutes. Add the rice and water and stir. Bring to a simmer, cover, and cook until the water is just about absorbed, about 15 minutes. Stir in the shrimp, cover again, and cook until the shrimp turn pink, 3 to 5 minutes. Garnish with the reserved bacon and parsley and serve.

ALTERNATIVE FISH FOR THIS RECIPE:
Shucked clams or oysters; crayfish or scallops. Adjust the cooking times accordingly.

SHRIMP SOUP WITH GARLIC

Makes 4 servings
Time: 45 minutes
Wonderful winter food.

12 to 16 large shrimp, about 1 pound, with shells on
8 cups any fish or chicken stock, preferably a rich one (pages 40–41)
¼ cup olive oil
8 cloves garlic, peeled
4 thick slices French or Italian bread
1 teaspoon ground cumin

Salt and freshly ground black pepper to taste
Minced fresh parsley for garnish

Shell the shrimp. Simmer the shells with the stock while you continue with the recipe.

Heat the olive oil over medium heat in a large casserole. Add the garlic and cook, stirring, until it is golden brown. Remove and set aside to cool. Brown the shrimp in the olive oil, 6 to 8 at a time, over medium-high heat. Remove and turn the heat to medium-low. Brown the bread in the oil on both sides; it will take 3 to 4 minutes per side. Remove the slices.

Strain the stock into the casserole and bring to a simmer. Add the cumin, salt, and pepper, and let the flavors mingle for a few minutes over low heat. Chop the garlic coarsely and return it to the pot. Place a quarter of the shrimp and a piece of bread in each of four bowls. Top with some of the broth and garnish with parsley. Serve immediately.

SHRIMP MARINARA

Makes 4 servings
Time: 30 minutes
A tried and true dish, still a favorite in old-style Italian restaurants throughout the country. With fresh herbs, it's a revelation.

2 tablespoons olive oil
1 tablespoon minced garlic
4 cups canned (don't drain them) or fresh tomatoes, chopped
½ cup fresh basil leaves, chopped
1 teaspoon minced fresh oregano or marjoram or ¼ teaspoon dried
½ teaspoon freshly ground black pepper
Salt to taste
1 pound linguine or spaghetti
1 ½ pounds medium to large shrimp, peeled

Start the water for the pasta. In a large skillet, heat the oil over medium-low. Add the garlic and cook, stirring occasionally, until golden. Add the tomatoes, raise the heat to medium-high, and let bubble, stirring occasionally, for about 10 minutes. Add half the basil, the oregano, pepper, and salt. Stir and taste for seasoning. Reduce the heat to medium and let simmer while you cook the pasta.

Just before the pasta is done, add the shrimp to the sauce; cook until the shrimp are firm and pink, about 5 minutes. Remove 3 or 4 shrimp from the sauce and set aside. Drain the pasta, toss with the sauce, and top with the remaining basil and the reserved shrimp. Serve immediately.

ALTERNATIVE FISH FOR THIS RECIPE:
Chunks of blackfish, catfish, precooked conch, dogfish, eel, grouper, lobster, monkfish, precooked octopus, squid, or swordfish; clams, mussels, or oysters. Adjust the cooking times accordingly.

SHRIMP À LA GREQUE

Makes 4 servings
Time: 30 minutes
A standard in the house of my good friend Semeon, who is a great cook. Fast, easy, and great with bread.

6 tablespoons olive oil
1 tablespoon minced garlic
1 ½ cups chopped fresh or canned (drained if canned) tomatoes
½ cup dry white wine
2 tablespoons minced fresh parsley
½ teaspoon crushed dried marjoram or oregano
1 teaspoon salt
Freshly ground black pepper to taste
1 ½ pounds large shrimp, peeled
4 ounces fresh feta cheese, cut into ½-inch cubes

Heat the oil in a 10- or 12-inch skillet over medium heat. Add the garlic, lower the heat to medium-low, and cook, stirring occasionally, until it colors. Add the tomatoes, wine, 1 tablespoon of the parsley, the marjoram, salt, and pepper. Cook over medium-high heat, stirring occasionally, until the sauce is the thickness of a light puree.

Add the shrimp and continue to cook until they turn pink, about 5 minutes. Add the feta and stir very gently, trying to keep the delicate cheese from crumbling too much. Garnish with the remaining parsley and serve immediately.

ALTERNATIVE FISH FOR THIS RECIPE:
Same as for Shrimp Marinara (page 269).

BAKED SHRIMP WITH TOMATOES AND PARSLEYED BREAD CRUMBS

Makes 4 servings
Time: 30 minutes
This simple dish requires some judgment. Ideally, you will have lovely, juicy tomatoes to moisten the bread crumbs. If your tomatoes are dry, you'll have to use a little more butter or fewer bread crumbs.

¼ cup (½ stick) butter, more or less
¾ cup unseasoned bread crumbs (preferably fresh and coarse, but packaged are acceptable)
½ cup minced fresh parsley
2 cloves garlic, minced
Salt and freshly ground black pepper to taste
1 pound medium to large shrimp, peeled
12 thick slices ripe tomato

Preheat the oven to 450°F. Melt about half the butter over medium heat in a 10- or 12-inch nonstick skillet, then toss in the bread crumbs, parsley, and garlic. Cook until the bread crumbs are nicely browned, stirring occasionally, and the mixture is fragrant. Turn off the heat and let it cool a bit.

Spread 1 teaspoon or so of the remaining butter around the bottom of an 8- or 9-inch-square baking dish, then arrange the shrimp in the dish. Cover with about half the bread crumb mixture, then arrange the tomatoes on top. Sprinkle with the remaining bread crumbs and dot with the remaining butter. Bake until the shrimp are pink and hot, 8 to 12 minutes (depending on the size of the shrimp).

ALTERNATIVE FISH FOR THIS RECIPE:

Fillets of blackfish, bluefish, catfish, cod, dogfish, flatfish, grouper, haddock, mackerel, ocean perch, pollock, rockfish, sea bass, red snapper, tilefish, turbot, weakfish, or wolffish; crayfish or scallops. Adjust the cooking times accordingly.

ROAST SHRIMP WITH ORANGE AND TARRAGON

Makes 4 servings
Time: 20 minutes
A less-is-more dish, with a wonderful marriage of flavors.

3 tablespoons flavorful olive oil
4 sprigs fresh tarragon or ½ teaspoon dried
1 to 1 ½ pounds large shrimp, peeled
½ cup fresh orange juice
Zest of 1 orange, finely minced
Salt and freshly ground black pepper to taste

Preheat the oven to 450°F. When it is hot, warm 2 tablespoons of the olive oil in a baking pan on top of the stove, then add the tarragon; return to the oven until the tarragon begins to sizzle. Add the shrimp, then sprinkle with the orange juice and zest, salt, pepper, and the remaining olive oil. Roast until the shrimp turns pink, about 10 minutes.

ALTERNATIVE FISH FOR THIS RECIPE:
Crayfish or scallops.

SHRIMP SALAD ITALIAN STYLE

Makes 3 to 4 servings
Time: 30 minutes
Essential in flavor, this is worlds away from American shrimp salad.

8 cups Flavorful Fish and Vegetable Stock (page 40) or water plus the following 8 ingredients:
Salt and freshly ground black pepper to taste
1 medium-size onion, cut in half but unpeeled
3 cloves garlic, lightly crushed and peeled
1 medium-size carrot, cut into chunks
½ bunch fresh parsley
2 bay leaves
1 tablespoon distilled or other vinegar
½ cup dry white wine
2 pounds medium to large shrimp, shells on
½ bunch fresh parsley, stems removed and minced
Fruity olive oil
Fresh lemon juice
Lemon wedges

Bring the stock to a boil or simmer together the water and the following eight ingredients over medium heat for about 10 minutes. Add the shrimp and simmer until they begin to turn pink, 2 to 3 minutes. Turn off the heat and let the shrimp cool in the water for 10 minutes.

Shell the shrimp (strain and reserve the stock for another use), toss with the minced parsley and a few tablespoons of olive oil, and season with salt and pepper. Add some lemon juice and serve the salad with lemon wedges.

ALTERNATIVE FISH FOR THIS RECIPE:
Same as for Seafood Salad Adriatic Style (page 49).

SHRIMP SALAD WITH CAPERS:
Cook the shrimp as directed above. Mix with 1 small red onion, minced, 1 clove garlic, minced, 2

tablespoons capers, ½ cup minced fresh parsley leaves, ½ cup extra virgin olive oil, fresh lemon juice or any good vinegar, and salt and freshly ground black pepper to taste.

SHRIMP SALAD WITH ARUGULA "PESTO":

Cook the shrimp as directed above. Wash and dry 2 cups arugula and remove any tough stems. Place in a food processor or blender with 1 teaspoon salt, 1 clove garlic, 2 tablespoons walnuts or pine nuts, and ¼ teaspoon freshly ground black pepper. Add ¼ cup olive oil and pulse until minced. With the motor running, add ½ to ¾ cup additional olive oil. Taste for seasoning. Serve the shrimp with tomato wedges and the sauce.

POTTED SHRIMP

Makes 8 servings
Time: 20 minutes, plus time to chill
We all have weaknesses that can't be explained; here's one of mine. It's an English dish, and far from the most important recipe in this book. Nevertheless, I love it. Please try it if you're ever lucky enough to get a batch of fresh shrimp.

1 pound fairly small shrimp, shells on
1 cup (2 sticks) butter
2 teaspoons fresh lemon juice
Pinch freshly grated nutmeg
Pinch ground mace (optional)
¼ teaspoon cayenne pepper
Salt and freshly ground black pepper to taste

Bring a large pot of salted water (seawater is ideal) to a boil. Toss in the shrimp and, 1 minute later, start tasting them; they'll cook very quickly. Drain them immediately and peel when they're cool. Cut them into little bite-size pieces.

Melt ½ cup of the butter over medium heat; stir in the shrimp, lemon juice, nutmeg, mace, cayenne, salt, and pepper, and turn off the heat. Divide the shrimp among small bowls or place in a nice crock.

Melt the remaining butter over very low heat. Skim the foam off the top, then carefully pour the clarified butter over the shrimp, leaving the butter solids in the pan. Refrigerate immediately.

Serve chilled or slightly warmed as a spread (traditionally on brown bread).

ALTERNATIVE FISH FOR THIS RECIPE:

Char, crabmeat, lobster meat, or salmon. Adjust the cooking times accordingly.

SKATE

Latin name(s): *Raja* genus, a score or so of species.
Other common names: Ray, rajafish.
Common forms: Whole (rarely); "wings" only, skinned (best) and unskinned (undesirable).
General description: Relative of the shark with delicious meat. A unique fish unlike any other in form or treatment, skate is usually poached initially, after which it may be cooked in other ways.
For other recipes see: Crab (skate meat can be used in any crabmeat recipe).
Buying tips: There are two: Skate should smell sweet; as with shark, a whiff of ammonia indicates spoilage has begun. Additionally, you should never buy skate with the skin on—it's inedible, and taking it off is almost as challenging as skinning an eel.

There are several kinds of skate, but the only difference that matters to us is size. All have much in common with sharks: tough, inedible skin; a circulation system that makes it important to ice the fish down immediately after capture to prevent the development of ammonia; firm, mild flesh that sits on cartilage rather than bone; and immense popularity in Europe and Asia. But although skate is plentiful off both East and West coasts, it has yet to catch on here—I've seen boatloads destined for New Bedford for processing before being sent to their ultimate destination: Europe. Because domestic demand for skate is low, the fish remains inexpensive, especially when you consider just how good it is.

Many people soak skate in a vinegar-and-water solution before cooking, but this treatment is unnecessary if the skate is fresh and good smelling. (If the smell of ammonia is faint, don't worry about it; it will disappear during cooking. If it's strong, it isn't necessarily a problem, but the fish won't be fun to deal with.)

Each of the skate's two flat, tapered wings (actually pectoral fins) contains two layers of meat separated by one of cartilage. Raw fillets are difficult to come by, although practiced knife-wielders can cut them. And although some people eat the cartilage (moist cooking softens it considerably; it isn't that tough to begin with, and in small fish can be eaten with no trouble), it's best to cook skate wings quickly, then remove the layers of meat from the cartilage before serving what is, in effect, a fillet.

If you chill the fillets, they become quite firm, and can be sautéed, broiled, deep-fried, or served in salads. Steaming, broiling, and even grilling are all good alternatives to poaching.

Finally: The long-held rumor that skate wings are often stamped out to be sold as imitation scallops is a complete falsehood. Not only does skate not resemble scallops, but this process would be so expensive that the resulting meat would cost more than even bay scallops.

SKATE WITH BLACK BUTTER

Makes 2 servings
Time: 20 minutes

Skate au buerre noir is the classic French preparation for skate, and remains one of the best. The initial poaching, or one similar to it, is also the basis for most other skate recipes.

1 skate wing, 1 to 2 pounds, skinned
Court Bouillon (page 41) or a mixture of 8
 parts water to 1 part distilled vinegar
Salt to taste
1 whole onion (optional)
1 bay leaf (optional)
1 tablespoon capers, lightly crushed
2 tablespoons minced fresh parsley
¼ cup (½ stick) butter
1 tablespoon red wine vinegar

Place the skate in a deep, wide saucepan or skillet and add court bouillon to cover. Salt the water well and add the onion and bay leaf. Bring to a boil, skim off any foam, lower the heat to medium-low, and poach the skate until you can easily lift the meat off the cartilage at the wing's thickest point, about 10 minutes. Remove the skate, drain it, and place it on a hot platter. If you like, you can lift the top half of the meat with a broad spatula, remove the cartilage, and replace the meat (it's not as difficult as it sounds). Top the fish with the capers and parsley.

During the last 5 minutes of the poaching, prepare the buerre noir: Heat the butter over medium-high heat. Watch it carefully: After it foams it will turn golden and then darken; just when it becomes brown, take it off the heat and drizzle it over the skate. Rinse the saucepan with the vinegar and pour that over everything. Serve instantly.

SKATE WITH OLIVE OIL AND VINEGAR:
 Warm an equal amount of olive oil instead of the butter; increase the vinegar to 2 tablespoons.

STEAMED SKATE WITH SCALLIONS AND SESAME OIL

Makes 4 servings
Time: 40 minutes

Although I love skate au buerre noir, this recipe is more current and, I think, more interesting. Happily, you can make either.

1 skate wing, 2 to 3 pounds, skinned
1 tablespoon high-quality soy sauce
⅓ cup peanut oil
1 tablespoon sesame oil
½ cup minced scallions, both green and white
 parts

Rub the skate wing all over with the soy sauce, then steam on a rack above boiling water until the meat can be easily separated from the cartilage, about 15 minutes. During the last few minutes of cooking, heat the peanut oil over medium-high heat, just until it begins to smoke; turn off the heat and add the sesame oil. When the skate is done, sprinkle it with the scallions and drizzle the oil mixture over it.

ALTERNATIVE FISH FOR THIS RECIPE:
 Fillets of grouper, salmon, red snapper, tilefish, or wolffish. Adjust the cooking times accordingly.

SAUTÉED SKATE OVER MESCLUN

Makes 4 servings
Time: 40 minutes plus chilling time

This contemporary salad can be prepared in stages, making it ideal for an elegant lunch.

1 poached skate (without the buerre noir,
 above)
6 to 8 cups assorted lettuces and other greens,
 well washed and dried
½ cup olive oil, more or less

Flour for dredging
2 large shallots, minced
½ cup dry white wine
Juice of 1 large lemon

Remove the poached skate from its water and allow to cool. Lift the meat from the cartilage in pieces as large as possible. Place on a plate, cover, and refrigerate for several hours or overnight.

Arrange the greens on a platter. Cut the skate, if necessary, into six to eight "steaks." Heat a 10- or 12-inch nonstick skillet over medium-high heat. Add 2 to 3 tablespoons of olive oil to the pan and, when it is hot (a pinch of flour will sizzle), dredge the skate in the flour and cook quickly, just until browned on both sides. Do this in batches, without crowding, adding olive oil as necessary; as the steaks are done, remove them to a warm oven.

When all the skate is cooked, add the shallots to the pan; stir briefly, then add the wine. Reduce by half, add 1 tablespoon of lemon juice and turn off the heat. Dress the greens with the remaining lemon juice and olive oil to taste. Top with the hot skate steaks and pour the pan juices over all. Serve immediately.

ALTERNATIVE FISH FOR THIS RECIPE:

Fillets of blackfish, grouper, rockfish, red snapper, or wolffish. Do not poach any of these first.

BROILED OR GRILLED SKATE WITH WINE BUTTER

Makes 4 servings
Time: 30 minutes

Skate can be broiled or grilled easily and successfully; try this for starters. Then try broiling or grilling skate in any of the recipes for swordfish or salmon.

1 cup dry red wine
One 1-inch piece fresh ginger, peeled
1 clove garlic, lightly crushed and peeled
1 skate wing, about 2 pounds, skinned
Salt and freshly ground black pepper to taste
2 tablespoons butter
Minced fresh parsley for garnish

In a small saucepan, boil together the wine, ginger, and garlic until the liquid is reduced to about ¼ cup; this will take 15 to 20 minutes. Meanwhile, preheat the broiler or grill (the fire should not be too intense) and season the skate wing with salt and pepper.

When the wine is reduced, stir in the butter. If you're broiling, place the skate wing on a lightly buttered broiling pan and brush with half the wine butter; if you're grilling, brush it with the wine butter first, and put the buttered side down. Broil or grill 4 to 5 inches from the heat source until lightly browned, 7 to 8 minutes. Turn carefully, brush again with wine butter, and cook until the thickest part of the wing separates easily from the cartilage. Remove from the heat and serve at once.

Note: Occasionally, a large skate wing will cook too rapidly in a broiler for this method to be effective. If that happens, move the skate 8 inches or more from the source of the heat, or bake at 450°F for 15 minutes, then broil just to crisp up each side.

ALTERNATIVE FISH FOR THIS RECIPE:

Steaks of any firm-fleshed fish: Grouper, salmon, swordfish, or tuna are best.

SKATE SALAD WITH APPLES AND APPLE VINAIGRETTE

Makes 4 servings
Time: 45 minutes including poaching the skate

6 tablespoons olive oil
2 to 3 tablespoons mild cider vinegar
1 teaspoon Dijon mustard
Salt and freshly ground black pepper to taste
¼ teaspoon dried tarragon or several leaves fresh, minced
6 cups mixed greens, washed and dried
1 poached skate (without the buerre noir, page 274), cooled enough to handle
2 crisp, tart apples, peeled, cored, and cut into julienne strips

Whisk the oil, vinegar, and mustard together. Season with salt and pepper and add the tarragon. Divide the greens among four plates. Remove the skate from the cartilage and top the greens with it and the julienned apples. Drizzle some of the dressing over all and serve.

ALTERNATIVE FISH FOR THIS RECIPE:

Poach any firm thin, white fillet—especially dogfish, which is closely related to skate—for this dish.

SMELT

Latin name(s): *Osmerus mordax*, *Retropinna retropinna*, and others.
Other common names: Sparling, candlefish, cucumberfish, icefish.
Common forms: Whole; headed and gutted.
General description: Small, narrow fresh or saltwater fish, usually six to eight inches long and weighing just a few ounces; silvery on the sides with olive-green back.
For other recipes see: Anchovy, butterfish, sardines, whitebait.
Buying tips: Smelt should be shiny and bright; bruising should be minimal, and the smell sweet.

"Smelt," like "sardine" or "whitebait," is a name given to a variety of fish that are sold in the same way and, for culinary purposes, are interchangeable. Some smelts are more flavorful than others. Some taste like cucumbers; note the common name above. Some are oilier than others, and were used in candlemaking, as another common name indicates. Some are freshwater, some live in bays. But all are small, silvery fish with a central backbone that can be easily removed before or after cooking; it can also be eaten, especially if you have smaller specimens.

Smelt are most often sold headed and gutted, but if you buy whole ones, make a small cut just behind the top of the head, then pull the head down and back; most of the innards will come out with the head. Using your fingers and running water, pull and rinse away the little that remains.

BONELESS DEEP-FRIED SMELTS

Makes 2 to 4 servings
Time: 30 to 45 minutes, including cleaning

If smelts are small enough, their soft bones are less crunchy than the crisp coating of these fish. But if they're over three inches long, you might want to remove the backbone, a simple if somewhat time-consuming process. It's worth it. Try serving these crispy smelts with Spicy Pepper Sauce for Fried Fish (page 42) or Sicilian Pesto Dipping Sauce (page 296).

1 to 1 ¼ pounds smelts, the smaller the better, headless and gutted
Milk
Vegetable for deep-frying
2 cups all-purpose flour for dredging
Salt and freshly ground black pepper to taste
Lemon wedges

To bone the smelts, run your thumb along the belly flap, tearing the fish open all the way to the tail. Then grab the backbone between your thumb and forefinger and pull it out gently. This is easier than it sounds; stay with it and after five fish you'll be an expert. As you finish each fish, drop it into a bowl of ice water.

Heat the oil to 350°F to 370°F. (If your fryer doesn't have a thermostat, or you don't have a frying thermometer, drop a small piece of bread in the oil; it should sink, then rise to the top and begin bubbling away.) Drain the fish and return them to the bowl; cover with milk. Put the flour in a plastic bag and season it well.

Plan to cook the smelts in two or three batches, depending on the size of your fryer. They don't spatter much, so you may be tempted to cram them in, but if you want crisp fish you shouldn't fry more than a fistful or so at a time. Remove some smelts from the milk, toss in the bag with the flour, and drop them into the oil. Stir to make sure they don't stick together, then cook until golden brown, 3 to 4 minutes. Drain on paper towels and serve immediately, with lots of lemon, or keep warm while you cook the remainder.

ALTERNATIVE FISH FOR THIS RECIPE:

Cut-up pieces of blackfish, catfish, dogfish, flat-fish, or ocean perch; chunks of crayfish, lobster, or shrimp; shucked hard-shell clams, mussels, or oysters. Adjust the cooking times accordingly.

SMELTS FRIED WITH PEANUTS AND NORI

Makes 2 to 4 servings
Time: 30 minutes
Even crunchier and more flavorful than the recipe above.

Vegetable oil for deep-frying
1 sheet nori seaweed (available in Asian markets and health food stores)
½ cup roasted peanuts
Salt if needed
1 pound smelts, the smaller the better, headless and gutted
Flour for dredging
2 large eggs, lightly beaten
Lemon wedges

Heat the oil to 350°F to 370°F. Toast the nori by running it a couple of inches above an open flame several times (alternatively, toast it on a cookie

sheet in a low oven until brittle, about 10 minutes.) It will become brittle. Break it into large pieces and, in a food processor, crumble it with the peanuts (do not puree). Salt the mixture if the peanuts were unsalted.

Rinse and dry the smelts. Dredge them in the flour, shaking off any excess, then dip them in the egg, then roll them in the peanut-nori mixture. Plan to cook the smelts in two or three batches, depending on the size of your fryer. While they fry, stir occasionally to make sure they don't stick together, then cook until golden brown, 3 to 4 minutes. Drain on paper towels and serve immediately, with lots of lemon, or keep warm while you cook the remainder.

ALTERNATIVE FISH FOR THIS RECIPE:

Cut-up pieces of blackfish, catfish, dogfish, flat-fish, or ocean perch; chunks of crayfish, lobster, or shrimp; shucked hard-shell clams, mussels, or oysters. Adjust the cooking times accordingly.

HERBED SMELTS IN BUTTER

Makes 4 servings
Time: 30 minutes

1 ½ pounds smelts, heads off and gutted
1 recipe any herb butter (page 44), softened
2 tablespoons butter
2 tablespoons olive or peanut oil
Flour for dredging
2 large eggs, beaten
Bread crumbs for dredging, seasoned with the same herb you've chosen for the butter
Salt and freshly ground black pepper to taste
Lemon wedges

If the smelts are large, fillet them as in Boneless Deep-fried Smelts (page 277), leaving the sides attached, if possible, by the flap on skin on their back. If they are small, just a couple of inches or so, you probably won't mind eating the bones. Drain the fish and dry them. Put a little dab of herb butter in the center of each fish and close it up, or spread one fillet with a bit of the butter and lay another on top of it.

Heat a 12-inch nonstick skillet over medium-high heat for 3 to 4 minutes. Add the plain butter and oil and, when the butter foam subsides, begin to roll the smelts in the flour, shaking off any excess, dip in the egg, roll in the bread crumbs, and add to the pan. You'll need to do this in at least two batches. Season as they cook and adjust the heat so they sizzle but don't burn (some of the herb butter will run out of the fish, but don't let it bother you).

Turn once, after about 3 to 4 minutes. The smelts are done when nicely browned on both sides. Serve with some of the pan juices spooned over, and lemon wedges on the side.

ALTERNATIVE FISH FOR THIS RECIPE:

Sardines. (Of course almost any fish can be breaded, sautéed, and topped with herb butter; but only with small fish can you make these "sandwiches.")

SMELTS WITH GARLIC:

Add 1 tablespoon minced garlic to the bread crumbs or the herb butter. When the smelts are finished cooking, sauté 1 teaspoon minced garlic in the remaining fat. Garnish with minced fresh parsley or the herb of your choice.

SNAIL

Latin name(s): *Littorina littorea*.
Other common names: Periwinkle, winkle, cockle, sea snail.
Common forms: Whole, live.
General description: Small (under one inch) sea snail with brown, gray, tan, or multicolored shell, found mostly in the North Atlantic.
For other recipes see: Clams (soft-shell), conch, mussels, shrimp.
Buying tips: Snails must be live (or cooked or frozen) when you buy them; they move slowly, but they do move, so don't buy them if they don't; they'll start smelling pretty bad after they die, so that's a giveaway. Some are washed before you buy them, which is a nice feature.

These are not the garden or field snails of Europe, which are relatively large and sold in cans, but the familiar citizens of the North Atlantic coast, black dots seen by the thousands at low tide everywhere. All snails, however, have this in common: They move slowly, they cook slowly, and you will eat them slowly, one by one, usually with a pin or a toothpick. This is slow food at its slowest.

You can often buy snails in a fish market, especially if you're in a neighborhood where Asian, Italian, or Portuguese people shop. But the famous "winkle" of London streets has become a stranger to most American tables, and it's too bad. Snails will never become a ubiquitous item—they're not easy to harvest by the millions, which is what it would take, and they must be shipped live, which is costly—but you can gather enough for a meal in minutes, and they're as tasty as clams or oysters.

European snails are larger and sandier, and must undergo a time-consuming process of purging and cleaning before they are ready to cook. New York restaurateur Tony May, in his info-packed gem *Italian Cuisine*, begins his recipe with "Put the live snails into a wicker basket lined with grape or fig leaves (lettuce can be used) with some crustless bread which has been soaked in water . . ." Others would have you sprinkle the snails with bread crumbs and let them sit for a day or two.

With periwinkles, thankfully, the task is much easier. (There is one distinct advantage to eating snails in Europe, however: You're far more likely to find someone else willing to cook them for you.) James Beard recommended a simple soaking in warm water. I prefer cool water, with some cornmeal added; see the first recipe, on the next page.

STEAMED SNAILS

Makes 2 servings
Time: About 90 minutes

You can have these just for fun, as an appetizer or a leisurely lunch—it takes a while to eat them, and they're not especially filling. You can also cook them, chill them, and serve them as part of a larger spread, such as Seafood Salad Adriatic Style (page 49).

1 pound or more snails
½ cup cornmeal
2 tablespoons distilled or wine vinegar
2 cloves garlic, smashed and peeled
1 medium-size onion, sliced
2 tablespoons olive oil
½ cup dry white wine
Several sprigs fresh thyme
½ cup roughly chopped fresh parsley
Salt and freshly ground black pepper to taste

Soak the snails in water to cover mixed with cornmeal for about 30 minutes, stirring occasionally. Change the water a couple of times (you don't need to add more cornmeal) over the course of the next 30 minutes, mixing with your hands and rinsing as you do so. Then put the snails in a pot, cover with clean water and the vinegar, and bring to a boil. Simmer for a few minutes over medium heat, then remove a snail from the pot. Using a pin, try to pull the snail from its shell; if the operculum (the hard, shell-like disk at the end of the meat) falls off and the snail comes out easily, the snails are done. If not, continue cooking for a few more minutes.

When the snails are done, drain them, then return them to the pot with the remaining ingredients. Cover and steam for about 10 minutes, then drain and serve. Eat with a pin or toothpick.

SNAILS WITH GARLIC BUTTER:
After boiling the snails with the vinegar (make sure they are all done), serve them with melted butter to which you have added minced garlic and salt to taste.

MARINATED SNAILS:
Increase the quantity of snails to about 5 pounds. After boiling the snails with the vinegar (make sure they are all done), remove them all from their shells (discard the operculums), and mix them with 1 cup white wine vinegar, 1 cup water, ½ cup olive oil, 2 bay leaves, several sprigs fresh thyme and/or dill, and 1 tablespoon salt. Marinate for at least 1 hour, or overnight; drain and eat with bread.

SNAILS WITH AÏOLI:
Prepare as directed in the original recipe and serve cold, with aïoli (page 43). These are best as part of a larger spread of cold shellfish.

SAUTÉED SNAILS

Makes 4 appetizer or 2 main course servings
Time: 90 minutes, including purging time

Cooking and eating snails take patience, but I've never been sorry when I've spent my time peacefully preparing and consuming good food.

4 pounds snails, purged as directed above
2 tablespoons distilled or wine vinegar
½ cup olive oil
1 tablespoon minced garlic
Salt and freshly ground black pepper to taste
½ cup unseasoned bread crumbs
½ cup minced fresh parsley

Put the snails in a pot, cover with clean water and the vinegar, and bring to a boil. Simmer for a few minutes over medium heat, then remove a snail from the pot. Using a pin, try to pull the snail from its shell; if the operculum (the hard, shell-like disk at the end of the meat) falls off and the snail comes out easily, the snails are done. If not, continue cooking for a few more minutes.

When they're done, drain them well. Warm the olive oil in a large skillet, then add the garlic; cook, stirring, over medium-low heat until the garlic colors. Raise the heat to medium-high and toss in the snails, salt, and pepper. Cook, stirring, for about 3 minutes. Add the bread crumbs and continue to cook and stir until they brown nicely. Toss in the parsley and serve. Eat slowly (you'll have no other choice), with a pin.

ALTERNATIVE FISH FOR THIS RECIPE:

Hard-shell clams or mussels (no precooking for either).

SAUTÉED SNAILS WITH ANCHOVIES:

Mash 4 or 5 anchovy fillets (rinsed if salted) into the oil while you're heating the garlic. Add 1 or 2 sprigs fresh rosemary and ½ cup dry white wine to the skillet along with the snails. Garnish with minced fresh basil in place of the parsley.

RED SNAPPER

Latin name(s): *Lutjanus campechanus.*
Other common names: Mexican snapper, Caribbean red snapper, Florida snapper.
Common forms: Whole fish, fillets, steaks.
General description: One of the great firm, white-fleshed fish, ranging from three pounds to thirty (three to eight pounds are most common); all-purpose, with lovely, delcious skin.
For other recipes see: Blackfish, bluefish, butterfish, carp, catfish, cod, croaker, dogfish, flatfish, grouper (especially), haddock, halibut, mackerel, mako shark, monkfish, ocean perch, pollock, pompano, porgy, rockfish, salmon, sea bass, striped bass, swordfish, tilefish, weakfish, whiting, wolffish.
Buying tips: A tough one, since not all "snappers" are actually red snappers, and the differences are significant (see below). In any case, judging freshness isn't difficult—whole fish should look great and smell great (check for red gills and unbruised flesh); fillets should gleam, and have minimal gaping. Snappers are often sold gutted; ask the fishmonger to scale them.

There are more "snappers"—and more names for snappers—than for any other fish commonly sold in our markets, with the possible exception of rockfish. On the West Coast, red rockfish is legally sold as "Pacific red snapper." Other fish with red or pink or red and yellow skin, in and out of the snapper genus, are passed off as snapper. Some—especially those of the *Lutjanus* genus—are almost interchangeable with red snapper; others don't even come close. This wouldn't be so much of an issue if red snapper were not so expensive; you don't want to pay five dollars a pound for a whole fish that weights four pounds and be disappointed by texture or flavor.

Unfortunately, few consumers have the ability to distinguish between true red snapper and the impostors. I'm suspicious if fillets have been skinned or if the skin isn't truly red. Real red snapper is deep red on top, fading to rosy pink near the belly, and it is often silvery. The fins are also red. As always, if you trust your fishmonger, you should be getting red snapper when you pay for it (it doesn't hurt to ask, just for emphasis).

Having said all of this, if you do get true red snapper (and the odds aren't all that bad; at least half of the fish that sells as snapper is, indeed, red snapper), you will be pleased: It's a meaty, delicious fish that responds well to all cooking techniques.

GRILLED WHOLE RED SNAPPER WITH GARLIC SAUCE

Makes 2 servings
Time: 60 minutes or less
A two-pound red snapper is the perfect size for broiling or, if you have a fish basket, grilling. Eliminate the olive oil marinade if you're pressed for time.

1 whole red snapper, about 2 pounds, scaled and gutted, with head on
½ cup flavorful olive oil
Salt and freshly ground black pepper to taste
2 tablespoons minced garlic
2 tablespoons sherry vinegar, more or less
2 tablespoons minced fresh parsley

Rinse the fish and make several shallow cuts on each side, from top to bottom. Rub the fish liberally with some of the olive oil, then lay it in a baking pan or dish; let it sit for 30 minutes—in the refrigerator if it's a warm day—or so.

Start a charcoal fire or preheat the broiler or a gas grill (the fire should be medium-hot). Sprinkle the fish with salt and pepper. Place the remaining olive oil and the garlic in a small saucepan over low heat. If broiling, place the fish in a nonstick baking pan, about 4 to 6 inches from the source of heat. If grilling, use a fish basket (see page 26). Broil or grill until nicely browned on one side. Turn carefully.

When the garlic is very lightly browned, turn off the heat and add most of the vinegar and some salt and pepper. Taste for balance and add more vinegar if necessary. Stir in the parsley.

The fish is done when nicely browned on both sides (peek in one of the cuts you made and make sure it's cooked through to the bone; if not, move it a little farther from the heat and cook another few minutes). Serve it by scooping sections off the bone and sprinkling them with the sauce.

ALTERNATIVE FISH FOR THIS RECIPE:
Pompano, rockfish, salmon, sea bass, or tilefish. Adjust the cooking times accordingly.

GRILLED RED SNAPPER WITH GREEN VINAIGRETTE:
Whisk together 6 tablespoons olive oil, 2 tablespoons fresh lemon juice or good white wine vinegar, salt and pepper to taste, 1 teaspoon Dijon mustard, 1 teaspoon capers, and ½ cup chopped fresh parsley spiked with basil, tarragon, thyme, or other fresh herbs. Pass at the table with the grilled fish.

WHOLE RED SNAPPER ROASTED WITH TOMATOES

Makes 4 servings
Time: 45 minutes

Snapperlike fish (grouper and rockfish are among these) are roasted all over the world. Here's a basic recipe, with variations.

One 3-pound red snapper, scaled and gutted, head on
Salt and freshly ground black pepper to taste
1 tablespoon ground cumin
½ teaspoon cayenne pepper or to taste
2 tablespoons olive oil
1 tablespoon minced garlic
½ cup minced cilantro (fresh coriander)
2 cups roughly chopped tomatoes, fresh or canned (drained)
1 cup any fish or chicken stock (pages 40–41), dry white wine, or water
1 lemon, cut into thin slices

Preheat the oven to 400°F. Rinse the fish and make several shallow cuts on each side, from top to bottom. Rub the fish with the salt, pepper, cumin, and cayenne. Pour half the olive oil into a baking dish, then lay the fish on it. Top the fish with the remaining oil, the garlic, and half the cilantro. Spread some of the tomatoes over the fish and the rest around it. Pour the stock around the fish.

Roast for a total of 30 to 45 minutes, basting occasionally with the pan juices, until the fish is done (you can peek in one of the cuts down to the center bone; the flesh should be white and opaque throughout). Garnish with the remaining cilantro and lemon slices and serve with the pan sauce.

ALTERNATIVE FISH FOR THIS RECIPE:

Cod, croaker, grouper, mackerel, pompano, porgy, rockfish, sea bass, striped bass, tilefish, or weakfish. Adjust the cooking times accordingly.

RED SNAPPER ROASTED IN THE STYLE OF VERACRUZ:

Begin as directed above, then rub the fish with a mixture of 2 tablespoons fresh lime juice, 1 teaspoon chili powder, salt, and pepper. Heat 2 tablespoons good lard or vegetable oil over medium heat, then add 1 cup minced onions and cook, stirring, until softened; add 1 tablespoon minced garlic and cook 1 minute more. Stir in ¼ cup minced cilantro (fresh coriander), 1 teaspoon chili powder, and 2 cups chopped tomatoes (canned are fine; drain them first). Cook until the tomatoes break down, about 10 minutes. Top the fish with this sauce and bake, basting, as directed above. Garnish with minced cilantro.

RED SNAPPER ROASTED WITH ONIONS:

Begin as directed in the original recipe, then rub the fish with 1 tablespoon fresh lemon juice, then a mixture of 1 tablespoon chopped fresh mint (or 1 teaspoon dried), salt, pepper, and 1 teaspoon minced garlic. Melt 3 tablespoons butter over medium heat, then add 2 cups sliced onions and cook, stirring occasionally, until softened. Stir in 1 cup chopped fresh mint and ½ cup fish or chicken stock, wine, or water. Top the fish with this mixture and bake, basting, as directed above. Garnish with mint sprigs.

RED SNAPPER ROASTED WITH CHICK-PEAS:

Begin as directed in the original recipe, then rub the fish with 1 tablespoon fresh lemon juice, then a mixture of 1 teaspoon minced garlic, ½ teaspoon cayenne pepper, 1 tablespoon olive oil, and 1 teaspoon paprika. Mix 2 cups cooked chick-peas (drained if canned) with 1 tablespoon minced garlic, ½ cup minced fresh parsley or cilantro (fresh coriander), and 1 tablespoon fresh lemon juice or any good vinegar. Put half the chick-peas in the bottom of a baking pan and lay the fish on them. Sprinkle the remaining chick-peas over all. Pour ½ cup chick-pea cooking liquid (or the liquid from the can), fish or chicken stock, dry white wine, or water into the pan and bake, basting, as directed above. Garnish with minced cilantro or parsley.

RED SNAPPER ROASTED WITH FENNEL:

Begin as directed in the original recipe, then rub the fish with 1 tablespoon olive oil. Mix together 2 bulbs fennel, chopped, ½ cup unseasoned bread crumbs, ½ cup chopped fresh parsley, ½ cup olive oil, salt, and pepper. Put some of this mixture in the snapper's body cavity and some in the cuts in the flesh. Spread 2 tablespoons olive oil on the bottom of a baking pan. Lay the fish on it, then spread the remaining fennel mixture over it. Drizzle with a little additional olive oil and about 1 teaspoon balsamic vinegar. Roast without basting. Garnish with fennel sprigs.

RED SNAPPER FILLETS WITH LEMON RICE

Makes 2 servings
Time: 60 minutes

Short-grain rice is essential for this dish; don't try it with long-grain, which is not sticky enough.

1 cup short-grain rice
1 ½ cups water
1 teaspoon salt
¼ cup (½ stick) butter
Lots of freshly ground black pepper
1 tablespoon minced garlic
Juice of 1 ½ lemons
2 red snapper fillets, 4 to 6 ounces each, scaled
1 tablespoon vegetable or olive oil
½ lemon, sliced

Rinse the rice in several changes of water; place it in a saucepan with the water and salt; bring to a boil, cover, and simmer over low heat until the water is absorbed, about 12 to 15 minutes. Turn off the heat and let the rice sit, covered.

Heat half the butter over medium-high heat in a 10- or 12-inch nonstick skillet; when the foam subsides, spoon in the cooked rice. Toss and stir it to break up lumps, add more salt to taste, lots of pepper, about half the garlic, and most of the lemon juice. Cook, stirring frequently, for about 5 minutes; remove it from the pan to a plate and cool.

When the rice is cool enough to handle, press a thick layer of it onto each fillet; the rice will hold together and will stick to the fish. Wipe out the skillet and heat it over medium-high heat. When it's hot, add the remaining butter and the oil. Cook the remaining garlic, stirring for 1 minute or so, then push to one side and put the fillets in the pan, rice-coated side facing up. Cook undisturbed, until nearly done (you'll see the fillets turning white), 5 to 6 minutes. Scoop up the now-browned garlic and place it atop the fillets. Carefully turn the fillets over, allowing the rice to brown lightly for 1 to 2 minutes. Serve, rice side up, sprinkled with a few drops of lemon juice and topped with the lemon slices.

ALTERNATIVE FISH FOR THIS RECIPE:

Fillets of blackfish, dogfish, grouper, ocean perch, or rockfish. Adjust the cooking times accordingly.

COURT BOUILLON, VERSION I

Makes 4 servings
Time: 60 minutes
Not to be confused with the basic fish simmering stock (page 41), this is the single-fish stew of Guadeloupe and Martinique. For the related court-bouillon, New Orleans style, see the following recipe.

4 firm-fleshed steaks cut from a large red snapper or one 4-pound red snapper, scaled, gutted, head on, and cut into 4 to 8 pieces
2 cups water
½ cup fresh lime juice
Salt
¼ cup olive or peanut oil
1 cup chopped shallots, scallions (both green and white parts), or a mixture of both
1 tablespoon minced garlic
1 jalapeño or other hot pepper, deveined, seeded, and chopped
1 ½ cups chopped tomatoes, fresh or canned (drained)
1 bay leaf
¼ cup chopped fresh parsley
½ teaspoon minced fresh thyme or ¼ teaspoon dried
Freshly ground black pepper to taste
Lime wedges

Marinate the fish in the water, lime juice, and 1 tablespoon or so of salt, making sure the fish is completely covered, for about 30 minutes, refrigerated if the weather is warm. Drain.

Heat the oil in a large skillet over medium heat and cook the shallots, about two thirds of the garlic, and the jalapeño, stirring occasionally, until soft. Add the tomatoes and herbs, season with salt and pepper, and cook, stirring, for 5 minutes. Drain the fish and add it, along with ½ cup of its marinade if the mixture seems dry. Bring to a boil, cover, and simmer over low heat until the fish is done, about 10 minutes. (Red snapper is white, opaque, and tender when cooked.)

Remove the fish, add the remaining garlic, and reduce the mixture slightly by boiling for a few minutes. Spoon over the fish and serve over rice, with lime wedges.

ALTERNATIVE FISH FOR THIS RECIPE:

Steaks, fillets, or chunks of blackfish, croaker,

grouper, halibut, mako shark, monkfish, pollock, porgy, rockfish, sea bass, striped bass, weakfish, whiting, or wolffish. Adjust the cooking times accordingly.

COURT BOUILLON, VERSION II

Makes 4 servings
Time: 45 minutes
The New Orleans version.

2 tablespoons good lard or vegetable oil
2 tablespoons all-purpose flour
1 cup chopped onion
½ cup chopped scallions, both green and white parts (or more onion)
1 tablespoon minced garlic
1 bay leaf
½ teaspoon ground allspice or several allspice berries, crushed
1 teaspoon minced fresh thyme or ½ teaspoon dried
¼ cup chopped fresh basil (optional)
½ cup minced fresh parsley
½ teaspoon cayenne pepper or to taste
Salt and freshly ground black pepper to taste
2 cups chopped tomatoes, fresh or canned (not drained)
1 cup dry red wine
2 cups any fish or chicken stock (pages 40–41) or water
One 3-pound red snapper, gutted, scaled, beheaded, and cut into 4 to 8 pieces
2 tablespoons fresh lemon juice

First make a roux: Heat the lard in a large saucepan over medium heat; when it is hot, add the flour and stir constantly until it is nicely browned, 4 to 5 minutes. Add the onion, scallions, garlic, and seasonings (reserve half of the parsley for garnish) and cook, stirring, until the onion softens. Add the

tomatoes and cook 10 minutes. Add the wine and stock and simmer for 5 minutes to allow the flavors to blend. Add the snapper and poach over medium-low heat for 5 to 8 minutes, until it is barely cooked through. (Red snapper is white, opaque, and tender when done.) Add the lemon juice, garnish with the parsley and serve in bowls, with crusty bread.

ALTERNATIVE FISH FOR THIS RECIPE:
Steaks, fillets, or chunks of blackfish, croaker, grouper, halibut, mako shark, monkfish, pollock, porgy, rockfish, sea bass, striped bass, weakfish, whiting, or wolffish. Adjust the cooking times accordingly.

JOHNNY EARLES' RED SNAPPER FILLETS WITH TOASTED PECAN BUTTER

Makes 4 servings
Time: 20 minutes
My friend Johnny's restaurant, Criolla's, is the best in the Florida panhandle. This is one of the dishes that brought him national recognition.

½ cup unbleached all-purpose flour
¼ teaspoon cayenne pepper
¼ teaspoon ground thyme
1 tablespoon paprika
Salt to taste
¼ cup peanut or vegetable oil
½ cup milk
4 good-sized red snapper fillets, about 6 ounces each, scaled
¼ cup (½ stick) butter
⅔ cup pecan halves
Salt and freshly ground black pepper to taste
Juice of ½ lemon
2 tablespoons minced fresh parsley

Mix together the flour, half the cayenne, and the thyme, paprika, and salt in a bowl. Heat the oil in a 12-inch skillet (preferably nonstick) over medium-high heat until it is good and hot (a pinch of flour will sizzle). Put the milk in a bowl. Dip the fillets, one by one, in the milk; dredge them in the seasoned flour, then put them in the pan. Cook over high heat, turning once, until nicely browned on both sides; total cooking time will be 5 to 6 minutes. (Red snapper is white, opaque, and tender when cooked.)

Remove the fish to a platter and keep warm; wipe out the pan and immediately melt the butter in it over medium heat. Add the pecans, the remaining cayenne, salt, and pepper, and cook, stirring frequently, until the pecans are lightly browned and fragrant, 3 to 5 minutes. Add the lemon juice and parsley. Spoon a portion of nuts over each fillet and serve immediately.

ALTERNATIVE FISH FOR THIS RECIPE:

Fillets of blackfish, catfish, cod, dogfish, grouper, haddock, pollock, rockfish, salmon, sea bass, tilefish, or wolffish. Adjust the cooking times accordingly.

RED SNAPPER FILLETS EN PAPILLOTE

Makes 6 servings
Time: 60 minutes

There are few cooking methods as fun as this one, which has the added advantage of being virtually foolproof. Since all of the fish's essences are locked within the package, moistness is guaranteed. And seasonings can be minimal, so the flavor of the fish shines.

The following is a basic recipe with a number of suggested variations; it's sometimes fun to make several different combinations at the same meal, so each serving is a surprise. If you do that,

cut the fillets in half, so each diner gets two packages.

6 red snapper fillets, 4 to 6 ounces each, scaled and cut in half
1 large potato, sliced as for chips
2 large ripe tomatoes, cut into ¼-inch-thick slices
Salt and freshly ground black pepper to taste
24 fresh basil leaves
2 tablespoons olive oil, more or less

Preheat the oven to 450°F. Tear off a 1-foot-square piece of aluminum foil (the more traditional parchment paper is, of course, acceptable). Place a thin layer of potato slices, roughly the same size as the fillet, on the foil; top with a piece of fish, a slice of tomato, salt and pepper, basil, and a drizzle of oil. Seal the package and repeat the process with the other pieces.

Place all the packages in a large baking dish and bake for about 30 minutes (the snapper will be white, opaque, and tender when done). Serve the closed packages, allowing each diner to open his or her own at the table.

ALTERNATIVE FISH FOR THIS RECIPE:

Cod, haddock, ocean perch, rockfish, salmon, striped bass, or tilefish. Adjust cooking times accordingly.

RED SNAPPER EN PAPILLOTE WITH SPINACH:

Use a bed of well-washed spinach with any tough stems removed rather than potatoes; top with sun-dried tomatoes rather than fresh; use tarragon (sparingly) in place of basil. Bake 15 to 20 minutes

RED SNAPPER EN PAPILLOTE WITH BROCCOLI:

Use a bed of small broccoli florets; top with fresh or canned tomatoes; substitute butter for the olive oil. Bake 20 to 25 minutes.

RED SNAPPER EN PAPILLOTE WITH
ROOT VEGETABLES:

Use a bed of thinly sliced carrots, celery, and
well-washed leeks; top with minced shallots and
fresh parsley; use butter instead of olive oil. Bake
25 to 30 minutes.

RED SNAPPER EN PAPILLOTE WITH
TOMATOES AND HERBS:

Use a bed of chopped fresh tomatoes; top with a
variety of minced fresh herbs; sprinkle with a few
drops of dry white wine instead of the olive oil.

RED SNAPPER EN PAPILLOTE WITH
CARROTS AND ZUCCHINI:

Use a bed of julienned carrots and zucchini,
sprinkled with a few drops of balsamic vinegar; top
with olive oil, chopped fresh tarragon, and a thin
slice of lemon.

PAN-FRIED RED SNAPPER FILLETS
KOREAN STYLE

Makes 2 servings
Time: 20 minutes

2 tablespoons sesame seeds
1 teaspoon minced garlic
4 scallions, minced
1 teaspoon sesame oil
1 tablespoon high-quality soy sauce
¼ teaspoon cayenne pepper or to taste
Salt and freshly ground black pepper to taste
¾ pound red snapper fillets (2 to 4 fillets),
    scaled
3 tablespoons peanut or vegetable oil

Toast the sesame seeds in a dry pan over medium
heat, shaking occasionally, until they darken and
begin to pop, about 5 minutes (or microwave for
2 or 3 minutes). Mix half of them with the garlic,
half the scallions, the sesame oil, soy sauce,
cayenne, salt, and pepper. Coat the fillets with

this mixture, and allow them to sit while you heat
the oil.

Heat the oil in a 10- or 12-inch nonstick skillet
over medium heat until it shimmers. Carefully add
each of the fillets. Cook until lightly browned and
opaque all the way through, about 3 minutes; cook
and brown the other side. Serve immediately, garnished with the reserved scallions and sesame
seeds.

ALTERNATIVE FISH FOR THIS RECIPE:

Catfish, dogfish, flatfish, haddock, ocean perch,
sea bass, or wolffish. Adjust the cooking times
accordingly.

SNAPPER FILLETS STEAMED ON
ROOT VEGETABLES

Makes 4 servings
Time: 40 minutes
Use a food processor or mandoline to julienne the
vegetables.

2 tablespoons butter
¼ cup minced onion
1 teaspoon minced garlic
½ cup julienned carrots
¼ cup peeled and julienned parsnip
¼ cup peeled and julienned potato
¼ cup peeled and julienned turnip
½ cup julienned celery
½ cup minced fresh parsley
Salt and freshly ground black pepper to taste
2 tablespoons balsamic or sherry vinegar
½ cup any fish or chicken stock (pages 40–41)
    or water
4 red snapper fillets, 4 to 6 ounces each, scaled

In a 12-inch skillet that can later be covered, melt
the butter over medium heat. Add all the vegetables and cook gently until they begin to wilt, about
10 minutes. Stir in half the parsley, some salt and

pepper, and the vinegar. Cook, stirring, still over medium heat, until most of the vinegar has evaporated, 2 or 3 minutes. Add the stock and let boil for 1 to 2 minutes.

Lay the snapper fillets on top of the vegetables, season them, cover the pan, and lower the heat slightly. Steam until the fillets are done, 6 to 8 minutes (the fillets will be white, opaque, and tender). Sprinkle with the remaining parsley and serve.

ALTERNATIVE FISH FOR THIS RECIPE:

Fillets or steaks of blackfish, catfish, cod, dogfish, grouper, haddock, ocean perch, pollock, rockfish, tilefish, or wolffish. Adjust the cooking times accordingly.

BROILED RED SNAPPER FILLETS WITH HERB-TOMATO BUTTER AND ONION CONFIT

Makes 4 servings
Time: 60 minutes
This is a more complex recipe than most of the others in this book, but it's worth the extra time. Be sure that the fish has its skin on (be equally sure it's been scaled); it will be delicious.

6 tablespoons (¾ stick) butter
4 large onions, halved and thinly sliced
1 tablespoon sugar
Salt and freshly ground black pepper to taste
2 shallots, minced
½ cup dry white wine
2 medium-size tomatoes, chopped, fresh or canned (drained)

4 teaspoons minced mixed fresh herbs, such as chives, chervil, tarragon, basil, cilantro, or parsley, in any appetizing combination
2 tablespoons olive oil
4 red snapper fillets, 4 to 6 ounces each, scaled
Minced fresh parsley for garnish

Melt 4 tablespoons (½ stick) of the butter in a large skillet and cook the onions, stirring occasionally, over medium heat until they are very soft, 20 to 30 minutes. Add the sugar, salt, and pepper and cook a few minutes longer, until they are brown and sweet. Keep warm.

In a small saucepan, melt the remaining butter over medium heat. Add the shallots and cook, stirring occasionally, until soft; add the wine and reduce to about 2 tablespoons. Add the tomatoes and herbs, raise the heat to high, and cook 5 minutes, stirring occasionally. Put through a strainer or puree in a blender or food processor; keep warm.

Heat the olive oil in a 12-inch nonstick skillet over medium-high heat until it shimmers. Dry the fillets and place them in the oil one at a time, skin side down. Cook over high heat until the top is almost opaque, about 5 minutes; season with salt and pepper. Turn the fish and cook the flesh side for just 1 minute. To serve, spoon some of the onion compote onto a plate, top with a fillet, and drizzle with a bit of the tomato butter. Garnish with the parsley and serve.

ALTERNATIVE FISH FOR THIS RECIPE:

Haddock, ocean perch, rockfish, or tilefish, all preferably with skin on. Adjust cooking times accordingly.

SPOT

Latin name(s): *Leiostomus xanthurus*.
Other common names: Porgy, oldwife, croaker.
Common forms: Whole.
General description: Popular mid-Atlantic panfish, with a dark spot behind its gill cover; skin is edible.
For other recipes see: Butterfish, croaker, mackerel, mullet, pompano, porgy, sea bass.
Buying tips: As with any whole fish, spot should be buried in ice (with ice separating individual fish), and have red gills, bright skin, and no bruising. The smell should be sweet.

This small panfish, rarely as much as a pound in weight, is similar to croaker, but often somewhat oilier and more strongly flavored; this is not necessarily a disadvantage, since some spot taste quite rich and buttery.

PAN-FRIED WHOLE SPOT

Makes 2 servings
Time: 20 minutes
The basic panfish recipe. Best—I think—with peanut oil.

2 to 4 spot, ¾ pound each, gutted, scaled, and heads off
2 cups milk
Vegetable, olive, or peanut oil for frying
Fine cornmeal for dredging
¼ teaspoon cayenne pepper
1 teaspoon salt
½ teaspoon freshly ground black pepper
Lemon wedges

Soak the spot in the milk while you heat a 12-inch skillet (preferably nonstick) over medium-high heat for 3 to 4 minutes. Pour enough oil into the pan to cover the bottom to a depth of at least ⅛ inch. When the oil is hot (a pinch of cornmeal will sizzle) dredge the fish in the cornmeal, patting to help the meal adhere. Put the fish in the pan (you can probably fry only two at a time). Mix together the cayenne, salt, and black pepper, and sprinkle some of this over the fish.

When the fish have browned nicely on the bottom, turn them and sprinkle with the salt and peppers on the other side. Continue frying until browned. The fish are done when the inside contains no trace of pink and the flesh pulls easily from the bone when tugged with a fork. Serve immediately, with lemon wedges.

ALTERNATIVE FISH FOR THIS RECIPE:
Butterfish, croaker, or porgy.

SQUID

Latin name(s): *Illex illecebrosus*, *Loligo peallei*, Atlantic coast; *Loligo opalescens*, Pacific coast; dozens world-wide.

Other common names: Calamari, inkfish.

Common forms: Fresh, whole and cleaned; frozen, cleaned, rings, and steaks.

General description: Tubelike cephalopod perfect for stuffing when whole, good fried, sautéed, braised, or poached when cut up; care must be taken not to over- or undercook.

For other recipes see: Clams, conch, octopus, scallops, shrimp.

Buying tips: Check the color: purple to white is acceptable, brown is not. The smell should be clean and sweet (spoiled squid smells particularly foul), and the skin should shine. Frozen squid is usually quite good, as long as there is no evidence of freezer burn. See below for more details.

Ten years ago squid rarely was sold outside of Italian and Asian neighborhoods, and it has been only recently that adventuresome restaurants have begun adding it, carefully, to their menus. But although squid, like octopus, elicits squeamishness, almost everyone becomes converted eventually. Squid is inexpensive (one reason chefs like it), low in fat (less than 1 percent), and in little danger of extinction—the supply is extensive off of both East and West coasts.

This underappreciated shellfish with an internal skeleton has other advantages: Like shrimp, squid freezes well, and can be defrosted and refrozen with little loss in flavor or texture. Frozen squid, typically cleaned before freezing, is available in supermarkets all over the country, frequently for less than two dollars a pound. Fresh squid can be purchased in the Northeast from winter through summer and on the West Coast in early summer and late winter.

Squid is easy to cook, and more versatile than the ubiquitous fried calamari would lead you to believe. Although its flavor is mild, squid has a sweet, nutty character that manages to permeate most dishes in which it is featured.

There are two potential difficulties in preparing squid, both of which can be readily overcome. The first is cleaning: Although time spent on each individual squid is minimal, working your way through a few pounds is time-consuming. The solution here is to buy cleaned squid. (At one time, you could chat or read the newspaper as the local fishmonger cleaned it for you. Alas, those days are gone, at least in my neighborhood.) If you choose to clean squid yourself, be aware that it may be cleaned and cut up hours in advance; I store it wrapped in a kitchen towel in a bowl or on a plate, refrigerated.

Once cleaned, the only trick that remains in serving delicious squid involves timing. When undercooked, squid has a rubbery texture. But when it spends more than a couple minutes in pot or pan, it becomes as tough as beef jerky. Long, slow cooking retenderizes it. This explains the saying, prevalent in the seafood trade: "Cook squid 20 seconds or 2 hours." That oversimplification points in the right direction: When cooking squid over high heat, it is usually done within a minute or so. Perfection varies with the species, the time of year, and the storage conditions. But, generally speaking, stir-fried, sautéed, or fried squid quickly loses its rubbery texture. Although it doesn't become soft, it becomes tender in the same way that a properly cooked lobster claw, shrimp, or piece of sirloin becomes tender. Cook it as you would pasta, and taste it every minute or so; the instant it loses its rawness, turn off the heat and serve.

In braised dishes, squid performs much more predictably. After thirty minutes to an hour of cooking (again, depending on the squid itself), toughness is no longer a concern. However, care should be taken not to cook longer than necessary because, when the squid has lost all of its water (about two thirds of its total weight), it can become quite dry.

A word about serving size: One quarter to one half pound of squid per person is sufficient for quickly cooked dishes. But shrinkage is so significant when you braise or stew squid that you should figure a good half pound of raw squid per person in such recipes. In any case, if you begin with fresh, uncleaned squid, assume that 25 percent or more of the original weight will be lost in cleaning.

To Clean Whole Squid for Sautéing, Stir-frying, Deep-frying, etc.

Squid loses 25 to 30 percent of its weight during cleaning, so begin with a little over two pounds of whole squid to obtain one and a half pounds of cleaned squid. Medium (five to eight inches) and large (over eight inches) squid are easier to clean, have a higher ratio of meat to innards, and therefore yield more meat after cleaning than small squid. Squid about eight inches long (measure the body only) are best for most recipes.

Begin by grasping each squid's head where it enters the body (reach into the body a little if possible). Pull off the head and, with it, as much of the innards as possible (don't worry about getting all of it here; for many recipes, you can open the bodies for cleaning).

Just above the squid's eyes is a hard ball (called the beak) that creates a slight bulge. Cut the tentacles above that bulge. Discard the head and innards and reserve the tentacles. (This step really isn't worth it if you are saddled with really small squid, under four inches or so—just pull out the head, innards, and tentacles, and toss the whole mess.)

With your fingers, peel off the mottled purple skin. It usually comes off in one or two pieces. Don't bother with the skin that remains on the "wings"—no one will see it on the plate. And don't fret about bits of skin that hang tough; this ethereal membrane virtually disappears during cooking.

Using a thin-bladed knife (such as a small boning knife), slit the squid bodies open lengthwise. Remove the quill (the hard, translucent cartilage that runs the length of the body) if it didn't come out with the head and innards. Using the dull edge of the knife, scrape any remaining innards from the squid.

Rinse the tentacles and bodies and dry well before proceeding with your recipe. Cleaned squid can be kept, well wrapped and refrigerated (preferably on ice), for a day or so.

To Clean Whole Squid for Stuffing

Follow the directions for cleaning squid for sautéing, above, with these changes:

When pulling out the head, get your thumb and first and/or second fingers deep into the body. Most of the innards will come out cleanly. Then reach into the body with two fingers and grasp the quill and any remaining innards; pull them out (this step is troublesome with very large squid, because few of us have 10-inch-long fingers). A

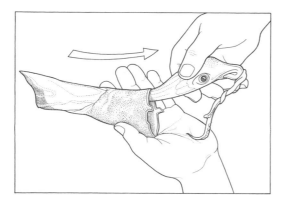

Pull out the head of the squid; most of the entrails will come along with it.

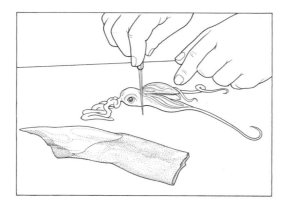

Cut the head just below the beak (the hard round ball found inside); discard, reserving tentacles.

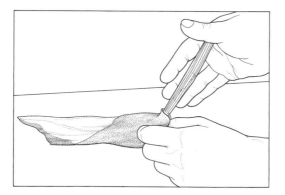

Reach into the body and remove the hard, transparent quill and any remaining innards.

dull teaspoon may be used on any innards that prove stubborn. Rinse out the squid's interior. If you've done a perfect job, the squid's body will hold water, but it doesn't matter much as long as any leaks are small.

GRILLED SQUID SALAD WITH GREENS

Makes 4 servings
Time: About 60 minutes, using cleaned squid
This is a great summer salad, when greens and squid are fresh, and it makes a tasty finish to an all-fish dinner. Try it following Monkfish in the Style of Veal (page 174).

1 pound large fresh squid
¼ cup high-quality soy sauce
6 to 8 cups assorted greens
Juice of 1 large lemon
½ cup fruity olive oil, more or less
1 teaspoon sesame oil

Clean the squid, cutting it open as shown on this page. Soak it in the soy sauce while you ready a charcoal or preheat a gas grill and wash the greens. When you're ready to cook, thread the skewers through the squid two or three times so that they will lie flat on the grill. Skewer the tentacles separately.

Grill the squid very quickly, on the hottest part of the grill; it should take no more than 60 seconds per side to become lightly browned (if it takes longer than 90 seconds per side, it will begin to become tough). Dress the greens with the lemon juice and olive oil, then cut up the squid and scatter it atop the salad. Sprinkle with the sesame oil and serve.

DEEP-FRIED CALAMARI WITH THREE DIPPING SAUCES

Makes 8 appetizer or 4 main course servings
Time: 20 to 40 minutes, using cleaned squid

Squid can be fried with a light batter, cornmeal, or flour. Batter smothers the squid, and I prefer flour to cornmeal—it is easy, produces a light coating, and gives sufficient crunch. Its one drawback is that the final color is relatively pale, but adding a bit of baking soda to the flour helps it brown. Any dipping sauce can be used for squid, but these three are among the best.

This is the kind of dish that is best to serve to friends who don't mind standing around the kitchen nibbling while you cook; it's pointless to try to make an elegant presentation out of it, or even to bring it into the dining room. Squid must be bone-dry before frying, or you and your kitchen will be attacked by spattering oil (if you have a covered fryer, such as that made by DeLonghi, use it).

2 pounds large whole squid, cleaned and cut up, or 1 ½ pounds cleaned squid, cut up
Vegetable oil for deep-frying
3 cups unbleached all-purpose flour, more or less
Salt and freshly ground black pepper to taste
1 tablespoon baking soda (optional)

Rinse the squid in several changes of water and cut it into ¼-inch rings. Cut tentacles in half lengthwise if they are big. Shake off excess water in a strainer (or, even better, a salad spinner). Lay a clean kitchen towel flat on a table and spread the squid evenly over it. Cover with another clean towel and roll the towels up together with the squid inside. Let sit for a few minutes while the oil is heating. (Squid may be cleaned early in the day and refrigerated, wrapped in the towels.)

Preheat 3 or 4 inches of the oil to 350°F. Season the flour liberally with salt and pepper, add the baking soda, and place the flour in a bowl near the sink. Have a strainer handy.

When the oil is ready (if your fryer doesn't have a thermostat, or you don't have a frying thermometer, drop a small piece of bread in the oil; it should sink, then rise to the top and begin bubbling away), remove about a quarter of the squid from the towels (more if your fryer is a big one, less if it is small; a quart of oil can handle two good handfuls of squid) and toss it into the flour. Move the squid around until it is well coated with flour and shake off the excess. Transfer the squid to a strainer and, holding the strainer above the sink, shake off more flour.

Place the squid in the frying basket and carefully lower it into the hot oil. Unless the fryer has a cover, stand back. Squid is done when golden, 2 to 3 minutes; do not overcook. Drain quickly in the frying basket, then on paper towels. Serve immediately with one or more of the dipping sauces, and fry the remaining squid in batches.

SESAME DIPPING SAUCE

Makes about ½ cup

This sauce may be varied by changing the proportions of garlic, ginger, or vinegar. Just be sure to keep tasting.

¼ cup high-quality soy sauce
1 tablespoon sesame oil
1 ½ teaspoons rice or other light vinegar
1 clove garlic, minced
1 tablespoon peeled and grated fresh ginger or 1 teaspoon ground
½ teaspoon sugar
1 tablespoon sesame seeds, toasted until brown in the oven (5 to 10 minutes at 350°F), a dry sauté pan (3 to 4 minutes, shaking the pan, over medium heat), or microwave (1 minute at high power; stir and nuke 1 more minute if necessary)

Combine all the ingredients and stir briefly to blend. Taste; if the mixture is too strongly flavored (which it may be if your soy sauce is very salty), add water, 1 tablespoon at a time, until the flavor is to your liking.

SICILIAN PESTO DIPPING SAUCE

Makes about 1 cup
A terrific pasta sauce, Sicilian pesto is not used frequently enough in other roles. Try the leftovers, if any, atop polenta.
1 cup chopped, very ripe tomatoes (good quality canned plum tomatoes, drained thoroughly, are acceptable)
1 teaspoon balsamic vinegar
2 tablespoons fruity olive oil
Salt and freshly ground black pepper to taste
2 tablespoons minced fresh basil
1 clove garlic, smashed

Place all the ingredients except the garlic in a broad-bottomed bowl and mash together well, using a fork or potato masher (do not puree). Add the garlic, stir, and let rest at room temperature for 1 or 2 hours before using. Remove the garlic before serving.

LEMON-TABASCO DIPPING SAUCE

Makes ½ cup
Simple as it is, this is the cleanest and most refreshing sauce to serve with fried squid. Take it easy on the hot sauce, and leave the bottle on the table so heat freaks can get their fill.

½ cup fresh lemon juice
Tabasco sauce to taste
Salt to taste

Combine and stir.

"BLASTED" SQUID WITH GINGERED CABBAGE

Makes 4 servings
Time: 30 minutes, using cleaned squid
Like the "blasted" shrimp on page 263, this technically should be called squid à la plancha, after the Spanish style of cooking seafood on a very hot surface with little or no oil. But blasted is more like it—once the cabbage is cooked (and there's no reason not to cook it in advance) this is a 10-minute dish: 8 for preheating the skillet, 2 for cooking.

2 tablespoons olive oil
1 small head Savoy cabbage, about 1 ½ pounds, shredded and chopped
1 tablespoon minced garlic
Salt and freshly ground black pepper to taste
About a dozen tiny squid, cleaned, or 1 pound larger squid, cleaned and cut into pieces
Juice of 1 lemon
Minced fresh parsley for garnish

Heat the olive oil in a large skillet over medium heat and cook the cabbage, stirring occasionally. When it is limp but not mushy, add the garlic, salt, and pepper, and cook another 2 minutes, stirring occasionally. Remove to a platter and keep warm.

Heat a 12-inch nonstick skillet over high heat until very hot, about 5 minutes. Sprinkle the bottom of the pan liberally with salt. Place only as many squid in the pan as will fit without crowding (you probably will need to do this in two batches; salt the pan again before cooking the second batch). Do not lower the heat. Turn after about 2 minutes and cook the other side for 1 minute. Place the squid atop the cabbage and drizzle with the lemon juice; sprinkle with the parsley and serve.

SAUTÉED SQUID STEAKS WITH GARLICKY GREENS

Makes 4 servings
Time: 40 minutes

This is sort of the minute steak of the fish world, sold—always frozen—by only a few companies. It's essentially the body of large Pacific squid, opened up, cleaned, and mechanically tenderized (the process consists of little more than puncturing the steak with small needles). I've had the Grippa brand, and like it very much; treat it the way you would veal scallops, cooking it, if anything, for a bit less time. Leftovers of this dish make great sandwiches (see the recipe for Grouper Sandwich with Spinach on page 136).

1 pound dark greens, such as collards or kale
5 tablespoons olive oil
1 teaspoon minced garlic
1 clove garlic, crushed and peeled
4 squid steaks, about 1 to 1 ½ pounds, thawed
Flour for dredging
1 large egg, lightly beaten in a bowl
Unseasoned bread crumbs for dredging
Salt and freshly ground black pepper to taste
Minced fresh parsley for garnish
2 lemons, cut into wedges

Set a large pot of water to boil while you wash the greens. Salt the water; when it boils, add the greens and simmer over medium heat until the stems are tender (cooking time depends on the thickness of the stems but could be as little as 2 minutes or as long as 10). Drain the greens; when they're cool enough to handle, squeeze them dry and chop them, stems and all.

Heat about half the olive oil in a 10-or 12-inch nonstick skillet over medium-high heat. Cook the greens, stirring briskly until well mixed with the oil. Add the minced garlic and cook another 2 minutes, stirring. Remove the greens to a serving platter and keep warm.

Heat the remaining oil over medium heat in the same skillet. Cook the garlic clove for a couple of minutes, stirring occasionally, while you prepare the squid. Dredge each steak in the flour, tap off the excees, then dip in the egg and dredge in the bread crumbs. Cook the steaks quickly over medium-high to high heat, until lightly browned on both sides, seasoning as you cook; total cooking time should be less than 2 minutes per steak. Place the cooked squid atop the greens and garnish with parsley. Serve with lemon wedges, squeezing fresh lemon juice over the squid and greens.

SPICY SQUID SAUTÉED WITH POTATOES AND TOMATOES

Makes 4 servings
Time: 30 minutes, using cleaned squid

3 tablespoons olive oil
4 dried hot peppers or to taste
1 tablespoon minced garlic
3 medium-size starchy potatoes, peeled and cut into ½-inch dice (about 2 cups)
3 medium-size fresh tomatoes, roughly chopped, or 3 or 4 canned plum tomatoes, with their juice
Salt and freshly ground black pepper to taste
1 sprig fresh tarragon or ¼ teaspoon dried
½ cup minced fresh parsley
Water or any fish or chicken stock (pages 40–41) as needed
1 pound squid meat, cut into cubes, from steaks or cleaned tubes and tentacles

Heat the olive oil in a 12-inch nonstick skillet over medium-high heat. Add the dried peppers and garlic and cook, stirring occasionally, until the garlic colors slightly. Add the potatoes, raise the heat to high, and cook, stirring occasionally, until the potatoes brown a bit, 5 to 10 minutes. Add the tomatoes and stir. Lower the heat to medium-low, add the salt, pepper, tarragon, and most of the parsley, and stir. The mixture should not be completely dry; if it is, add ½ cup or so of water or stock. Cover and cook until the potatoes are almost tender, about 10 minutes.

Add the squid, stir, and cook until it is tender, 3 to 5 minutes. Taste for salt and pepper, sprinkle with the remaining parsley, and serve.

ALTERNATIVE FISH FOR THIS RECIPE:
Precooked conch or octopus; shrimp or scallops. Adjust cooking times accordingly.

VARIATION:
You can turn this into a large, filling, one-dish meal by adding 4 cups chopped tomatoes, 2 cups stock or water, and ½ pound broken bits of pasta to the potatoes. Add water as necessary, cook until the pasta and potatoes are very soft (not al dente in this case), and then add the squid.

STIR-FRIED SQUID WITH BASIL AND GARLIC

Makes 4 servings
Time: 15 minutes, using cleaned squid
This dish is amazingly quick and easy to make, especially if you purchase cleaned squid. The delicious basil-garlic combination (fresh basil is essential) comes through beautifully here, so although there is some red pepper, the dish should not be too hot. I like this best over rice, with the pan juices (the rice should be fully cooked before beginning to cook the squid, since this dish is done so quickly).

2 pounds whole squid or 1 ½ pounds cleaned squid
½ cup loosely packed basil leaves
2 tablespoons plus 1 teaspoon (optional) peanut oil
4 ½ teaspoons minced garlic (about 4 or 5 large cloves)
⅛ teaspoon red pepper flakes or to taste
1 teaspoon salt or to taste

Dry the squid well, using cloth or paper towels. Cut vertically through the group of tentacles if it is large; otherwise, leave whole. Cut the squid bodies into rectangles, diamonds, or squares, with no dimension greater than 1 inch. The pieces should be fairly uniform in size.

Wash and dry the basil. If the leaves are large, chop coarsely into pieces about the same size as the squid. If time permits, mix the squid, basil, and the teaspoon of peanut oil in a bowl. Cover and refrigerate for 1 hour or so. (This is far from essential, but helps the flavor of the basil permeate the squid.)

When you're ready to cook, have all the ingredients ready—including a serving dish and rice, if any. Remove the squid from the refrigerator. Mix together the squid and the basil if you haven't already done so. Preheat a wok (or a large sauté pan) over high heat until smoking.

Lower the heat to medium and add the remaining peanut oil to the wok. Swirl it around and add the garlic. Stir once or twice. As soon as the garlic begins to color—about 15 seconds—return the heat to high and add the squid-basil mixture. Stir quickly and add the red pepper. Stir frequently but not constantly until the squid becomes opaque, less than 1 minute. Begin tasting the squid and continue to taste frequently until it is tender, between 1 and 3 minutes. Season with salt and stir. Turn off the heat and serve, with pan juices, over rice.

ALTERNATIVE FISH FOR THIS RECIPE:
Shrimp, pieces of monkfish or mako shark (cook a bit longer), or scallops.

STIR-FRIED SQUID WITH TOMATOES AND BLACK BEANS

Makes 4 servings
Time: 30 minutes, using cleaned squid

I like to use frozen squid steaks for this because it simplifies the process greatly. You can, of course, use whole squid, fresh or frozen, following the general directions given on page 293 and in the preceding recipe.

3 or 4 squid steaks, thawed (about 1 pound)
2 tablespoons high-quality soy sauce
1 tablespoon fermented black beans (available in Asian markets)
2 tablespoons dry sherry
1 large onion, cut into rings
3 tablespoons peanut oil
1 tablespoon minced garlic
1 teaspoon peeled and minced fresh ginger
3 or 4 scallions, cut into 1-inch lengths, with some of the green
3 medium-size ripe tomatoes, peeled, seeded, and roughly chopped
½ teaspoon chili paste (available in Asian markets), Tabasco, or any other hot sauce, or to taste (optional)
Salt and freshly ground black pepper to taste

Cut the squid into small pieces and soak in the soy sauce while you get everything else ready. Soak the black beans in the sherry at the same time.

Place the onions rings, dry, in a 12-inch nonstick skillet or a wok. Turn the heat to high and cook, without stirring, until the onions begin to char. Stir once or twice, cook until they brown some more, then slowly add the oil. Cook, still over high heat, until the onions soften. Remove with a slotted spoon. Add the garlic, ginger, and scallions to the pan; cook for 30 seconds. Add the squid; cook and stir for 1 minute. Add the tomatoes; cook and stir for another minute. Add the black beans, the onions, and the hot sauce. Stir, taste for salt and pepper, and serve immediately, over rice.

ALTERNATIVE FISH FOR THIS RECIPE:
Precooked conch or octopus; shrimp or scallops. Adjust cooking times accordingly.

SQUID IN SPICY RED SAUCE

Makes 4 servings
Time: 45 minutes, using cleaned squid

This can be used as a sauce for pasta, or as a simple main course.

½ cup olive oil
3 cloves garlic, quartered
3 dried hot peppers or ½ teaspoon cayenne pepper or to taste
3 cups chopped tomatoes (drain if canned)
2 pounds large whole squid, cleaned and cut up, or 1 ½ pounds cleaned squid, cut up
⅓ cup minced fresh parsley for garnish

Heat the olive oil over high heat in a 10- or 12-inch skillet until almost smoking; add the garlic and hot pepper and brown the garlic slightly. Turn off the heat; when the mixture has cooled down a bit, add the tomatoes and crush them, raising the heat to medium. Add the squid and stir. Cook over fairly medium-high heat until the squid is tender but not dry, 30 minutes or more. Sprinkle with the parsley and serve over pasta or with good bread.

ALTERNATIVE FISH FOR THIS RECIPE:
Shrimp and/or scallops (cook 3 to 4 minutes only), tenderized octopus (see entry), or a combination.

OVEN-BRAISED SQUID WITH WINE, CINNAMON, AND GARLIC, SERVED WITH POTATO CROUTONS

Makes 4 servings
Time: 2 hours or less

This dish exudes a heady aroma of cinnamon and garlic that will make your mouth water. Use a bone-dry but sturdy white wine, such as a good Sauvignon Blanc. The stew may be prepared a couple of hours early, but it really starts to lose its distinctive aroma if it sits around much longer than that.

¼ cup olive oil
½ cup cloves garlic (1 or 2 heads), peeled
2 pounds squid, cleaned and rinsed, the bodies cut into ½-inch rings, the tentacles split if large
1 teaspoon paprika
1 tablespoon all-purpose flour
½ teaspoon ground cinnamon
½ teaspoon dried tarragon
½ teaspoon freshly ground black pepper or to taste
½ cup chopped fresh parsley
1 cup very dry white wine
1 pound starchy potatoes (3 or 4 medium-size), such as Russet or Idaho
Salt to taste

Preheat the oven to 350°F. Heat 2 tablespoons of the olive oil over medium-low heat in an oven-proof pot (I use a pot that can be brought to the table). Add the garlic and cook, stirring occasionally, until the cloves barely begin to color. Add the squid and stir briefly.

Still over medium-low heat, sprinkle on the paprika and flour and stir well. Add the cinnamon, tarragon, and pepper, and stir to blend. Reserve about 2 tablespoons of the parsley and add the rest to the pot along with the wine; stir, raise the heat to medium-high and bring to a boil. Stir once more, cover, and place in the oven.

Meanwhile, boil (20 to 40 minutes, depending on size) or microwave (5 to 8 minutes) the potatoes until a knife pierces them fairly easily; they will not be fully cooked. Peel as soon as they are cool enough to handle. Cut into ¼-inch dice.

Heat the remaining 2 tablespoons of olive oil in a 10- or 12-inch nonstick skillet over a medium-high flame. When the oil shimmers, add the potatoes and cook, stirring briskly until brown and crisp all over, 10 to 15 minutes. Remove from the oil with a slotted spoon, salt lightly, and set aside.

When the squid has cooked for 1 hour, remove it from the oven and stir. It will have shrunk considerably. If it is swimming in a good deal of liquid, remove the cover. If not, leave the cover on the pot. Return the squid to the oven for another 30 minutes. The stew is done when the squid is tender and the garlic is of a spreadable consistency. Sprinkle it with parsley and the potato croutons (or pass the croutons at the table), and serve with lots of crusty bread.

BRAISED STUFFED SQUID

Makes 4 servings
Time: 1 hour, using cleaned squid

Since squid shrinks significantly during cooking, it is important not to overstuff it. Squid may be stuffed a couple of hours before cooking as long as they are iced in the interim. They can also be cooked a few hours in advance, covered, and gently reheated.

Stuffed squid makes an impressive first course. Slice the bodies diagonally into pieces about ½ to ¾ inch wide, and serve with a teaspoon or two of drained cooking liquid and a nice garnish. Stuffed squid is also a fabulous topping for pasta.

3 tablespoons plus 1 teaspoon olive oil

⅓ cup pine nuts (chopped walnuts may be substituted)

8 whole squid, with bodies about 8 inches long, cleaned, washed, and dried (about 1 ½ pounds)

1 teaspoon minced garlic

6 anchovy fillets, minced

⅓ cup minced fresh parsley

2 tablespoons freshly grated Parmesan (optional)

⅓ cup dry white wine

½ cup fresh bread crumbs, lightly browned in a 350°F oven 8 to 10 minutes

Salt and freshly ground black pepper to taste

3 dried hot peppers

3 cloves garlic, peeled

1 ½ cups drained canned plum tomatoes, chopped

2 teaspoons minced fresh rosemary or ½ teaspoon dried

Heat the teaspoon of olive oil in a small sauté pan over medium heat, then add the pine nuts. Cook, stirring occasionally, until lightly browned, 2 to 3 minutes. Put ¼ cup of the nuts in a small bowl, reserving the remainder for garnish.

Chop the tentacles of the squid finely; no piece should be larger than a pea. Add them to the nuts, along with the minced garlic, half the anchovies, ¼ cup of the parsley, the Parmesan, wine, and 1 tablespoon of the olive oil. Stir to combine. The mixture should be fairly wet.

Add bread crumbs as needed to make a stuffing that is neither soupy nor dry. Season with pepper. As with any stuffing, this one should be tasted for seasoning. Sauté 1 teaspoon or so in a few drops of oil. Despite the anchovies and cheese, it may need salt. Additional pepper, garlic, anchovies, or cheese may also be added; the flavors of each of these should be present.

Stuff the squid bodies with this mixture, using your fingers and a teaspoon. Each body should get about 2 teaspoons of the mixture. *Do not overstuff* (squid shrinks a lot more than turkey). Close the openings with one or two toothpicks (round ones are less likely to break than flat ones). Set aside.

Over a medium flame, heat the remaining 2 tablespoons of olive oil in a pot large enough to hold all the squid in one layer (this is not as difficult as you might think—the squid will shrink significantly as soon as it hits the hot oil). Add the hot peppers and garlic cloves and stir occasionally until the garlic is good and brown. Remove the peppers and garlic and discard. Add the remaining anchovies and stir briefly. Add the stuffed squid and brown on both sides (raising the heat if necessary), about 1 minute per side.

Add the tomatoes and rosemary, reduce the heat to low, cover, and set a timer for 15 minutes. Don't worry if things appear dry; after the timer goes off, the squid will be sitting in a puddle of bubbling sauce. Make sure no piece is sticking to the bottom of the pan, reduce the heat a bit further, and recover.

Fifteen minutes later, remove the cover and stick a toothpick into one of the squid. It should penetrate easily (if not, recover and cook 10 more minutes). Remove the cover, raise the heat to medium, and reduce the sauce—with the squid still in the pan—for about 10 minutes. Remove the squid from the pan and let it sit 5 minutes or so as you continue to reduce the sauce.

To serve as a first course, slice each squid into ½-inch diagonals, top with 1 or 2 teaspoons of sauce, and garnish with the reserved nuts and parsley. Serve either one or two squid per person.

To serve as a main course, toss the remaining sauce with a pound of cooked pasta. Top each serving with several slices of stuffed squid, and garnish with the nuts and parsley.

SQUID STUFFED WITH GARLICKY GREENS:
Use garlicky sautéed greens, such as those for

Sautéed Squid Steaks with Garlicky Greens, page 297, or Grouper Sandwich with Spinach, page 136. Cook as described above.

Squid Stuffed with Polenta:

Use freshly made polenta, seasoned with parsley, Parmesan, salt, lots of black pepper, and butter. Sauté the squid in butter and proceed as above.

Squid Stuffed with Porcini:

Use a mixture of 1 tablespoon rehydrated cèpes (porcini), 1 tablespoon minced garlic, ½ to ¾ cup bread crumbs, 2 tablespoons minced parsley, and 1 tablespoon olive oil. Cook as described above.

Squid Stuffed with Vegetables:

Use chopped fresh vegetables—carrots, celery, onion, tomatoes—sautéed in olive oil until soft and combined with the bread crumbs to bind to make about 1 cup or a bit more. Moisten with olive oil and/or lemon juice. Use tomato sauce as described above or, after browning, simmer in a mixture of stock and white wine, seasoned with bay leaf, garlic, thyme, and parsley.

Squid Stuffed with Rice and Raisins:

Combine 1 tablespoon minced scallions, 1 tablespoon minced parsley or mint, 1 tablespoon pine nuts, 1 tablespoon raisins or currants, about 1 cup cooked white rice, salt and pepper to taste, and a pinch cinnamon. Cook as in Squid Stuffed with Vegetables.

QUICK-POACHED SQUID WITH CILANTRO AND SAFFRON COCONUT CREAM

Makes 4 servings
Time: 40 minutes, using cleaned squid

This light dish has considerable visual appeal. If saffron is used (turmeric is an inferior but acceptable substitute), if the squid is cleaned and skinned well (using precleaned squid eliminates half the work), and if care is taken not to brown the onions,

the result is alabaster squid in a brilliant yellow sauce flecked with green cilantro and chopped red tomatoes.

As in the stir-fry recipe (page 298), cooking time varies with the squid's natural tenderness; 5 minutes is average, but it could take as little as 2 or as many as 10. Again, I recommend frequent tasting, beginning as soon as the squid becomes opaque, which happens within a minute or so of adding it to the sauce. Undercooking is preferable to overcooking; if the squid begins to toughen, get it off the stove.

2 pounds large whole squid, cleaned and cut up, or 1 ½ pounds cleaned squid, cut up
1 cup unsweetened grated dried coconut
⅛ teaspoon saffron, measured after crumbling a few threads, or turmeric
2 cups boiling water
3 tablespoons peanut oil
1 large onion, cut in half and then into slices about ⅛ inch thick
1 tablespoon peeled and minced fresh ginger
1 teaspoon garlic, minced with 1 teaspoon coarse salt
¼ teaspoon cayenne pepper or to taste
½ cup minced cilantro (fresh coriander)
2 fresh plum tomatoes, cut in half, seeds scooped out, and cut into ¼-inch dice
Salt to taste

Cut the squid into diamonds, rectangles, or squares, no longer than 1 to 1 ½ inches. Place in a bowl, cover, and refrigerate until ready to cook.

Put the coconut and saffron in a blender and pour the boiling water over them. Holding the top of the blender firmly closed with a folded towel (I once painted a ceiling purple with blueberry soup, so I may be a bit overcautious, but please be careful), blend for 10 or 15 seconds. Let sit for 10 minutes or so, then pour the liquid through a fine strainer into a bowl, pressing on the coconut to extract as much cream as possible. There should be almost 2 cups.

In a 10- or 12-inch skillet heat the oil over medium heat. Add the onion and cook, stirring, until the half rings separate, soften slightly, and become translucent. Adjust the heat so the onion does not brown, and proceed to the next step before it softens too much.

Add the ginger, garlic-salt mixture, and cayenne to the onion and cook over medium-low heat, stirring, for about 5 minutes. Add 1 ½ cups of the coconut cream and raise the heat to medium. Bring to a gentle boil, add a bit more than half of the cilantro, and cook, stirring occasionally, until the sauce is slightly reduced, 5 to 10 minutes.

Drain the squid of any accumulated liquid and add it, along with the tomatoes, to the sauce. Cook over medium heat, stirring occasionally. The mixture may look dry at first, but as the squid cooks it will release some liquid.

Begin tasting the squid when it becomes opaque. Continue to taste frequently until it is tender, about 5 minutes. When done, add the remaining cilantro and season with salt. Turn out onto a large platter full of steaming rice (basmati is best in this instance) and serve immediately.

ALTERNATIVE FISH FOR THIS RECIPE:

Shrimp or scallops; chunks of blackfish, grouper, monkfish, or wolffish.

TRICOLOR SQUID SALAD

Makes 4 servings as a light lunch or 8 appetizer servings
Time: 30 minutes, using cleaned squid
This easy salad has eye appeal and, unlike many others, showcases the squid's delicate flavor. It can be made a day or two in advance—and, indeed, benefits from sitting for at least a few hours—but the parsley should not be added until just before serving.

The only trick here lies in boiling the squid to tenderness, which takes a watchful eye. It is not unlike cooking capellini pasta, which has a tough core one second and is mushy the next. Here, the squid can go from a raw mushiness to fairly tough in less than a minute. As in other squid recipes, tasting during cooking is important.

2 medium-size carrots, peeled
1 pound cleaned squid, the bodies cut into ¼-inch rings, the tentacles split lengthwise
⅓ cup minced red onion
4 ½ teaspoons fresh lemon juice
2 to 3 tablespoons fruity olive oil
Salt and freshly ground black pepper to taste
½ cup minced fresh parsley

Shred the carrots, using the finest grating blade of a food processor or a hand grater. (If you do not have a tool that will shred them, cut them into a fine julienne and parboil for one minute.)

Start with a pasta pot full of furiously boiling water, and keep a stopwatch handy. Have ready a colander, a big bowl of ice water, and a small saucer of cold water. Add the squid, all at once, to the pot. Stir once and start the stopwatch; begin tasting the squid after 30 seconds have elapsed (it doesn't matter if the water returns to the boil): pull a piece from the water, dip it into the cold water, and taste. At first it will be a bit raw and rubbery, but that quality will soon disappear. Remove it from the heat the instant it becomes tender, even if it is only 30 seconds after you added it to the pot. If the squid is cooked any longer, it will begin to toughen.

Drain the squid and immediately plunge it into the ice water. When it's cool, drain it again and mix it with the carrots and onions in a bowl. Add the lemon juice and 2 tablespoons of the olive oil and stir; there should be just enough dressing to make the salad glisten. Add more olive oil if necessary.

Stir, taste, and add salt and pepper as needed.

Cover and refrigerate for several hours or as long as 2 days; the squid will become more succulent as it sits. Stir occasionally. Add the parsley just before serving, taste, and correct the seasoning.

ALTERNATIVE FISH FOR THIS RECIPE:
Precooked conch or octopus.

CLASSIC SQUID SALAD

Makes 4 servings as a light lunch or 8 appetizer servings
Time: 30 minutes, using cleaned squid

The technique here is the same as that for the preceding recipe; the final flavor is different. This is the standard calamari salad of East Coast Italian restaurants.

1 ½ pounds cleaned squid, the bodies cut into ¼-inch rings, the tentacles split lengthwise
1 medium-size carrot, shredded
2 stalks celery, diced
½ teaspoon finely minced garlic
3 tablespoons minced fresh parsley
2 tablespoons minced fresh mint
2 tablespoons white wine vinegar
5 tablespoons fruity olive oil
Juice of 1 lemon
Salt and freshly ground black pepper to taste

Cook the squid as instructed in the preceding recipe. When it is cool, place it in a bowl, and add the carrot, celery, garlic, parsley, and mint. Add the vinegar, olive oil, and lemon juice and stir; add salt and lots of pepper. Taste for seasoning and adjust for olive oil, lemon (the dressing should be rather acidic), salt, or pepper as needed. Serve at room temperature.

ALTERNATIVE FISH FOR THIS RECIPE:
Precooked conch or octopus.

SQUID AND BLACK BEAN SALAD WITH CILANTRO

Makes 6 servings
Time: About 2 hours

When fresh corn is in season, add a cup or so of quickly sautéed kernels for more flavor and color.

1 ½ cups dried black beans
1 pound cleaned squid, cut into bite-size pieces
Salt and freshly ground black pepper to taste
1 medium to large onion, peeled
2 tablespoons any vinegar
¼ cup chopped cilantro (fresh coriander) leaves for garnish, the stems reserved for the stock
⅓ cup chopped red onion
2 medium-size red bell peppers, stemmed, deveined, and chopped
½ cup vinaigrette, made with 3 parts olive oil and 1 part lemon juice
1 tablespoon ground cumin or to taste

Wash and pick over the dried beans. Soak overnight in cold water to cover, or boil for 2 minutes in water to cover and soak for 2 hours. Drain, place in a large pot with water to cover, and cook, over medium heat, until tender but not mushy, 1 hour or more. Drain and set aside.

Place the squid in a a pot along with the salt, pepper, the whole onion, vinegar, cilantro stems, and water to cover. Bring to a boil and simmer until the squid is tender, about 30 minutes. Leave the squid in the stock to cool.

Remove the squid and reserve the stock for use in risotto or soup. Mix together the squid, beans, and the remaining ingredients. Taste for seasoning, and garnish with the minced cilantro leaves.

STRIPED BASS

Latin name(s): *Morone saxatilis*.
Other common names: Rockfish, greenhead.
Common forms: Whole (usually quite small and farm-raised), fillets or steaks (usually large and wild).
General description: Popular sport fish with firm, meaty, pinkish flesh; now being farm-raised in California and elsewhere; skin is edible.
For other recipes see: Blackfish, bluefish, carp, cod, dogfish, grouper, monkfish, ocean perch, pollock, rockfish, salmon, sea bass, red snapper, swordfish, tilefish, wolffish.
Buying tips: Color of fillet should be fairly uniform, and show no evidence of browning or drying. Whole fish should be gorgeous; check the gills to make sure they're bright red.

Traditionally, striped bass was a midsize sport fish. Keepers ran to several pounds, and big fish—over three feet long—were real prizes. In many places these days, stripers come in two sizes: small and large. That's because much of the depleted and endangered striped bass population has been protected, and fish as large as thirty inches are often returned to the water. So, in areas where sport fishing is common, you may see five-pound fillets in fish stores, and nothing smaller (of course, you can ask for a piece of the fillet).

Small fish (actually hybrids of striped and white bass) are from fish farms, and are a couple of pounds at most. At the time of this writing (1993) they are quite expensive, as are all farm-raised fish in the first few years of development. They're also not nearly as flavorful as their wild cousins. You can expect the flavor and the price to be more favorable as the years go by.

The popularity of striped bass comes not only from its fighting ability, but from its unusual texture and flavor. It's a meaty, strong-flavored fish, but not an especially oily one—sort of a cross between bluefish and monkfish—a combination not found elsewhere. It can substitute for milder fish, like cod, as well as for stronger fish. It also provides one of the few easily grilled fillets, which makes it especially beloved in the beach communities in which it is caught.

BASIC GRILLED STRIPED BASS

Makes 4 servings
Time: 40 minutes

Striped bass yields one of the few fish fillets that is firm enough to grill without a basket (although using one won't hurt). And, since the skin does not make especially good eating, you can leave the scales on to give the fish even more structural integrity.

The garlic in this dish is optional; striped bass has plenty of flavor on its own.

One 1 ½-pound center-cut striped bass fillet, of fairly uniform thickness (about 1 inch)
2 tablespoons olive oil
1 clove garlic, minced (optional)
Salt and freshly ground black pepper to taste
Lemon wedges

Preheat a gas grill or broiler or start a charcoal or wood fire; it should be very hot, and the grate should be clean. Drizzle the flesh of the fish with the olive oil, and sprinkle it with the garlic, salt, and pepper.

When the fire is ready, grill the fish, flesh side down, about 5 minutes, inserting a metal spatula between the fish and the grill every 2 minutes or so to prevent sticking. Turn the fish and grill another 5 minutes, again making sure the fish doesn't stick. Check for doneness—the fish will still be firm and juicy, but will have lost its translucence, and a thin-bladed knife will pass through it fairly easily—and serve immediately (skin side down) with lemon wedges.

ALTERNATIVE FISH FOR THIS RECIPE:
Blackfish, eel, grouper, monkfish, swordfish, or tuna. Adjust the cooking times accordingly.

GRILLED STRIPED BASS WITH A RELISH OF SHERRIED GARLIC AND NECTARINES

Makes 4 servings
Time: 90 minutes

Sherried garlic is a wonderful ingredient, one I use all the time—on pizza, in rice, as a garnish. If you don't have the time to make it, substitute some finely chopped mild onion or shallot; but if you do, you won't regret the time and work.

30 to 40 cloves garlic
1 cup sherry vinegar or a mixture of sherry vinegar and inexpensive wine vinegar
3 tablespoons olive oil
Salt to taste
¼ cup dry sherry
2 very ripe nectarines
Juice of 1 lime
2 tablespoons minced cilantro (fresh coriander)
1 recipe Basic Grilled Striped Bass (see left)

Peel the garlic (it's fine to crush it lightly to make peeling easier). Place it in a small saucepan with the vinegar and olive oil; bring to a boil and cook over medium-low heat until almost all of the liquid has evaporated, about 30 minutes. Salt lightly and add the sherry; continue to cook until the garlic is swimming in a syrupy liquid, about 10 more minutes.

Pit and coarsely chop the nectarines. Place them in a bowl with the lime juice and crush lightly with a fork. Add 1 to 2 tablespoons of the sherried garlic and mash again. Add the cilantro, stir, and let sit while you prepare the fish. Serve the bass with the cool relish.

ALTERNATIVE FISH FOR THIS RECIPE:
Same as for Basic Grilled Striped Bass.

JOURFISH JAMAICAN STYLE

Makes 2 servings
Time: 30 minutes

I learned this recipe in a bar in Jamaica, where I had gone to discover the secret of goat's head soup. This made the trip worthwhile; the soup was only fair.

One ¾-pound striped bass fillet, skinned
Flour for dredging
¼ cup peanut or vegetable oil
¼ cup dry white wine
1 cup unsweetened shredded coconut
1 scallion, minced
½ cup any fish or chicken stock (pages 40–41)
Juice of 1 lime
½ cup cubed ripe papaya or cantaloupe
½ teaspoon dried thyme or 1 teaspoon minced fresh
Salt and freshly ground black pepper to taste
Minced fresh parsley for garnish

Dust the fillet lightly with flour. Heat a 10- or 12-inch nonstick skillet over medium-high heat for 3 or 4 minutes. Add the oil and, when it is hot (a pinch of flour will sizzle) raise the heat to high and brown the fish quickly, about 1 minute per side.

Add the wine to the pan, and let it bubble away for 20 seconds or so, still over high heat. Add the remaining ingredients except the parsley, reduce the heat to medium-low, and continue to cook, uncovered. If the sauce seems a bit thick, add a little chicken stock or coconut milk. Turn the fish once in the sauce during cooking; it will be done 5 to 7 minutes after the sauce begins to bubble, depending on the thickness of the fillet (a thin-bladed knife will pass through the fish with little resistance when it is done). Serve immediately, garnished with the parsley.

ALTERNATIVE FISH FOR THIS RECIPE:
Blackfish, grouper, halibut, mahi-mahi, monk-fish, rockfish, red snapper, swordfish, or wolffish. Adjust the cooking times accordingly.

BRAISED STRIPED BASS WITH ZUCCHINI AND LIGHTLY PICKLED ONIONS

Makes 4 servings
Time: About 60 minutes

A spicy striped bass dish that is great with a rice spiked with raisins, orzo, and/or chopped nuts.

1 medium-size zucchini
Salt
1 large Spanish or other sweet onion
⅓ cup white or white wine vinegar
½ cup dry white wine
½ teaspoon crushed red pepper or chili-garlic paste (available in Asian markets)
One 1 ½-pound striped bass fillet, skinned
½ cup olive or peanut oil
Flour for dredging
2 or 3 cloves garlic, minced
3 plum tomatoes, fresh or canned (drained if canned)
2 or 3 sprigs fresh thyme or ½ teaspoon dried
Freshly ground black pepper to taste

Rinse the zucchini and cut it into ½-inch-thick slices. Place it in a colander and sprinkle liberally with salt. Cut the onion in half and cut each half into slices; separate the slices into rings. Soak the rings in a bowl with the vinegar, wine, and hot pepper. Let the zucchini and onion sit for about 20 minutes before continuing.

Rinse the fish and dry it well between paper towels. Heat a 12-inch nonstick skillet over medium-high heat for 3 to 4 minutes. Add ⅓ cup of olive oil to the pan, dredge the fillet quickly in the flour, shake off the excess, and put it in the oil. Brown the fish, about 3 minutes. Turn and brown the other side. Turn off the heat and remove the fish to a plate.

Wipe out the pan (carefully; it is hot). Return it to the stove, over medium-high heat, and add the remaining oil. Rinse the zucchini and squeeze it in a dish towel to extract excess liquid. Add it to the oil, raise the heat to high, and add the garlic. Brown the zucchini, then turn the slices. Lift the onions from their marinade (do not discard), and add them to the pan. Stir once or twice, then cover and cook over medium heat for 3 minutes. Remove the cover and stir. Add the reserved marinade, raise the heat to high, and let it bubble away for 1 to 2 minutes. Add the tomatoes, crushing them with a fork, and the thyme. Cook, stirring occasionally, for 2 to 3 minutes. Taste the sauce for salt and pepper. Nestle the fish fillet in the sauce, cover the pan, and cook until the fillet offers little resistance when pierced with a thin-bladed knife, 5 minutes or so. Serve immediately.

ALTERNATIVE FISH FOR THIS RECIPE:
Blackfish, grouper, mahi-mahi, or monkfish. Adjust the cooking times accordingly.

CRISPY PAN-FRIED STRIPED BASS WITH SPICY GARLIC SAUCE

Makes 3 to 4 servings
Time: 20 minutes
Striped bass has a delicious, sturdy flavor, so it stands up to this sauce better than most other fish. I love this dish, especially at lunch.

½ cup peanut oil, more or less, plus 1 tablespoon
One 1- to 1½-pound striped bass fillet, skinned
Flour for dredging
1 large egg
1½ tablespoons minced garlic
1 teaspoon peeled and minced fresh ginger
1 tablespoon dry sherry
½ cup any fish or chicken stock (pages 40–41)
1 tablespoon high-quality soy sauce
¼ teaspoon chili-garlic paste (available in Asian markets) or hot sauce or to taste

Heat a 10- or 12-inch nonstick skillet over medium-high heat for 3 to 5 minutes. Add enough oil to cover the bottom to a depth of ⅛ inch or more. When the oil shimmers, toss a pinch of flour into it; if it sizzles, the pan is ready.

Dredge the fillet in the flour, then dip it into the egg, then back into the flour. Place it in the oil and raise the heat to high. Cook about 4 minutes, regulating the heat so the fish browns but does not burn. Turn it carefully and brown on the other side, again for about 4 minutes. Pierce the fish with a thin-bladed knife; when the knife passes through the fillet easily, the fish is done. Remove the pan from the heat and transfer the fish to paper towels to drain.

Working quickly, wipe the pan clean (carefully; it's still hot), return it to the stove over high heat, and add the tablespoon of oil. Place the garlic and ginger in the oil, stir, and let cook 15 seconds. Add the sherry; it will bubble away almost immediately. Add the stock and let it bubble for 30 seconds or so; add the soy sauce and cook for another few seconds. Add the chili-garlic paste, stir, turn off the heat, and pour the sauce over the fish. Serve immediately, with rice.

ALTERNATIVE FISH FOR THIS RECIPE:
Blackfish, bluefish, grouper, or mahi-mahi. Adjust the cooking times accordingly.

STURGEON

Latin name(s): *Acipenser transmontanus* and other species of the *Acipenser* genus.
Other common names: Hackleback, green sturgeon, white sturgeon, etc.
Common forms: Steaks, fillets, whole fish (rarely).
General description: Farm-raised fish with ivory-colored, boneless fillets and meaty steaks. Excellent veal substitute; very mild-flavored. Skin is tough and inedible.
For other recipes see: Swordfish, tuna.
Buying tips: Almost all sturgeon sold in this country is farm-raised, and quite expensive. Be sure the flesh glistens nicely; the odor should be sweet and may be slightly muddy.

Sturgeon is best known for its eggs which, when salted, make caviar. But the meat of sturgeon is also valuable for its veallike texture and mild flavor. Like salmon, sturgeon is anadromous, born in fresh water but spending much of its life at sea. And, like salmon, it has not thrived in the face of humans' incursions into its living areas. But more and more sturgeon is being raised in tanks in California, with encouraging results.

The differences between these tame creatures and those of the wild are profound: Wild sturgeon grow to several hundred pounds; the farm-raised beasts are "harvested" at about fifteen to twenty pounds. In the wild, sturgeon live for decades, and sometimes centuries; farm-raised fish are granted just a few years of life.

Still, farm-raised sturgeon have enough in common with their cousins to make them welcome additions to the kitchen: Like sharks and a number of other ancient fish (the sturgeon has been around for 200 million years), it relies on cartilage to retain its torpedolike body shape. Its flesh is an ivory white, firm enough to cut into scallops like veal and

sauté or grill, yet tender enough to cut with a fork. It's also a little on the fatty side, which makes it ideal for smoking (see the recipe for Smoked Sablefish, page 225), the form in which it has most often been found in recent years.

There are three problems with sturgeon. One is its flavor, or lack thereof; this is about as mild-flavored a fish as you can find. Another is its availability; although it is becoming increasingly common, you may have trouble finding it. Finally, like other farm-raised fish in the early stages of development, sturgeon can be expensive. Plan to spend about eight dollars a pound for fillets or steaks.

There's little you can do about the price, except buy smaller amounts of the fish (its sturdiness makes it ideal for stir-fries, so you can easily stretch a pound to feed four or more people). As for finding it, there is at least one mail-order source: Gerard and Dominique Seafood, in Seattle, Washington (800-858-0449). And the neutral flavor can be seen as an asset; much like veal, sturgeon provides a wonderful palette for your creative efforts.

PAN-FRIED STURGEON WITH THYME BUTTER

Makes 3 to 4 servings
Time: 20 minutes

One 1- to 1 ¼-pound sturgeon fillet
6 tablespoons (¾ stick) butter
1 large shallot, minced
Salt and freshly ground black pepper to taste
6 to 8 sprigs fresh thyme
Flour for dredging

Using a thin boning or fillet knife, cut ¼-inch-thick scallops from the fillet (see illustration, page 24). Heat a 10- or 12-inch nonstick skillet over medium-high heat for a few minutes. Meanwhile, melt 3 tablespoons of the butter in a small saucepan; add the shallot, salt, pepper, and 5 or 6 sprigs of the thyme and simmer over low heat while you cook the sturgeon.

Add 1 tablespoon of the remaining butter to the skillet, raise the heat to high and, when the foam subsides, dredge some of the sturgeon scallops in the flour. Cook until lightly browned on both sides, 2 to 3 minutes per side. Adding butter to the pan as necessary, cook all the scallops, keeping the done pieces warm in a low oven.

Remove the thyme from the butter and, still over low heat, stir in 2 more tablespoons of butter, 1 tablespoon at a time. Spoon a little of the thyme butter over the sturgeon, decorate with the remaining thyme sprigs, and serve, passing the remaining thyme butter at the table.

ALTERNATIVE FISH FOR THIS RECIPE:
Scallops cut from salmon; medallions of monkfish.

CRISP SAUTÉED STURGEON WITH PARMESAN CRUST

Makes 3 to 4 servings
Time: 20 minutes

One of the rare exceptions to my "no cheese with fish" rule.

One 1- to 1 ¼-pound sturgeon fillet
½ teaspoon salt
1 clove garlic
1 tablespoon minced fresh parsley
1 cup freshly grated Parmesan cheese
1 cup unseasoned bread crumbs
2 to 4 tablespoons olive oil
Chopped fresh parsley for garnish
Lemon wedges

Using a thin boning or fillet knife, cut ¼-inch-thick scallops from the fillet (see illustration, page 24). Mince together the salt, garlic, and parsley, and mix them with the cheese and bread crumbs. Heat a 12-inch nonstick skillet over medium heat for about 3 minutes; add 2 tablespoons of olive oil, and continue to heat until it shimmers. Dredge the sturgeon scallops in the bread crumb mixture and cook over medium-high heat until browned, about 2 minutes per side. Don't crowd the pan; you'll have to cook them in batches. As the scallops finish, keep them warm in a low oven. When they're all done, sprinkle with the chopped parsley and serve with lemon wedges.

VARIATION:
When the scallops are done, add 3 tablespoons of butter to the pan; cook over medium-high heat until the butter browns lightly, then add 2 tablespoons fresh lemon juice, 2 tablespoons capers, and ¼ cup chopped fresh parsley. Cook another 30 seconds or so, then spoon some of the sauce over each scallop and serve.

STURGEON WITH TUNA SAUCE

Makes 6 servings
Time: 30 minutes, plus time to chill
This is a cold dish, and a wonderful one. You can make it days in advance, and it just keeps getting better and better.

Court Boullion (page 41) or water, seasoned with a little thyme, whole peppercorns, salt, white wine, and distilled or other vinegar
One 2-pound sturgeon fillet
1 recipe Anchovy Mayonnaise (page 336), made with 6 to 8 anchovies
1 clove garlic, peeled
3 tablespoons capers, with a little of their juice
One 6 ½-ounce can tuna, preferably the dark Italian kind
½ cup olive oil, more or less
Sprinkling fresh lemon juice
Chopped fresh parsley for garnish

Bring an 1 to 2 inches of court boullion or seasoned water to a boil in a large, deep skillet that can later be covered. Cut the sturgeon fillet in two if necessary to fit it in the pot. Lower the heat to a simmer over medium heat, place the fillet in the liquid, cover the skillet, and cook, undisturbed, for 5 minutes. Turn off the heat and let the fish sit in the liquid. Remove the tail end of the fillet after 5 minutes and allow the thicker end of the fillet to rest for an additional 5 minutes. Ice down the fish, drain it, dry it with paper towels, and keep it cool.

With the mayonnaise still in the blender or food processor, add the garlic and capers and process until smooth. Add the tuna (drained, if it was packed in water or soy oil; with its oil, if packed in olive oil) and process until blended but not completely smooth. By hand, blend in enough olive oil to soften the mayonnaise and reduce it to the consistency of yogurt.

Using a thin boning or fillet knife, cut ¼-inch-thick scallops from the fillets (see illustration, page 24); there will be at least twelve. Layer a few on an attractive serving dish, cover with some of the sauce, and continue to make layers of sturgeon and sauce until both are used up. Cover and refrigerate from 1 hour to 2 to 3 days before serving.

When ready to serve, sprinkle with a little fresh lemon juice and top with chopped parsley.

A SIMPLER VARIATION:

Slice the poached sturgeon while it is still warm. Dress it with the best olive oil you can find, a little bit of lemon juice, some salt and pepper, and, if you like, a few minced fresh thyme leaves. Chill and serve cold.

BRAISED STURGEON WITH ONIONS AND CÈPES

Makes 4 to 6 servings
Time: 45 minutes
Braising is a traditional European approach to this meaty fish, and one that works nicely. It has the added advantage of giving you a little leeway in cooking time; even slightly overcooked fish will be moist. I prefer butter in this dish, for its richness of flavor, but olive oil is an acceptable substitute.

¼ cup (½ stick) butter or olive oil
4 or 5 medium to large onions, cut into rings
2 or 3 medium-size carrots, thinly sliced
½ cup any fish or chicken stock (pages 40–41) or water
¼ cup dried cèpes (porcini mushrooms; available in specialty or Italian markets)
Salt and freshly ground black pepper to taste
4 or 5 sprigs fresh thyme or 1 teaspoon dried
Four to six 1-inch-thick sturgeon steaks, about 4 to 6 ounces each

In a large skillet that you can later cover, melt the butter over medium heat. Add the onions and carrots and cook until the onions become tender, about 10 minutes. Heat the stock and soak the mushrooms in it for at least 10 minutes. When the onions soften, turn up the heat a little to brown them a bit.

Chop the mushrooms if they are large and strain the stock through a double layer of paper towels if it contains sand. Add both to the onion-carrot mixture and cook over medium-high heat until most of the liquid evaporates. Add the salt, pepper, and thyme. Sprinkle the fish steaks with salt and pepper, and lay them atop the onions. Cover, turn the heat to medium-low, and cook, basting occasionally with the pan juices, until done, about 20 minutes (the fish will become white and readily loosen from its center cartilage when prodded with a fork).

ALTERNATIVE FISH FOR THIS RECIPE:

Choose from a wide variety of steaks: Cod, grouper, halibut, salmon, swordfish, tilefish, or tuna. Take care not to overcook the more delicate fish.

GRILLED STURGEON WITH CAPERS AND TOMATOES

Makes 4 servings
Time: 30 minutes

¼ cup olive oil
2 tablespoons minced garlic
2 tablespoons capers
2 cups roughly chopped fresh or drained canned tomatoes
Salt and freshly ground black pepper to taste
½ cup minced fresh basil
Four 1-inch-thick sturgeon steaks, 4 to 6 ounces each

Start a gas or charcoal grill. Heat 2 tablespoons of the olive oil over medium heat in a 10-inch skillet and add the garlic; cook, stirring, until lightly colored, then add the capers. Cook 15 seconds; add the tomatoes, salt, and pepper and cook over medium-high heat until thick, about 10 minutes. Add half the basil, stir, and cook 1 minute more. Keep warm.

Brush the sturgeon with the remaining olive oil and sprinkle with salt and pepper. Grill until lightly browned on both sides, a total of 8 to 10 minutes; the fish will be stark white throughout. Serve immediately, covered lightly with sauce; garnish with the remaining basil.

ALTERNATIVE FISH FOR THIS RECIPE:

Steaks of grouper, large mackerel, marlin, striped bass, swordfish, or tuna.

SWORDFISH

Latin name(s): *Xiphias gladius*.

Other common names: None.

Common forms: Steaks (almost exclusively); skin is tough and inedible.

General description: Large fish (can weigh several hundred pounds) found in all of the world's oceans. Usually sold fresh in warm weather, frozen in colder months.

For other recipes see: Grouper, halibut, mahi-mahi, mako shark, monkfish, rockfish, salmon, red snapper, tuna.

Buying tips: The flesh should be gleaming and bright, with tight swirls. Browning and gaping are dead giveaways to fish that is going bad.

One of the original substitutes for "real" steak, swordfish became increasingly popular as a "heart-healthy" restaurant meal through the eighties. And it's a fish people love to grill at home, because it stays in one piece and doesn't stick to the grill. Swordfish doesn't quite rank with salmon and tuna for versatility, but, as long as it is not overcooked, it is just as delicious and even juicier when prepared simply.

Swordfish freezes well, and the chances are good that much of what you buy in the colder months will have been frozen. Just make sure that the fish smells good, and that the flesh is tightly closed (not "gaping"), and the quality will probably be fine. Contrary to the claims of many fishmongers, swordfish from one part of the world is not inherently better than that from any other; how the fish was treated after the catch is far more important.

BASIC GRILLED SWORDFISH

Makes 2 servings
Time: 45 minutes, including marinating

Nothing simpler, few things better. The marinade just gives a bit of tang to the browning crust; you could eliminate it, and brush the grilling fish with a bit of olive oil or soy sauce if you prefer. Or, skip it entirely. See Basic Grilled Tuna (page 329) for more variations.

One 1-inch-thick swordfish steak, weighing about 1 pound
Juice of 1 lime
2 tablespoons high-quality soy sauce
Lime or lemon wedges

Start a wood or charcoal fire or preheat a gas grill or broiler; the grill should be quite hot, and the grill grate clean. Soak the steak in the lime juice and soy sauce for 15 to 30 minutes, if desired. Grill the fish about 3 inches from the source of heat. Turn when nicely browned, about 4 to 5 minutes, then cook an additional 4 to 5 minutes. Check the fish for doneness by peeking between the layers of flesh with a thin-bladed knife—when the knife meets little resistance and no translucence remains, the swordfish is done. Serve immediately, with lime or lemon wedges.

ALTERNATIVE FISH FOR THIS RECIPE:

Steaks of mahi-mahi, mako shark, salmon, or tuna; eel or monkfish. Adjust the cooking times accordingly.

GRILLED SWORDFISH WITH
MUSTARD SAUCE:

Brush the fish lightly with olive oil, then sprinkle with salt and pepper. Omit the lime juice and soy sauce. Grill as directed above. Mix together ¼ cup olive oil, 3 tablespoons Dijon mustard, ¼ cup minced shallots, 2 tablespoons chopped fresh parsley, 2 tablespoons fresh lemon juice, salt, and pepper. Drizzle the steak with a bit of this, then pass the rest at the table. (This dish is great with boiled potatoes.)

GRILLED SWORDFISH WITH CORN AND TOMATO RELISH

Makes 4 servings
Time: 30 minutes
Make this dish only in late summer; without good corn and tomatoes, it's pointless.

Four 1-inch-thick swordfish steaks, about 6 ounces each (or cut a large steak into pieces)
3 tablespoons extra virgin olive oil
Salt and freshly ground black pepper to taste
4 ears corn, stripped of their kernels
2 large fresh ripe tomatoes, cored and roughly chopped
½ cup minced fresh basil

Preheat a gas grill or broiler or start a charcoal or wood fire; the fire should be quite hot. Brush the swordfish with 2 tablespoons of the olive oil and

season it with salt and pepper. Heat a 12-inch non-stick skillet over medium-high heat for 3 to 4 minutes. Add the remaining oil, then the corn. Cook, stirring, over high heat until lightly browned, 1 to 2 minutes. Add the tomato and the basil, cook 30 seconds more, then turn off the heat. Season with salt and pepper.

Grill the fish about 3 inches from the source of heat. Turn when nicely browned, about 4 or 5 minutes, then cook an additional 4 or 5 minutes (reduce the cooking time if you are using small steaks). Check the fish for doneness by peeking between the layers of flesh with a thin-bladed knife—when the knife meets little resistance and no translucence remains, the swordfish is done. Serve with the relish.

ALTERNATIVE FISH FOR THIS RECIPE:
Same as for Basic Grilled Swordfish (page 313).

LIME-GRILLED SWORDFISH WITH CUMIN VINAIGRETTE

Makes 4 servings
Time: 30 minutes

Zest of 1 lime, minced
1 clove garlic, minced
¼ cup fresh lime juice
Salt and freshly ground black pepper to taste
Four 1-inch-thick swordfish steaks, about 6 ounces each (or cut a large steak into pieces)
½ cup olive oil
½ teaspoon ground cumin
1 tablespoon capers
1 tablespoon minced fresh parsley

Preheat a gas grill or broiler or start a charcoal or wood fire; the fire should be quite hot. Mix together the lime zest and garlic with just enough of the lime juice to form a paste. Add salt and pepper, and rub the swordfish steaks lightly with the paste.

Grill the fish about 3 inches from the source of heat. Turn when nicely browned, about 4 to 5 minutes, then cook an additional 4 to 5 minutes. As the fish cooks, mix the remaining lime juice with the olive oil, cumin, capers, and parsley; season with salt and pepper, then taste to see whether more lime juice is needed. Check the fish for doneness by peeking between the layers of flesh with a thin-bladed knife—when the knife meets little resistance and no translucence remains, the swordfish is done. Serve the fish with a bit of the vinaigrette over each steak.

ALTERNATIVE FISH FOR THIS RECIPE:
Same as for Basic Grilled Swordfish (page 313).

GRILLED WASABI SWORDFISH WITH SPINACH AND SOY

Makes 4 servings
Time: 45 minutes
Wasabi, the dried horseradish used in sushi, is extremely hot; be very careful when handling it. Keep the powder in a closed container, where it will remain potent practically forever.

1 ½ teaspoons wasabi powder (available in Asian markets)
1 tablespoon water
1 tablespoon sesame seeds
1 pound fresh spinach, well washed and tough stems removed
2 tablespoons best-quality shoyu or tamari (Japanese soy sauce)
Four 1-inch-thick swordfish steaks, about 6 ounces each, or 1 or 2 larger ones, cut up to make 4 steaks
Salt and freshly ground black pepper to taste
Juice of ½ lemon
2 scallions, finely minced

Build a hot charcoal or wood fire, or preheat a gas grill or broiler until it is as hot as you can make it. Set a large pot of water to boil. Mix together the wasabi and water and set aside for a few minutes. Toast the sesame seeds: Heat them, dry, in a small skillet over medium heat, shaking occasionally, until they darken and begin to pop, about 5 minutes.

When the water boils, plunge the spinach into it and cook just for 1 to 2 minutes. Remove it and place in a bowl of ice water. Drain (squeezing it dry in your hands or a kitchen towel), chop, and mix it with 1 tablespoon of the soy sauce and half the sesame seeds; spread on a platter.

Using a knife or small spatula, spread the wasabe on the swordfish. Sprinkle with a little salt and pepper and grill about 4 minutes per side. Check for doneness by peeking between the layers of flesh with a thin-bladed knife—when the knife meets little resistance and no translucence remains, the swordfish is done.

Lay the cooked fish atop the spinach. Drizzle with the remaining soy sauce and the lemon juice. Garnish with the remaining sesame seeds and the minced scallions, and serve.

ALTERNATIVE FISH FOR THIS RECIPE:
Same as for Basic Grilled Swordfish (page 313).

GRILLED SWORDFISH ROLLS
SICILIAN STYLE

Makes 4 servings
Time: 40 minutes

When you want to grill something a little more adventuresome, try this.

¼ cup raisins
Four ½-inch-thick swordfish steaks, about 4 ounces each
3 tablespoons olive oil
1 large onion, chopped
1 teaspoon minced garlic
2 anchovy fillets, rinsed if salted and minced
¼ cup pine nuts or coarsely chopped walnuts
1 cup unseasoned bread crumbs
⅓ cup freshly grated Parmesan
Salt and freshly ground black pepper to taste
4 bay leaves
2 tablespoons fresh lemon juice

Preheat a gas grill or broiler or start a charcoal fire; the fire should be quite hot. Soak the raisins in warm water to cover for about 20 minutes. Place each swordfish steak between two pieces of waxed paper and gently pound them until they are about ¼ inch thick.

Heat 2 tablespoons of the olive oil in a skillet over medium heat, then add the onion and cook, stirring occasionally, until soft. Add the garlic, anchovies, and pine nuts. Drain the raisins and add them to the skillet. Cook, stirring occasionally, about 3 more minutes. Add the bread crumbs and cheese and cook another 3 minutes. Turn off the heat and let cool slightly. Season with pepper and salt (carefully, since both the anchovies and Parmesan are salty).

Spread each swordfish steak with a portion of the mixture. Roll the steaks up and close each with a toothpick. Skewer the rolled steaks with a bay leaf between each one. Mix the remaining olive oil with the lemon juice and brush the rolls with this mix-ture. Grill, turning once and brushing occasionally, for a total of 8 to 10 minutes; the rolls will offer lit-tle resistance to a thin-bladed knife when done. Serve hot or at room temperature.

ALTERNATIVE FISH FOR THIS RECIPE:
Mahi-mahi or tuna. Adjust the cooking times accordingly.

SWORDFISH KEBABS

Makes 6 servings
Time: 1 hour

1 to 1 ½ pounds swordfish steaks, cut into 1-inch chunks
3 medium-size onions, quartered
6 medium to large mushrooms, quartered
6 bay leaves
6 slices bacon, cut into 3 or 4 pieces each
Salt and freshly ground black pepper to taste
1 teaspoon dried thyme, marjoram, oregano, mint, or fennel seeds
½ cup olive oil
Juice of 1 lemon

Thread the swordfish onto six skewers, alternating with pieces of onion, mushroom, bay leaf, and bacon. Lay the skewers on a platter and sprinkle with salt, pepper, and the herb of your choice. Drizzle with the olive oil and lemon juice and let sit for about 30 minutes, in the refrigerator if the weather is warm, turning occasionally. Start a char-coal or wood fire or preheat a gas grill or broiler; the heat should be intense. Grill or broil about 4 to 6 inches from the heat source, turning occasionally, for about 12 minutes; the bacon should be cooked but not crisp, the swordfish browned but still moist (try a piece). Serve immediately.

ALTERNATIVE FISH FOR THIS RECIPE:
Mahi-mahi, salmon, or tuna. Adjust the cooking times accordingly.

SWORDFISH WITH GARLIC-PARSLEY BUTTER

Makes 4 servings
Time: 20 minutes

This recipe has lots of options: Grill the swordfish, bake it, broil it, or sauté it. As long as it isn't over-cooked, it will be wonderful.

Four 1-inch-thick swordfish steaks, 6 to 8 ounces each, or 2 large ones, 1 pound or so each
Olive oil as needed
Salt and freshly ground black pepper to taste
¼ cup (½ stick) butter
1 tablespoon minced garlic
¼ cup minced fresh parsley
1 lemon, quartered

Preheat the oven to 500°F, preheat the broiler, start a charcoal or gas grill, or preheat a 12-inch nonstick skillet over medium-high heat. Brush the swordfish liberally with olive oil and season with salt and pepper.

To roast, place in a baking dish and bake for 8 to 12 minutes, depending on size.

To grill or broil, place the fish about 4 inches from the source of heat. Turn when nicely browned, about 4 to 5 minutes; cook an additional 4 to 5 minutes.

To sauté, cook the fish over high heat until nicely browned, 3 to 5 minutes per side.

With all the methods, check the fish for doneness by peeking between the layers of flesh with a thin-bladed knife—when the knife meets little resistance and no translucence remains, it's done.

While fish is cooking, melt the butter in a small saucepan over medium-low heat. Add the garlic and cook, stirring occasionally, until lightly browned; add the parsley and season with salt and pepper. To serve, spoon a little of the garlic butter over each steak; squeeze lemon juice over all and serve.

ALTERNATIVE FISH FOR THIS RECIPE:

Same as for Basic Grilled Swordfish (page 313).

SWORDFISH SANDWICHES WITH TOMATO-CAPER SAUCE

Makes 2 servings
Time: 20 minutes

A great sandwich, and not much more difficult to put together than a hamburger. You don't have to serve it as a sandwich, of course; leave the swordfish steak whole, increase the cooking time slightly, and it becomes a dinner or lunch entrée.

One 1-inch-thick swordfish steak, about ¾ pound
2 tablespoons olive oil
Flour for dredging
Salt and freshly ground black pepper to taste
1 teaspoon minced garlic
1 tablespoon capers, with a little of their vinegar
1 medium-size ripe tomato, cut into ½-inch dice
1 tablespoon fresh lemon juice
2 pita breads, cut in half, or any other bread you like

Preheat a 10- or 12-inch nonstick skillet over medium-high heat. Cut the swordfish into strips about ½ inch wide. Add the oil to the skillet. When the oil is hot (a pinch of flour will sizzle), dredge the swordfish steaks in the flour and cook them, seasoning on all sides with salt and pepper, until lightly browned and crisp all over, about 5 to 6 minutes total. Remove them from the skillet, and toss in the garlic, capers, and tomato. Cook briskly, stirring occasionally, until the tomato begins to liquefy, 1 to 2 minutes. Add the lemon juice, taste for salt and pepper, and turn off the heat. Make sandwiches with the swordfish and sauce.

ALTERNATIVE FISH FOR THIS RECIPE:

Mahi-mahi or tuna. Adjust the cooking times accordingly.

SPICY SWORDFISH CHUNKS WITH CUCUMBER

Makes 4 servings
Time: 45 minutes

Treated this way, cucumbers are not watery and mushy when cooked. Their crispness makes a nice foil for the tender swordfish and spicy sauce.

2 cucumbers
Salt
1 ½ pounds swordfish steaks, cut into 1 ½-inch cubes
½ cup white, rice, or cider vinegar
1 tablespoon curry powder
Freshly ground black pepper to taste
3 tablespoons peanut or vegetable oil
1 medium-size onion, chopped
2 or 3 fresh jalapeños or other hot peppers, deveined, seeded, and minced
1 tablespoon minced garlic
1 tablespoon peeled and minced fresh ginger
1 tablespoon sugar

Peel the cucumbers if they are not perfectly fresh; if they are, leave the peel on if you like. Cut them in half and scoop out the seeds with a spoon. Slice them thinly, put them in a colander, and sprinkle liberally with salt. Let them sit for 30 minutes; meanwhile, prepare the other ingredients.

Sprinkle the fish with a little of the vinegar, then with the curry powder, salt, and pepper; keep it cool.

Rinse the cucumbers briefly, then put them in a kitchen towel and wring all remaining moisture out of them. Heat the oil in a 12-inch skillet over medium heat; add the onion and cook, stirring, until it is soft. Add the jalapeños, garlic, ginger,

and sugar, and cook, stirring occasionally, for 2 minutes over medium-high heat. Add the cucumbers and cook another 2 minutes. Add the remaining vinegar and let bubble for 1 to 2 minutes. Add the swordfish and cook over medium heat, stirring, until the fish is almost cooked through, 4 to 5 minutes. Serve immediately, over rice.

ALTERNATIVE FISH FOR THIS RECIPE:

Mahi-mahi or tuna. Adjust the cooking times accordingly.

STIR-FRIED SWORDFISH WITH BROCCOLI

Makes 4 servings
Time: 30 minutes

2 cups broccoli florets
1 tablespoon peeled and minced fresh ginger
1 teaspoon minced garlic
2 tablespoons high-quality soy sauce
2 tablespoons dry sherry or rice wine
1 tablespoon cornstarch
1 pound swordfish steaks, cut into 1-inch cubes
2 tablespoons peanut oil
1 cup seeded and chopped red bell pepper
½ cup snow or snap peas, fine strings removed
½ cup minced scallions, both green and white parts
1 cup any fish or chicken stock (pages 40–41)
1 teaspoon sesame oil
Minced cilantro (fresh coriander) for garnish

Parboil or microwave the broccoli until it is barely tender. Combine the ginger, garlic, soy sauce, sherry, and cornstarch; add the swordfish and stir to blend. Marinate for about 20 minutes, in the refrigerator if the weather is warm; drain and reserve the marinade.

Heat a wok or 12-inch nonstick skillet over high heat for 5 minutes; add half the peanut oil and heat until it smokes. Toss the fish in the oil and stir-fry until it browns lightly, 2 to 3 minutes. Remove the swordfish and wipe the wok or skillet clean.

Reheat the wok or skillet, add the remaining oil, and stir-fry the pepper and broccoli over high heat for about 2 minutes. Add the snow peas and scallions and stir. Add the fish, marinade, and stock. Bring to a boil; the sauce will thicken slightly. Stir in the sesame oil and serve over rice, topped with minced cilantro.

ALTERNATIVE FISH FOR THIS RECIPE:

Chunks of blackfish, grouper, lobster, mahi-mahi, mako shark, monkfish, or salmon; shrimp. Adjust the cooking times accordingly.

ROAST GARLIC-STUDDED SWORDFISH WITH SALSA FRESCA

Makes 4 servings
Time: 20 minutes
You can grill the swordfish instead of roasting it; follow the directions for Basic Grilled Swordfish on page 313.

1 clove garlic, cut into tiny slivers
One 1-inch-thick swordfish steak, about 1 ½ to 2 pounds
2 tablespoons peanut oil
Salt and freshly ground black pepper to taste
1 recipe Salsa Fresca (page 209)

Preheat the oven to 500°F. With the aid of a boning knife, insert the garlic slivers into the middle of the steak. Brush the bottom of a baking pan with half the oil and lay the fish in it; brush the top of the fish with the remaining oil and sprinkle it with salt and pepper. Roast 10 to 15 minutes and check for doneness by peeking between the layers of flesh with a thin-bladed knife—when the knife meets little resistance and no translucence remains, the fish is done. Serve immediately, passing the salsa at the table.

ALTERNATIVE FISH FOR THIS RECIPE:
Tuna. Adjust the cooking time accordingly.

ROAST SWORDFISH WITH LEMON GRASS–MUSTARD SAUCE

Makes 4 servings
Time: 60 minutes
Like Roast Garlic-studded Swordfish with Salsa Fresca (preceding recipe) and Swordfish with Garlic-parsley Butter (page 317), this can be grilled. I prefer to roast it, though, because the baking pan retains all the delicious marinade and cooking juices.

1 tablespoon Dijon mustard
1 tablespoon chopped fresh lemon grass or 1 teaspoon ground dried (available in Asian markets)
1 tablespoon sugar
1 tablespoon high-quality soy sauce
1 tablespoon chopped garlic
2 tablespoons chopped shallot or onion
½ teaspoon freshly ground black pepper
1 tablespoon dry sherry
1 teaspoon sesame oil
One 1-inch-thick swordfish steak, 1 ½ to 2 pounds

Combine all ingredients except the swordfish in a food processor or blender; process until smooth. Spoon the mixture over the swordfish and marinate 20 to 30 minutes, in the refrigerator if the weather is warm. Preheat the oven to 500°F or start a grill. Roast 10 to 15 minutes and check for doneness by peeking between the layers of flesh with a thin-bladed knife—when the knife meets little resistance and no translucence remains, the fish is done. Serve immediately, spooning the pan juices over the fish.

ALTERNATIVE FISH FOR THIS RECIPE:
Mackerel, mahi-mahi, salmon, or tuna. Adjust the cooking times accordingly.

TILAPIA

Latin name(s): Various species of *Tilapia*.
Other common names: Mouthbrooder, St. Peter's fish, Nile perch.
Common forms: Whole.
General description: Freshwater fish popular in Asia, now being farm-raised here. Edible skin may be reddish, white, gray, or bluish.
For recipes see: Porgy, sea bass.
Buying tips: See below.

More and more, we're seeing tilapia in fish markets being sold as a substitute for red snapper and other whole fish. But every farm-raised tilapia I've ever had (and all the tilapia sold here is farm-raised) has had an undesirable, muddy flavor. I avoid this fish when I see it, and recommend that you do also.

TILEFISH

Latin name(s): *Lopholatilus chamaeleonticeps*.
Other common names: Ocean whitefish, blanquillo.
Common forms: Whole, fillets, steaks (rarely).
General description: Wonderfully versatile yellow-spotted Atlantic fish from one to ten pounds with firm, white flesh and delicious skin.
For other recipes see: Blackfish, bluefish, carp, catfish, cod, dogfish, grouper, haddock, halibut, mackerel, mako shark, monkfish, ocean perch, pollock, rockfish, sea bass, red snapper, striped bass, turbot, weakfish, whiting, wolffish.
Buying tips: Good tilefish is lovely—colorful, bright, and alive-looking. The yellow spots fade and eyes become increasingly dull with age. In addition, there are the more common and reliable indicators: the gills, which should be red, the flesh, which should be firm, and the smell, which should be of seawater.

Long Beach, New Jersey, is known—in Long Beach at least—as "The Tilefish Capital of the World," but tilefish are found up and down the East Coast. Because they are a deep-water fish, they are rarely caught in droves and so are hardly a staple of fish markets anywhere (except, perhaps, Long Beach).

They are, however, a fish to be bought whenever possible. You might think of tilefish as a less expensive red snapper: It's firmer than cod, with snow white, large-flaked flesh. It's said that the diet of tilefish consists primarily of crabs and lobster; I don't know whether that's true, but it might explain why the flesh of tilefish is as firm and delicious as that of red snapper or any other first-class white-fleshed fish. Cook it whole whenever possible; fillets are great too.

GRILLED WHOLE TILEFISH WITH TARRAGON AND LEMON

Makes 4 servings
Time: About 30 minutes
You will need a grilling basket for this preparation; the long, thin kind specially designed for whole fish (see page 26) is best. Leaving the head on makes for a nicer presentation, but you can cut it off if the fish is too big.

One 3- to 4-pound tilefish, gutted and scaled, preferably with the head on
5 sprigs fresh tarragon
1 lemon, thinly sliced
Coarse salt

Preheat a gas grill or start a charcoal or wood fire; the fire should be medium-hot. Rinse the fish well, make three or four vertical slashes on each side, then place 1 sprig of tarragon and 2 lemon slices in the body cavity. Place the remaining tarragon and lemon in the slashes and on the outside of the fish—half on each side—and sprinkle all quite liberally with coarse salt. Sandwich the fish in the grilling basket.

Grill, turning occasionally, about 4 to 6 inches from the heat source, until dark brown on both sides, about 20 minutes total. (The fish is done when it is opaque clear down to the bone and flakes easily when prodded with a fork.) Remove the fish from the basket to a platter. Serve by spooning parts of the fish off the bone onto plates.

ALTERNATIVE FISH FOR THIS RECIPE:

Whole bluefish, mackerel, sea bass, red snapper, or striped bass. Adjust the cooking times accordingly.

ROASTED WHOLE TILEFISH WITH
TOMATOES AND LEMON

Makes 4 servings
Time: 60 minutes

This recipe shows what a first-class fish tilefish is. Its wonderful juices make the sauce and its delicious, firm meat holds up to the relatively long baking time. Serve it with bread, rice, or potatoes.

¼ cup olive oil
2 medium-size onions, sliced and separated into rings
4 sprigs fresh marjoram or oregano or 1 teaspoon dried
Salt and freshly ground black pepper to taste
4 medium-size ripe tomatoes, seeded and roughly chopped
3 cloves garlic, minced
½ cup minced fresh parsley
Juice of 1 lemon
One 2 ½- to 3-pound tilefish, scaled and gutted, with head on or off
½ cup unseasoned bread crumbs, more or less
1 lemon, thinly sliced

Preheat the oven to 425°F. Warm 2 tablespoons of the olive oil in a skillet. Add the onions and cook over medium-high heat, stirring frequently. When they begin to soften, add half the marjoram and some salt and pepper. Remove the onions from the heat when they are tender but not mushy, and let them cool.

Mix the tomatoes with the garlic, parsley, the remaining marjoram, and the lemon juice.

Rinse the fish and dry it. Add the cooled onions to the tomato mixture and enough bread crumbs to absorb most of the liquid from the tomatoes (don't make it too dry; the mixture should be quite creamy).

Cut four or five parallel slashes on each side of the tilefish. Put it in a baking pan large enough to hold it snugly (you might need to cut the fish's head off), rub the fish with the remaining olive oil, and lay it in the pan. Stuff the fish with some of the tomato-onion mixture, and spoon the rest of the mixture around and on top of the fish. Lay the lemon slices over all.

Roast the fish until the meat near the bone is no longer pink; start peeking in the slashes after about 20 minutes, although total cooking time is likely to be 30 to 35 minutes. Serve immediately.

ALTERNATIVE FISH FOR THIS RECIPE:

Whole bluefish, carp, grouper, sea bass, red snapper, striped bass, or weakfish. Adjust the cooking times accordingly.

BRAISED WHOLE TILEFISH
WITH SHALLOTS

Makes 4 servings
Time: 35 minutes

2 tablespoons butter
2 tablespoons olive oil
One 2- to 3-pound tilefish, scaled and gutted, with head on if possible

2 tablespoons minced shallots
1 cup dry white wine
Juice of ½ lemon
Salt and freshly ground black pepper to taste
Minced fresh parsley for garnish

Heat the butter and oil over medium-high heat in a 12-inch nonstick skillet. When the foam from the butter subsides, put the fish in the pan (remove the head and tail if necessary) and brown it on both sides, about 10 minutes total. Sprinkle the shallots into the skillet, add the wine, and let it bubble away for 1 to 2 minutes. Cover the pan, reduce the heat to low, and cook for about 20 minutes (or about 10 minutes per inch of the fish's thickness). Uncover, sprinkle with the lemon juice, season with salt and pepper, garnish with the parsley, and serve.

ALTERNATIVE FISH FOR THIS RECIPE:

Whole bluefish, carp, grouper, rockfish, sea bass, or red snapper. Adjust the cooking times accordingly.

SIMMERED WHOLE TILEFISH

Makes 4 servings
Time: 30 minutes

"Boiling," as it is equally accurately but less romantically called, was once a popular method for cooking whole fish. And it's still quite wonderful, especially if you have an impeccably fresh, firm-fleshed specimen. Tile, with its lobsterlike texture, it a prime candidate, but there are others (see below).

1 gallon Court Bouillon (page 41) or an equal amount of water combined with the following:
½ cup distilled or wine vinegar
1 medium-size onion
Several cloves unpeeled garlic
2 medium-size carrots, cut into chunks

Several sprigs fresh parsley
Handful coarse salt
2 bay leaves
One 3-pound tilefish, gutted and scaled, head on if possible

Bring the court bouillon or all the other ingredients, except the fish, to a boil. Lower the fish gently into the simmering liquid and cook about 15 minutes over medium heat. Remove it with a slotted spoon or strainer and check for doneness (cut a small slit at the thickest part and see whether any pinkness remains; if not, the fish is done). Return for further cooking if necessary; be careful not to overcook.

Drain on cloth or paper napkins or towels. Remove the skin if you like. Serve hot, cold, or at room temperature, with any of the following:

A light sprinkling of olive oil, fresh lemon juice, and minced fresh parsley
Green Sauce (page 144)
Pesto (page 41)
Parsley Pesto (page 208)
Creamy Pesto (page 76)
Garlicky Green Mayonnaise (page 236)
Anchovy Mayonnaise (page 336)
Dijon mustard

ALTERNATIVE FISH FOR THIS RECIPE:

Whole blackfish, carp, grouper, or red snapper. Adjust the cooking times accordingly.

BOILED FISH DINNER:

Poach several mild-flavored root vegetables in the court bouillon (if making a stock, simmer all the ingredients together for 45 minutes, then strain before adding the root vegetables)—peeled potatoes, carrots, parsnips, Jerusalem artichokes, etc.—until tender. Remove them and keep them warm in a low oven while you cook the fish.

TILEFISH FILLET WITH SCALLIONS

....

Makes 4 servings
Time: 20 minutes

Tilefish fillets are wonderful for braising; they hold their shape, texture, and moisture even if they're slightly overcooked.

2 tablespoons olive oil
2 tilefish fillets, preferably with skin on, about 1
½ to 2 pounds total
Salt and freshly ground black pepper to taste
Flour for dredging
2 cups chopped scallions or spring onions, green parts included
1 cup any chicken or fish stock (pages 40–41)
1 tablespoon high-quality soy sauce
Minced scallions, green and white parts for garnish

Heat a 12-inch nonstick skillet over medium-high heat for 3 to 4 minutes. Add the oil and raise the heat to high. Sprinkle the fish with salt and pepper, dredge in the flour, and brown for 2 minutes per side. Remove the fish and add the scallions; cook them, stirring occasionally, over high heat for 1 to 2 minutes, then add the stock and soy sauce. Let the liquid bubble away, then return the fish to the skillet, skin side down. Turn the heat down so that the liquid barely bubbles and cook the fish until it is tender and white, about 5 minutes. Serve immediately, garnished with minced scallions.

ALTERNATIVE FISH FOR THIS RECIPE:

Fillets of blackfish, carp, catfish, cod, dogfish, grouper, haddock, ocean perch, pollock, rockfish, red snapper, turbot, or wolffish. Adjust the cooking times accordingly.

BRAISED CURRIED TILEFISH:

Substitute onions for the scallions; add 1 tablespoon each peeled and minced fresh ginger and garlic along with the onions. Stir in 2 tablespoons fresh lime juice, 1 tablespoon curry powder, and 1 seeded, deveined, and minced jalapeño (optional) along with the stock and soy sauce. Cook as directed above; garnish with minced cilantro (fresh coriander).

TROUT

Latin name(s): *Salmo gairdneri* and others.
Other common names: Rainbow, brook, golden, brown, lake trout; salmon trout; char; steelhead.
Common forms: Whole, gutted (usually); split; fillets.
General description: Commercially available rainbow are a farm-raised version of the popular freshwater sport fish; other "trout" such as steelhead and char are best treated as salmon. As with salmon, skin is edible and delicious.
For other recipes see: Salmon.
Buying tips: Flesh should be shiny pink-orange; skin a brilliant gray. Smell should be fresh.

We could be singing the praises of trout for hours, for wild trout is as delicious a fish as there is, with pink, creamy, rich, flavorful flesh. But this is a book for shoppers, not one for fishermen. And the sad fact is that you can't buy wild trout in fish markets, and farm-raised trout is, by comparison, a tasteless and overrated fish.

Trout and salmon are closely related (there are seagoing trout and landlocked salmon) and there are some fish sold in markets as trout—most notably steelheads and char—that make wonderful eating. These are best treated as salmon, and cooked according to the recipes in that section. The recipes here are, of course, best with wild trout, but will also give good results with the farm-raised variety.

GRILLED TROUT WITH SAUSAGES AND PARSLEY PESTO

Makes 4 servings
Time: 30 minutes
Good, freshly caught trout can stand up to anything, even meat. This is loosely based on a dish I had in Provence.

4 small spicy sausages, any type
4 small whole trout, about ¾ pound each, gutted, heads on
Salt and freshly ground black pepper to taste
Parsley Pesto (page 208)

You can grill or broil the trout and sausage. If you choose to grill, oil a grilling basket (see page 26) and build a medium-hot charcoal or wood fire, or preheat a gas grill. Whether you grill or broil, keep the trout and sausages 4 to 6 inches from the heat source.

Grill or broil the sausages first; when they're nearly done, start the trout. Turn it frequently, and salt and pepper it as it cooks. When the skin blisters and the inside becomes pale in color—about 12 to 15 minutes—the fish is done. Serve it with the sausages and pesto.

ALTERNATIVE FISH FOR THIS RECIPE:
Butterfish, mackerel, pompano, or small salmon. Adjust the cooking times accordingly.

PAN-FRIED TROUT

Makes 2 servings
Time: 30 minutes

There are countless ways to pan-fry trout, from the simple to the complex. If you catch your own fish, the simplest is best. If you must rely on the relatively insipid farm-raised product, try one of the more flavorful variations.

2 whole trout, about ¾ pound each, gutted and split or filleted
1 cup oatmeal or cornmeal
¼ cup (½ stick) butter
Salt and freshly ground black pepper to taste
Minced fresh parsley for garnish

Rinse and dry the fish. If you're using oatmeal, grind it quickly in a food processor or blender so that it's almost as fine as coarse cornmeal.

Melt the butter over medium-high heat in a 12-inch nonstick skillet. When the foam subsides, dredge the fish in the meal, place in the pan, and raise the heat to high. Season with salt and pepper and cook on both sides until nicely browned and the interior turns white. Garnish with parsley and serve.

ALTERNATIVE FISH FOR THIS RECIPE:
Butterfish, croaker, mackerel, pompano, porgy, or small salmon. Adjust the cooking times accordingly.

TROUT WITH BACON:
Begin by cooking 4 slices of good bacon in a skillet. When the bacon is nice and crisp, remove it to a warm oven. Proceed as directed above, cooking the trout in the bacon fat. Garnish with the bacon slices.

MARINATED TROUT:
Thirty minutes before cooking, pour a mixture of ¼ cup olive oil, 1 tablespoon balsamic, sherry, or other flavorful vinegar, 1 minced shallot, and some salt and pepper over the fish. Turn the fish occasionally, dry it before cooking, then cook it in olive oil instead of butter.

TROUT WITH LEMON AND CUMIN:
Proceed as directed in the original recipe, using olive oil rather than butter and adding 1 tablespoon ground cumin to the dredging meal. When the fish are done, remove them to a warm oven. Cook, stirring, ¼ cup minced shallots or onion in the fat remaining in the pan over medium heat. When soft, add 1 teaspoon minced garlic, 2 tablespoons minced fresh parsley, 1 teaspoon ground cumin, and ½ cup red wine. Raise the heat to high and reduce the liquid to a glaze. Add 2 tablespoons fresh lemon juice and 2 more tablespoons wine. Reduce slightly, pour over the fish, garnish with additional minced parsley, and serve.

TROUT SIMMERED IN RED WINE

Makes 2 servings
Time: 30 minutes

2 tablespoons butter
¼ cup minced shallots
½ cup minced carrot
2 tablespoons all-purpose flour
Several sprigs of fresh thyme or ½ teaspoon dried
1 bay leaf
1 tablespoon minced fresh parsley
Salt and freshly ground black pepper to taste
1 ½ cups good red wine
2 whole trout, about ¾ pound each, gutted, heads on or off
Minced fresh parsley for garnish

Heat the butter over medium heat in a steep-sided 10-inch skillet. When it has melted, add the shallots and carrot and cook, stirring occasionally, until the shallots are soft. Add the flour and stir; add the thyme, bay leaf, parsley, salt, and pepper, stir, and cook for about 1 minute, then add the wine. Raise the heat a bit until the wine starts to bubble, then reduce it so that the wine simmers.

Add the trout to the skillet and simmer, turning once, for a total of about 10 to 12 minutes; the flesh will become tender and pale when the trout is done. Remove the trout and keep it warm; reduce the sauce over high heat until it is quite thick, then spoon it over the fish. Garnish with parsley and serve.

ALTERNATIVE FISH FOR THIS RECIPE:
Small salmon. Adjust the cooking times accordingly.

TROUT SIMMERED IN TOMATO SAUCE:
Substitute pureed tomatoes for the red wine and ¼ cup minced fresh basil for the thyme and bay leaf. Don't reduce the sauce quite as much.

ROAST TROUT WITH HERBS

Makes 2 servings
Time: 20 minutes

1 teaspoon minced fresh tarragon
1 tablespoon minced fresh parsley, plus extra for garnish
1 teaspoon minced garlic
2 tablespoons olive oil
1 tablespoon fresh lemon juice
Salt and freshly ground black pepper to taste
2 whole trout, about ¾ pound each, gutted, heads on
Lemon wedges

Preheat the oven to 450°F. Make a paste of the tarragon, parsley, garlic, oil, lemon juice, salt, and pepper, and rub this all over the fish. Place them in a baking pan and roast until they are done, without turning, a total of about 15 minutes (the flesh will flake easily when prodded with a fork). Serve, garnished with parsley and accompanied by lemon wedges.

ALTERNATIVE FISH FOR THIS RECIPE:
Butterfish, mackerel, pompano, or small salmon. Adjust the cooking times accordingly.

ROAST TROUT WITH SAGE:
Omit the tarragon, parsley, garlic, olive oil, and lemon juice. Make an herb butter using sage (page 44). Spread this all over the fish, sprinkle with salt and pepper, and roast, garnish, and serve as directed above.

TUNA

Latin name(s): *Thunnus thynnus* (bluefin); *T. albacares* (yellowfin), etc.
Other common names: Albacore, tunny, bonito, ahi, bigeye, bluefin, yellowfin, skipjack.
Common forms: Almost exclusively steaks, although some smaller skipjack may be filleted. Freezes well.
General description: Pale pink (albacore) to deep red (bluefin and yellowfin) meat, the most beeflike of all fish. Almost always sold without the skin, which is inedibly tough. Dark brown flesh is edible but stronger-tasting; those who find it too "fishy" may remove it before or after cooking.
For other recipes see: Blackfish, bluefish, eel, grouper, mackerel, mahi-mahi, mako shark, monkfish, pompano, salmon, red snapper, striped bass, swordfish.
Buying tips: Avoid fish with dry or brown spots, that which is uneven in color (with the exception of the naturally darker flesh, of course), that whose flesh reflects rainbows, or, of course, that whose smell is suspect.

In its canned form, tuna is the most popular fish in the United States. But it is the fresh fish—about 1 percent of the total sold—that is my primary concern. Only recently have we begun to appreciate the glories of fresh tuna. The best-known Italian recipe using tuna—*vitello tonnato*, cold roast veal with a tuna sauce—is made with canned fish. And James Beard wrote that tuna "is a fish that I think is better canned than fresh."

Sadly, Beard died before he could see the amazing things his disciples have done with fresh tuna: served raw and simply, made to mimic beef (which it does well), marinated, stuffed with herbs and roasted, and many more. The upshot is that many fishlovers, myself included, rank fresh tuna among their favorite fish.

Tuna are among the most impressive creatures on earth: They can swim fifty-five miles an hour, and they swim constantly—the majestic bluefin covers about 75,000 miles a year. As a result, they have a hefty appetite, and eat as much as 10 percent of their weight each day in order to maintain their high-pressured circulation system which feeds their body's main feature: muscle.

It is this muscle which makes such superb eating. Like sirloin steak, tuna is red, tender, flavorful, and better rare than well done. But unlike most beef, tuna is almost fat-free—less than 1 percent by weight.

There are several types of tuna in our markets; the relatively fatty bluefin is the tuna of choice, but yellowfin is far more common, less expensive, and almost as delicious. Skipjack, albacore, and a couple of others round out the list. All species migrate up and down the Atlantic and Pacific coasts, wintering in the south and becoming relatively plentiful in the north from late spring until late fall. (In years with mild winters, some Massachusetts fishermen catch tuna for Christmas dinner.) And with improved shipping and an increase in frozen product, tuna is available in much of the country year-round.

Don't shy away from frozen tuna. Ironically, this fish freezes so well that the best—and among the most expensive—"fresh" tuna, the so-called sushi grade, is gutted, iced, cut into loins, and blast frozen within an hour or two of the catch. These days, I don't eat much raw tuna at home. But if I'm sure of the source, I just cut it into cubes and serve it with the Ginger-Soy Dipping Sauce on page 154.

BASIC GRILLED TUNA

Makes 4 servings
Time: 1 hour, including marinating time

If ever a fish was meant to be grilled, it is tuna. If ever a dish was designed to appeal to beef lovers, it is grilled tuna. This simple method yields a crisp, simple steak, in some ways the most desirable way to eat tuna. For more elaborate preparations, see the variations and the succeeding two or three recipes.

⅓ **cup high-quality soy sauce (Japanese or domestic "shoyu")**
2 tablespoons olive oil
1 ½ to 2 pounds tuna, preferably in 1 steak
Ginger-soy Dipping Sauce (page 154; optional)
Lemon wedges (optional)

Mix the soy sauce and olive oil in a plate and marinate the tuna for 1 hour or less. Start a charcoal or wood fire—it should be quite hot—or preheat a gas grill or broiler and grill or broil the tuna about 4 inches from the heat source, basting occasionally with the marinade. Turn once, after about 5 minutes. Check for doneness by cutting into the steak with a thin-bladed knife; tuna should not be cooked well done, and will continue to cook a bit after you remove it from the grill. This will yield a crisp but slightly rare steak; cook longer if you prefer a darker steak, but be careful not to overcook. Serve with the sauce or lemon wedges.

<small>ALTERNATIVE FISH FOR THIS RECIPE:</small>

Thick, firm steaks of grouper, mahi-mahi, salmon, or swordfish; eel, monkfish, or shrimp (shells on). Adjust the cooking times accordingly.

<small>GRILLED TUNA WITH LEMON MARINADE:</small>

Add 2 tablespoons fresh lemon juice to the marinade and proceed as directed above. (You can reduce the olive oil to 1 tablespoon, or eliminate it entirely if you like.)

<small>GRILLED TUNA WITH MUSTARD:</small>

Do not marinate the tuna, but spread it with 2 tablespoons Dijon mustard before grilling.

<small>GRILLED TUNA WITH GINGER AND GARLIC:</small>

Add 1 tablespoon each minced fresh ginger and garlic to the original recipe.

<small>GRILLED TUNA WITH HERBS:</small>

Omit the olive oil and soy sauce. Rub the tuna with a mixture of 1 tablespoon grated or minced lemon peel, 1 teaspoon coarse salt, 1 large clove garlic, minced, and 2 tablespoons minced mixed fresh herbs, such as parsley, chives, basil, sage, thyme, and/or rosemary. Grill as directed above.

<small>GRILLED TUNA WITH MANGO-ONION RELISH:</small>

Omit the olive oil and soy sauce. Make a salsa with the chopped meat of 2 mangoes, ½ cup diced red onion, the juice of 2 limes, 2 tablespoons minced cilantro (fresh coriander), salt, and freshly ground black pepper. Brush the tuna lightly with olive or peanut oil, grill as directed above, and serve with the salsa.

GRILLED TUNA MARINATED WITH FRESH TOMATO SALSA

Makes 4 servings
Time: About 60 minutes
Just a tad more complicated than the recipes above.

1 cup loosely packed cilantro (fresh coriander) leaves
1 small red onion, diced
1 teaspoon ground cumin
Juice of 2 lemons
1 tablespoon olive oil
Salt and freshly ground black pepper to taste
1 large or 2 small tuna steaks, about 1 ½ pounds total
4 medium-size ripe tomatoes, roughly chopped
1 clove garlic, finely minced
Dash cayenne pepper or hot sauce or to taste

Mix together half the cilantro, the onion, cumin, lemon juice, olive oil, salt, and pepper. Marinate the tuna in this mixture for 1 hour or less (or more, refrigerated). Mix the remaining cilantro with the tomatoes, garlic, cayenne, salt, and pepper; let stand until ready to serve.

Start a charcoal or wood fire—it should be quite hot—or preheat a gas grill or broiler and grill or broil the tuna about 4 inches from the heat source, basting occasionally with the marinade. Turn once, after about 5 minutes. Check for doneness by cutting into the steak with a thin-bladed knife; tuna should not be cooked well done, and will continue to cook a bit after you remove it from the grill. This will yield a crisp but slightly rare steak; cook longer if you prefer a darker steak, but be careful not to overcook. Serve with the fresh tomato salsa.

ALTERNATIVE FISH FOR THIS RECIPE:
Same as for Basic Grilled Tuna (page 329).

SEMEON'S GRILLED ARUGULA-STUFFED TUNA STEAKS

Makes 4 servings
Time: 90 minutes, including marinating time
This is a gorgeous dish that seems to please everyone. The lime and pepper marinade complements the assertiveness of the arugula, which is somewhat tamed by a brief warming. Do not be intimidated by the creation of the pocket; it is easy, and takes just a minute.

Juice of 3 limes
¼ cup high-quality soy sauce
1 medium-size clove garlic, minced
1 teaspoon strong mustard
2 teaspoons peeled and finely minced fresh ginger or 1 teaspoon ground
½ teaspoon sesame oil
½ teaspoon coarsely ground black pepper
¼ cup dry white wine or water
1 tuna steak, no less than 1 ¼ inches thick, about 1 ½ pounds
1 small bunch arugula (about 1 cup leaves)

Mix together all the ingredients except the tuna and arugula; marinate the tuna in it for no more than 1 hour (less is fine); refrigerate if the weather is warm. Wash and pick over the arugula; remove woody stems.

Start a charcoal or wood fire—the fire should be quite hot—or preheat a gas grill or broiler. Remove the tuna from the marinade and dry it gently with paper towels. Toss the arugula with the marinade. Using a sharp, thin-bladed knife (a boning knife, for example), make a small incision halfway down any edge of the tuna steak. Insert the knife almost to the opposite edge of the steak, then move it back and forth, flipping it over and creating a large pocket. Be careful not to cut through the top, bottom, or opposite edge of the tuna, and try to keep the entry point small.

Stuff the pocket with the arugula, still drenched in marinade. If you've kept the pocket opening small, seal it with a toothpick; if it's more than 1 to 2 inches wide, use a couple of skewers. Grill the tuna, turning once, about 6 minutes per inch of thickness (if your steak is 1 ½ inches thick, for example, turn it after about 4 minutes and cook 4 to 5 minutes more). Serve, cut into quarters or ½-inch-thick slices.

ALTERNATIVE FISH FOR THIS RECIPE:
Swordfish. Adjust the cooking time accordingly.

GARLIC-STUFFED TUNA STEAKS:
Stuff the steaks with a mixture of ¼ cup minced garlic, ½ cup chopped scallions (green and white parts), 1 tablespoon olive oil, 1 tablespoon soy sauce (or shoyu), and ¼ teaspoon freshly ground black pepper. Let the mixture mellow in the fish while you prepare the grill. Baste lightly with a mixture of soy and oil (as in Basic Grilled Tuna, page 329) before and during grilling.

CHILE-STUFFED TUNA STEAKS:
Stuff the steaks with a mixture of ½ cup minced scallions (green and white parts), 1 medium-size red bell pepper, seeded and minced, ½ teaspoon minced garlic, 1 teaspoon minced fresh thyme (or ½ teaspoon dried), 1 jalapeño, seeded, deveined, and minced, salt, and freshly ground black pepper. Baste the tuna with melted butter as it cooks.

GRILLED TUNA STEAKS STUFFED WITH CILANTRO "PESTO"

Makes 4 servings
Time: 60 minutes
Like the preceding recipe, this is deceptively impressive. Once you master the simple technique, you can fill the pocket with any herb or vegetable mixture you like. Keep the marinating time short and you can start and finish this in an hour.

1 cup loosely packed cilantro (fresh coriander) leaves (substitute parsley for half the cilantro if you like)
2 medium-size cloves garlic, peeled
2 teaspoons coarse salt
½ cup extra virgin olive oil
Juice of ½ lime
Freshly ground black pepper to taste
1 very large fresh tuna steak, 1 ½ to 2 inches thick, about 2 pounds

Place the cilantro and garlic on a cutting board and sprinkle with the salt. Using an 8- or 10-inch chef's knife, chop the cilantro and garlic together until very fine (you can do this in a food processor, but it's not much easier, and you run the risk of ending up with a puree). Mix this in a bowl with the olive oil, lime juice, and pepper. Using a sharp, thin-bladed knife—such as a boning or fillet knife—make a small incision halfway down any edge of the tuna steak. Insert the knife almost to the opposite edge of the steak, then move it back and forth; the pocket need not be thick, but it should cover most of the steak. Be careful not to cut through the top, bottom, or opposite edge of the tuna, and try to keep the incision small.

Stuff the pocket with about three quarters of the "pesto," leaving behind most of the oil and some of the solids. If you've kept the pocket opening small, seal it with a toothpick; if it's more than 1 or 2 inches wide, use a couple of skewers. Marinate the fish in the remaining pesto while you preheat a gas grill or start a charcoal or wood fire; it should be quite hot.

Grill the tuna, turning once, about 6 minutes per inch of thickness (if your steak is 2 inches thick, for example, turn it after 6 minutes and cook 6 minutes more). Serve, cut into ½-inch-thick slices.

ALTERNATIVE FISH FOR THIS RECIPE:
Swordfish. Adjust the cooking time accordingly.

TUNA WITH POTATO CRUST

Makes 4 servings
Time: 30 minutes
Difficult as it may sound, this recipe requires more care than skill. Don't rush it and you'll be fine.

1 ½ pounds potatoes
1 large egg white
Salt and freshly ground black pepper to taste
2 tablespoons finely minced fresh chives
2 tablespoons all-purpose flour, plus extra for dredging
3 tablespoon olive or peanut oil
Two 1-inch-thick tuna steaks, ½ pound or more each
1 tablespoon chopped fresh parsley
Lemon wedges

Shred the potatoes, using the largest hole of a hand grater or the coarsest grating disk of a food processor. Drain them, squeezing to extract their liquid. Mix them with the egg white, salt, pepper, chives, and the 2 tablespoons of flour. If, upon standing, the mixture becomes watery, drain off excess water with a spoon.

Preheat a 12-inch nonstick skillet over medium-high heat. When it is good and hot—a drop of water will skip and evaporate—add the oil to the pan. Dredge one steak lightly in flour and pat a layer of the potato mixture onto each side; place the steak in the pan and repeat the process with the other steak, working quickly.

Cook until the potato coating is golden brown, 3 to 5 minutes. Turn and cook on the other side. Serve immediately, garnished with the parsley and accompanied by lemon wedges.

ALTERNATIVE FISH FOR THIS DISH:
Steaks of mahi-mahi, salmon, or swordfish.

TUNA VEAL STYLE

Makes 4 servings
Time: 20 minutes
In France and Italy, tuna has long been treated as if it were veal; here's how.

2 tablespoons butter
2 tablespoons olive oil
1 ¼ pounds tuna, cut into 8 thin "cutlets," about ¼ to 3/16 inch thick
Flour for dredging
2 large eggs, lightly beaten
Unseasoned bread crumbs for dredging
Minced fresh parsley for garnish
2 lemons, quartered

Heat the butter and oil in a 12-inch nonstick skillet over medium-high heat. When the butter foam subsides, dredge four of the cutlets in the flour, run them through the eggs, then dredge them in the bread crumbs. Put them in the skillet, turn the heat to high, and cook until browned on both sides, about 4 minutes total. Remove them to a warm platter or a low oven and repeat the process with the remaining cutlets. Garnish with parsley and serve with lemon wedges.

ALTERNATIVE FISH FOR THIS RECIPE:
Monkfish, salmon, or sturgeon. Adjust the cooking times accordingly.

TUNA PROVENCE STYLE

Makes 4 servings
Time: 20 minutes

The initial browning is important here; otherwise the tuna will become dull gray in appearance.

¼ cup olive oil
One 1 ½-pound tuna steak
Flour for dredging
4 cloves garlic, crushed and peeled
2 green frying peppers (the long, light green kind), seeded and chopped
3 medium-size ripe tomatoes, cored and chopped
Several sprigs fresh thyme or ½ teaspoon dried
Salt and freshly ground black pepper to taste
¼ cup good black olives (optional)
1 cup dry white wine
½ cup minced fresh parsley

Heat a 10- or 12-inch nonstick skillet over medium-high heat for 3 to 4 minutes. Add the oil and when it is hot (a pinch of flour will sizzle) dredge the tuna in the flour and brown it over high heat for about 2 minutes per side. Remove it to a warm plate and add the remaining ingredients to the skillet, reserving half of the parsley. Reduce the heat to medium and cook until the tomatoes break up, about 10 minutes. Return the tuna to the skillet and cook it in the sauce, turning once, until it is done, about 5 to 6 minutes (cut into the tuna; it should be slightly pink in the middle). Serve immediately, garnished with the reserved parsley.

ALTERNATIVE FISH FOR THIS RECIPE:
Mahi-mahi or swordfish. Adjust the cooking times accordingly.

TUNA AU POIVRE WITH ZINFANDEL AND SHALLOTS

Makes 4 to 6 servings
Time: 15 minutes

Another beeflike recipe—fast, easy, and convenient. Real zinfandel—as opposed to the pink stuff—has a spicy fruitiness that complements the black pepper and shallots nicely. But you can use any full-bodied red wine to finish this sauce.

2 teaspoons cracked black pepper, more or less
Coarse salt to taste
Two 1-pound tuna steaks
2 tablespoons butter
1 tablespoon minced shallots
1 sprig fresh tarragon or ⅛ teaspoon dried, plus additional fresh tarragon for garnish
¾ cup zinfandel or other good red wine

Press the pepper and salt into the tuna. Preheat a 12-inch nonstick skillet over medium-high heat for about 3 minutes and preheat the oven to 200°F. Add half the butter to the pan; when the foam subsides, turn the heat to high and add the tuna. Sear the steaks for about 3 minutes per side for rare tuna, a bit longer if you like it medium to well done; remove them to a platter and place the platter in the warm oven. Over medium heat, add the remaining butter to the pan along with the shallots. Stir until softened. Add the tarragon and wine, raise the heat to high, and let most of the liquid bubble away. Spoon the sauce over the steaks and serve, garnished with additional tarragon.

ALTERNATIVE FISH FOR THIS RECIPE:
Swordfish. Adjust the cooking times accordingly.

SPICE-CRUSTED PAN-FRIED TUNA

Makes 4 servings
Time: 20 minutes

You can find pan-fried tuna with a crisp crust throughout the Mediterranean—it's the rough equivalent of the chicken-fried steak you find in our own cattle country. Spicing up the crust with a bit of cayenne or wasabe powder makes it a little more fun.

Flour for dredging, divided into 2 bowls
½ teaspoon cayenne pepper or wasabe powder (available in Asian markets) or to taste
Salt and freshly ground black pepper to taste
3 tablespoons olive oil
3 tablespoons butter
4 small tuna steaks, 4 to 6 ounces each, about ¾ to 1 inch thick
1 large egg, lightly beaten
Minced fresh parsley for garnish
Lemon wedges

Heat a 12-inch skillet over medium heat. Season one bowl of flour with the cayenne, salt, and lots of black pepper. Add the olive oil to the pan; when it's hot, add the butter. When the butter foam subsides, dredge each steak first in the unseasoned flour, then in the egg, and finally in the seasoned flour; place it in the skillet. Cook over medium-high heat, rotating the steaks so they brown evenly, and turning after about 3 minutes. They will be medium-rare after about 6 minutes of cooking, overdone after 10. Garnish with parsley and serve with lemon wedges.

ALTERNATIVE FISH FOR THIS RECIPE:
Steaks or fillets of bluefish, grouper, halibut, mackerel, mahi-mahi, mako shark, monkfish, rockfish, red snapper, salmon, striped bass, swordfish, or wolffish. Adjust the cooking times accordingly.

HOT-AND-SOUR TUNA

Makes 2 to 3 servings
Time: 30 minutes

¼ cup olive oil
2 medium-size onions, thinly sliced
2 jalapeño peppers, deveined, seeded, and minced, or to taste
One 1-pound tuna steak
Flour for dredging
Salt and freshly ground black pepper to taste
2 tablespoons red wine vinegar
⅓ cup dry white wine
Minced fresh parsley for garnish

Heat the oil in a 12-inch nonstick skillet (which can later be covered) over medium-low heat; add the onions and jalapeños and cook, stirring occasionally, until the onion wilts; remove from the pan. Dredge the tuna in the flour; raise the heat under the same skillet to high and brown the tuna on both sides, about 4 minutes total. Return the onions and jalapeños to the pan and add the salt, pepper, vinegar, and wine. Cover, turn the heat to low, and cook for 5 more minutes. Remove the tuna and reduce the sauce if necessary. Spoon the sauce over the tuna, garnish with parsley, and serve.

ALTERNATIVE FISH FOR THIS RECIPE:
Swordfish. Adjust the cooking time accordingly.

PAN-SEARED TUNA WITH COSTA RICAN BROTH

Makes 4 servings
Time: 20 minutes

Another brainchild of Johnny Earles, chef-owner of Criolla's, in Grayton Beach, Florida.

3 cups any chicken stock (page 40)

⅓ cup fresh (cooked or uncooked) or frozen (thawed) corn kernels

½ cup cooked well-seasoned black beans (page 156) or canned black beans, drained

¼ cup chopped scallions, green and white parts

⅓ cup julienned fresh spinach, tough stems removed

¼ cup chopped cilantro (fresh coriander)

Juice of ½ lime

⅓ cup chopped tomatoes, fresh or canned

1 teaspoon pure chile powder, preferably from ancho chiles (available in specialty markets or by mail)

2 teaspoons chopped garlic

1 teaspoon chopped fresh parsley

Salt to taste

Two 2-inch-thick tuna steaks, 8 to 10 ounces each

2 tablespoons olive oil

Whole fresh chives for garnish

Preheat the oven to 400°F. Prepare the broth: Heat the stock and add the corn, beans, and scallions, then the spinach, cilantro, lime juice, and tomatoes. Keep warm while you cook the tuna.

Mix together the chile powder, garlic, parsley, and salt, and coat the tuna steaks with this mixture. Preheat a 10- or 12-inch nonstick skillet over medium-high heat for 3 to 4 minutes, add the olive oil, and sear the steaks for 1 minute on each side. Transfer the steaks to the oven; roast about 5 minutes for rare, 9 minutes for medium (there are only two ways to check for doneness: by feel, which takes practice, and by cutting into the steaks, which is not so dreadful).

For each serving, ladle a portion of broth into a deep bowl. When the tuna is done, slice each steak ½ inch thick—Earles cuts them into fans—and place in the bowls with the broth. Garnish each portion with two or three chives.

ALTERNATIVE FISH FOR THIS RECIPE: Mahi-mahi.

CHARRED TUNA SALAD WITH BEANS

Makes 4 servings

Time: 30 minutes, plus marinating and chilling (it's easiest to begin this dish the day before serving it)

Canned tuna with beans is a traditional and perfectly nice dish, if you can't get fresh tuna. But this is far superior. You might start this salad by grilling a little extra tuna when making one of the other grilled tuna recipes in this section.

One ½-pound tuna steak

½ cup extra virgin olive oil plus 2 tablespoons

Several sprigs fresh thyme or ½ teaspoon dried

1 medium-size red bell pepper

Juice of 1 large lemon

3 cups any cooked or canned white beans, cooled and drained

10 cherry tomatoes, halved

¼ cup diced shallots

12 to 15 good black or green olives, pitted and coarsely chopped

¼ cup minced fresh basil

¼ cup minced fresh parsley

Salt and freshly ground black pepper to taste

Mixed greens

Marinate the tuna in the 2 tablespoons of olive oil and the thyme while you preheat a gas grill or start a charcoal or wood fire; the heat should be intense. Grill the tuna 3 minutes per side. At the same time, grill the red pepper; cool and peel it (detailed instructions for grilling red peppers appear in Grilled Blackfish with Cumin-scented Red Pepper Relish, page 55), then cut into strips.

Cool the tuna, cover it with plastic wrap, and chill for several hours or overnight. Cut it into small cubes and toss it with the lemon juice, beans, and remaining olive oil while you prepare the other ingredients. Add the tomatoes, shallots, olives, and herbs to the tuna. Taste for salt and pepper, and correct the balance between olive oil and lemon juice, if necessary. Serve, topped with the strips of grilled red pepper, on a bed of greens.

ALTERNATIVE FISH FOR THIS RECIPE:
Pregrilled mackerel, mahi-mahi, salmon, shrimp, or swordfish.

SALADE NIÇOISE

Makes 4 servings
Time: 30 minutes, using pregrilled tuna
There are certain basics that are essential to salade Niçoise, and canned tuna is among them. But that doesn't mean it isn't better with fresh tuna (it is). Use the best olive oil you can get your hands on.

4 to 6 cups assorted salad greens, washed and dried
½ to 1 pound Basic Grilled Tuna (page 329) or grilled tuna from any other recipe
2 cups green beans, steamed for 2 minutes, rinsed, chilled, and cut in half if large (omit these if you're pressed for time)
1 cup good black olives, pitted
3 medium to large ripe tomatoes, cut into quarters or eighths
1 medium-size bell pepper, any color but green, seeded and cut into rings
6 anchovies (optional)
1 teaspoon capers (optional)
¼ cup good red wine vinegar, more or less
¾ cup olive oil, more or less
Salt and freshly ground black pepper to taste
1 small shallot, minced
1 teaspoon Dijon mustard

Arrange all the salad ingredients nicely on a platter—greens on the bottom, topped with the tuna, green beans, olives, tomatoes, and pepper, with the anchovies and capers sprinkled over the top. Or—less attractive but easier to serve—toss them all together.

Make the vinaigrette by adding most of the vinegar to the oil, along with the salt and pepper, shallot, and mustard. Stir and taste. Add more vinegar if necessary and adjust the seasoning. Stir or shake vigorously, drizzle about half the dressing over the salad, and serve, passing the remaining vinaigrette at the table.

ALTERNATIVE FISH FOR THIS RECIPE:
Pregrilled mackerel, mahi-mahi, salmon, shrimp, or swordfish.

COLD POACHED TUNA WITH ANCHOVY MAYONNAISE

Makes 4 to 6 appetizer servings
Time: 20 minutes, plus time to chill
It's important to keep the tuna rare in this dish; since it has a tendency to become slightly dry as it chills, overcooking would be ruinous. This also makes a wonderful change from canned tuna with bottled mayonnaise—the difference is vast.

Several sprigs fresh thyme or 1 teaspoon dried
10 black peppercorns
1 tablespoon salt
One 1-pound tuna steak
1 large egg
1 teaspoon Dijon mustard
6 to 8 anchovy fillets, with some of their oil
1 clove garlic, peeled
1 tablespoon red or white wine vinegar
Several grindings of black pepper
1 cup olive oil

Bring 2 inches of water to a boil in a pot big enough to hold the tuna. Lower the heat to a simmer and add the thyme, peppercorns, and salt. Gently place the tuna in the water and simmer 4 to 5 minutes for rare tuna (lift it from the water and press it with a finger; it should be elastic, neither mushy nor flaky). Plunge the tuna into ice water, adding ice until the tuna is cool. Dry it with paper towels and refrigerate.

To make the mayonnaise, put the egg, mustard, anchovies, garlic, vinegar, pepper, and a little of the oil in a food processor or blender. Process for about 10 seconds, then slowly add the remainder of the oil in a very thin stream. The mayonnaise is done when all the oil is added and it is creamy-thick. Taste for seasoning.

When ready to serve, slice the tuna thin, as you would a beefsteak, and serve it with a dollop of the mayonnaise.

ALTERNATIVE FISH FOR THIS RECIPE:

Mahi-mahi or swordfish. Adjust the cooking times accordingly.

TURBOT

Latin name(s): *Psetta maxima*, *Reinhardtius hippoglossoides*, and others.
Other common names: Greenland turbot.
Common forms: Steaks, fillets.
General description: Large (to ten pounds) flatfish not unlike halibut; skin is usually removed before eating.
For other recipes see: Catfish, cod, dogfish, flatfish, grouper, haddock, halibut, monkfish, ocean perch, pollock, rockfish, red snapper, striped bass, swordfish, tilefish, whiting, wolffish.
Buying tips: In addition to the usual guidelines with white-fleshed fish—avoid browning, gaping, or off-odors—see below.

There are, unfortunately, two turbots: those that are caught off the European coasts, and those from everywhere else. I say "unfortunately" because the European fish (*Psetta maxima*) are far superior, with firmer flesh and better flavor. Other turbot are not bad, but have soft, almost mushy flesh, almost like a second-rate halibut. The easiest way to tell the different in the store is by price: If the fish is inexpensive—say, under five dollars a pound—it's not European.

Recipes for one will work for the other; they are both, after all, mild, white-fleshed fish. But if you have the superior fish, you will know it.

TURBOT SIMMERED IN SOY BROTH

Makes 4 servings
Time: 20 minutes
Light and delicate, this is as perfect a lunch dish as you'll eat.

1 tablespoon peanut oil
1 or 2 turbot steaks or fillets, a total of about 1 ½ pounds

1 tablespoon minced garlic
1 tablespoon peeled and minced fresh ginger
1 teaspoon sesame oil
2 tablespoons high-quality soy sauce
½ cup Full-flavored Chicken Stock (page 40) or Flavorful Fish and Vegetable Stock (page 40)
¼ cup minced scallions, green and white parts

Heat a 12-inch nonstick skillet over medium-high heat for 3 to 4 minutes. Add the oil and raise the heat to high; sear the fish for 60 to 90 seconds on each side. Sprinkle the garlic and ginger around the fish, then drizzle the sesame oil over it. Add the soy sauce and stock to the skillet, bring to a boil, lower the heat to a minimum, and cover.

Cook 5 minutes, then remove the cover, raise the heat to high, and reduce the liquid by about half. Serve the fish over rice, with some of the sauce spooned over and garnished with the scallions.

ALTERNATIVE FISH FOR THIS RECIPE:

Catfish, cod, dogfish, haddock, halibut, ocean perch, rockfish, scallops, shrimp, red snapper, tilefish, or wolffish. Adjust the cooking times accordingly.

TURBOT EN PAPILLOTE

Makes 4 servings
Time: 45 minutes

Cooking in pouches is a great way to preserve the subtle flavor and intrinsic moisture of delicate fish. It's also easy; for variations, see Red Snapper en Papillote, page 288.

2 cloves garlic, slivered
Four 4- to 6-ounce pieces turbot fillet or 4 small steaks
Salt and freshly ground black pepper to taste
8 thick slices fresh tomato
8 fresh basil leaves
2 tablespoons pine nuts
1 tablespoon olive oil

Preheat the oven to 450°F. Tear off a 1-foot-square piece of aluminum foil (the more traditional parchment paper is, of course, acceptable). Place a bit of garlic on a piece of foil; top with a piece of fish, some salt and pepper, 2 slices of tomato, 2 basil leaves, some pine nuts, and the barest drizzle of oil. Seal the package and repeat the process with the remaining pieces of fish.

Place all the packages in a large baking dish and bake for about 30 minutes (the turbot will be white, opaque, and tender when done). Serve the closed packages, allowing each diner to open his or her own at the table.

ALTERNATIVE FISH FOR THIS RECIPE:

Fillets or steaks of catfish, cod, dogfish, flatfish, haddock, halibut, ocean perch, pollock, rockfish, red snapper, tilefish, or wolffish. Adjust the cooking times accordingly.

TURBOT WITH ONIONS, RAISINS, AND PINE NUTS

Makes 4 servings
Time: 30 minutes

A typical Catalonian preparation.

¼ cup raisins
1 cup dry (fino) sherry or dry white wine
3 tablespoons olive oil
One 1 ¼- to 1 ½-pound turbot fillet, in 1 or 2 pieces
Flour for dredging
Salt and freshly ground black pepper to taste
1 cup minced onion
½ cup pine nuts
3 or 4 sprigs fresh thyme or sage or ½ teaspoon dried

Soak the raisins in ¼ cup of the sherry while you cook the other ingredients.

Heat a 12-inch nonstick skillet over medium-high heat for 3 to 4 minutes; add 2 tablespoons of the oil and raise the heat to high. Dredge the fish lightly in the flour and brown it for about 2 minutes on each side, seasoning it with salt and pepper; remove it from the pan and keep it warm.

Add the remaining oil to the skillet and cook the onion over medium heat until softened, stirring occasionally. Drain and add the raisins, along with the pine nuts, and cook another 2 minutes. Season with salt and pepper and add the thyme and the remaining sherry. Return the fish to the pan and cook over medium-high heat until it has heated through and is opaque and tender. Serve immediately, with the onion mixture spooned over.

ALTERNATIVE FISH FOR THIS RECIPE:

Catfish, cod, dogfish, haddock, ocean perch, pollock, rockfish, red snapper, tilefish, or wolffish. Adjust the cooking times accordingly.

WEAKFISH

Latin name(s): *Cynoscion regalis* and others.
Other common names: Sea trout, speckled trout, gray trout, squeteague.
Common forms: Whole, fillets.
General description: A slender, basically gray but often multicolor fish, sometimes with spots, usually under five pounds, from the Atlantic and Gulf coasts, with soft white to slightly rosy flesh and edible skin.
For other recipes see: Catfish, cod, dogfish, flatfish, haddock, mackerel, ocean perch, pollock.
Buying tips: First, don't confuse weakfish with trout. Next, be aware that the flesh may be pinkish. Avoid fillets with graying or browning flesh, off odors, or excessive gaping. Whole fish should be quite alive-looking.

Weakfish—which are in no way related to trout, despite the insistence of mid-Atlantic cooks—are locally important, but don't have much of a national audience. They are, however, showing up in more and more supermarkets. This is an unusual fish with delicate flesh; the fillets flake so readily during cooking that they are almost as difficult to handle as those of flatfish. They are, however, quite delicious, as is the fish when it is cooked whole.

Weakfish are hardy; the term refers to the fish's mouth, which is easily torn by fishing hooks.

WEAKFISH AMANDINE

Makes 2 servings
Time: 20 minutes
Trout amandine is a classic. But since weakfish is often called, simply "trout"—especially in the Carolinas—this makes some kind of sense. In any case, it's tastier than any dish made with farm-raised trout.

¼ cup (½ stick) butter
¼ cup slivered blanched almonds
2 weakfish fillets, about 6 ounces each, skin on or off
Salt and freshly ground black pepper to taste
Flour for dredging
2 lemon wedges
Minced fresh parsley for garnish

Melt 1 tablespoon of the butter over medium heat in a small skillet; when the foam subsides, cook the almonds, stirring, until they start to brown, 2 to 3 minutes. Remove from the heat.

Heat a 12-inch nonstick skillet over medium-high heat for 3 to 4 minutes; add the remaining butter. Sprinkle the fillets with salt and pepper. When the butter foam subsides, dredge the fillets in the flour, shaking off the excess. Raise the heat to high and quickly cook the fish, about 2 to 3 minutes per side. Be very careful not to overcook, or the weakfish will start to fall apart.

Spoon a few slivered almonds over each fillet and drizzle with a little lemon juice. Garnish with parsley and serve.

ALTERNATIVE FISH FOR THIS RECIPE:

Fillets of catfish, cod, dogfish, flatfish, haddock, mackerel, ocean perch, pollock, pompano, rockfish, sea bass, red snapper, tilefish, turbot, or wolffish. Adjust the cooking times accordingly.

SPICY FRIED SPECKLED TROUT WITH GARLIC SAUCE

Makes 4 servings
Time: 45 minutes
Frying speckled trout is old hat in the South, but this preparation is hardly traditional.

1 tablespoon ancho or other pure chile powder (available in specialty markets or by mail)
2 tablespoons minced cilantro (fresh coriander)
1/2 teaspoon ground coriander
1/2 teaspoon ground cardamom
1/2 teaspoon dry mustard
1/2 teaspoon cayenne pepper
1/4 teaspoon freshly ground black pepper
1 teaspoon salt
1 tablespoon white wine or rice vinegar or fresh lemon juice
Peanut or vegetable oil as needed
Four 4- to 6-ounce weakfish fillets, skinned and cut in half
1 tablespoon minced garlic
1 tablespoon peeled and minced fresh ginger
1 tablespoon high-quality soy sauce
3/4 cup any chicken or fish stock (pages 40–41)
1 cup unbleached all-purpose flour

1 cup warm water
1 tablespoon cornstarch dissolved in 1/4 cup stock
Minced cilantro for garnish

Mix together the chile powder, cilantro, coriander, cardamom, mustard, cayenne, black pepper, salt, vinegar, and enough oil to make a paste. Spread this over the weakfish and let them sit on a rack while you proceed with the recipe.

Begin to heat about 1/2 inch of oil in a large, steep-sided skillet or deep-fryer over medium-high heat. Heat 1 tablespoon of oil in a small saucepan over medium-low heat and cook the garlic and ginger, stirring occasionally, until the garlic colors. Add the soy sauce and stock, simmer for about 5 minutes, and turn off the heat.

When the oil in the skillet is about 350°F (a pinch of flour will sizzle) mix together the flour and water to form a paste. One at a time, dip the fillets in this batter, then put them in the hot oil. Raise the heat under the skillet to high and cook the fish until crisp, about 3 minutes per side. Remove and drain on paper towels.

Heat the stock mixture until boiling, turn the heat to medium-low, add the cornstarch mixture, and stir until thickened. Serve the fish with some of this sauce spooned over it, garnished with cilantro.

ALTERNATIVE FISH FOR THIS RECIPE:

Fillets of catfish, dogfish, haddock, ocean perch, Atlantic pollock, rockfish, sea bass, red snapper, tilefish, or wolffish. Adjust the cooking times accordingly.

WEAKFISH ROASTED WITH TOMATOES AND CILANTRO

Makes 4 servings
Time: 30 to 40 minutes

One 3- to 4-pound weakfish, scaled and gutted,
  head on or off
Salt and freshly ground black pepper to taste
Olive oil
1 cup minced scallions, both green and white
  parts
1 teaspoon minced garlic
1 cup minced cilantro (fresh coriander)
3 cups seeded and diced tomatoes (canned are
  fine; drain them first)
½ cup dry white wine

Preheat the oven to 450°F. Cut three or four vertical gashes on each side of the fish, then sprinkle it with salt and pepper. Brush a baking pan with olive oil and lay the fish on it. Mix together all but 1 tablespoon of the scallions, the garlic, ¾ cup of the cilantro, and the tomatoes and season with salt and pepper. Stuff the fish with half of this mixture and spread the rest over the top. Pour the wine around the fish.

Roast for 20 to 30 minutes, basting occasionally with the pan juices. The fish is done when it begins to flake and is almost opaque clear to the bone. (Bear in mind that weakfish is slightly pink, so don't expect it to become stark white. Remember, too, that it flakes and overcooks easily.) Serve, spooning any remaining pan juices over the fish and garnishing with the reserved scallions and cilantro.

ALTERNATIVE FISH FOR THIS RECIPE:
  Whole bluefish, grouper, mackerel, porgy, rockfish, sea bass, or red snapper. Adjust the cooking times accordingly.

WHITEBAIT

Latin name(s): None (see below).
Other common names: Silverside, sand eel, herring, etc. (see below).
Common forms: Whole.
General description: Tiny, usually white or translucent fish, always eaten whole.
Buying tips: It's tough to judge these babies by anything other than smell; they're too small to inspect. If they smell fresh, they are.

Whitebait are baby fish, or very small ones, of almost any species. They are usually no more than an inch or two in length, and are eaten whole (head, guts, and all), usually fried. They have a rich, oily, almost gamy flavor, and most people who try them with an open mind find them delicious. Popular in almost every fish-loving country except the United States, whitebait deserve to be treated better here. I usually buy them in New York's Chinatown for about a dollar a pound. You cannot find a better bargain.

FRIED WHITEBAIT

Makes 2 or 3 servings
Time: 20 minutes
For fried fish lovers, there's nothing better than whitebait; it's all crunch and flavor. Like most fried food, they're best eaten while you're standing around in the kitchen.

1 pound whitebait
Vegetable oil for deep-frying
Unbleached all-purpose flour seasoned with salt and freshly ground black pepper for dredging

Salt to taste
Lemon wedges

Pick over the fish for debris; rinse if they seem dirty. Dry them well. Heat at least 2 inches of oil in a fryer or deep skillet to 375°F. Place the flour in a bag and add a handful of whitebait; shake well, then remove the fish and shake them to rid them of excess flour. Gently lower them into the oil—avoid crowding—and fry until browned, about 2 minutes. Drain and serve immediately, sprinkled with salt and lemon juice. While you're eating, fry the next batch.

WHITEBAIT IN THE STYLE OF ANGULAS

Makes 4 appetizer servings
Time: 15 minutes
It's difficult to get angulas—baby eels—in Spain, where they are popular (and quite expensive). It's nearly impossible here, although you may sometimes be offered them at better Spanish restaurants. But whitebait make a good substitute, especially since the dominant flavors here are of garlic and olive oil. Double the quantity of fish if you want a larger appetizer.

½ pound whitebait
¼ cup olive oil
10 slices peeled garlic (about 2 cloves)
1 dried hot red pepper
1 teaspoon salt

Pick over the fish for debris; rinse if they seem dirty. In a small, attractive skillet or flameproof ramekin, heat the oil, garlic, pepper, and salt over medium-high heat. Stir occasionally until the garlic browns very lightly. Add the whitebait, raise the heat to high, cook 1 minute, stirring once or twice; turn off the heat and serve immediately.

ALTERNATIVE FISH FOR THIS RECIPE:
Baby eels.

SARTAGNADO

Makes 4 to 6 appetizer servings
Time: 30 minutes

I'd heard about this odd fish cake, and spent three days searching Nice for it. No one, it seemed, knew of it, even though it was reportedly a Provençal specialty. Finally, in a seedy place behind a fish market, I found someone willing to make it for me. And it was wonderful, with the gutsy, fresh flavor of whitebait and good olive oil. Best of all, it's easy to duplicate at home, especially with a nonstick skillet.

1 pound whitebait
1 cup unbleached all-purpose flour, more or less, well seasoned with salt and freshly ground black pepper
½ cup olive oil, more or less
⅓ cup good red wine vinegar
Minced fresh parsley for garnish

Heat a 10- or 12-inch nonstick skillet over medium-high heat for 3 to 4 minutes. Pick over the fish for debris; rinse if they seem dirty. Put the flour in a plastic bag and shake the fish until they are lightly coated.

Put enough oil in the pan to coat the bottom well, and heat until it is shimmering and fragrant over medium-high heat. Add the fish, all at once, pressing them down with a wide spatula. Sprinkle with more salt and pepper and cook, shaking occasionally. The fish will not stick to the pan, but will stick to one another, forming a cake.

In 8 to 10 minutes, when the bottom of the cake is nicely browned (use your spatula to peek), slide it onto a plate. Cover this with another plate of equal size and invert the two. Add a little more oil to the pan and slide the cake back in. Cook another 8 to 10 minutes and slide onto a serving plate. Pour the vinegar into the pan; it will sizzle and reduce almost immediately. Drizzle it over the fish cake, garnish with parsley, cut into wedges, and serve.

WHITING

Latin name(s): *Merluccius bilinearis, M. merluccius*, etc.

Other common names: Hake, silver hake, kingfish, merluzzo, merlan, etc.

Common forms: Whole (usually), steaks, fillets (rarely).

General description: Silver-skinned, white-fleshed fish with pleasantly soft flesh and mild flavor. Often sold frozen; usually quite inexpensive. The thin skin is edible.

For other recipes see: Cod, croaker, flatfish, halibut, ocean perch, porgy, rockfish, sea bass, red snapper, or tilefish.

Buying tips: Unlike most fresh whole fish, even perfectly fresh whiting are quite limp and look very dead; don't let that bother you. Check the gills (they should be bright red) if they're whole, and the edges of the flesh if they've had their heads removed (there should be no browning or graying). Finally, the smell should be of seawater.

Whiting are slender fish with large eyes, wide mouths, and sharp teeth. They are caught worldwide and range from very small, almost smelt size, to four pounds and more. The price is almost always low, because the resource is widespread and the fish is not enormously popular; too many people insist on eating fillets, and too few fishmongers have mastered the rather complicated J-cut needed to remove all the bones from the whiting's oddly shaped skeleton.

But whiting is tender and sweet, and its central bone comes out almost effortlessly—bringing the entire skeleton with it—if you press on the cooked fish from the top with a fork. I love pan-fried whiting, which is a standard preparation, but this fish also takes well to baking.

WHITING BAKED IN WHITE WINE

Makes 4 servings

Time: 20 minutes

A very basic, lightning-quick recipe you can use for any small whole fish.

4 whiting, about 1 pound each, gutted and scaled, with heads on

1 cup dry white wine

1 tablespoon minced garlic

¼ cup olive oil

¼ cup capers

½ cup chopped fresh parsley

Salt and freshly ground black pepper to taste

Preheat the oven to its highest setting—550°F or so. Place the whiting in a baking dish, then sprinkle all the remaining ingredients over them, putting some in the fishes' cavities. Bake until the whiting flake when probed with a fork, about 10 minutes; don't overcook. Serve at once, pouring the pan juices over the fish.

ALTERNATIVE FISH FOR THIS RECIPE:

Butterfish, croaker, mackerel, porgy, rockfish, sea bass, red snapper, tilefish, trout, or weakfish. Adjust the cooking times accordingly.

WHITING BAKED WITH SHALLOTS AND HERBS

Makes 4 servings
Time: 30 minutes

The technique here is similar to that in Whiting Baked in White Wine (preceding recipe), with different results. This is a subtle preparation, perfect for this tender, moist fish. Make it when you can find big, whole whiting.

One 3- to 4-pound whiting, scaled, gutted, and beheaded
1 cup dry white wine
¼ cup chopped mixed fresh tarragon, parsley, dill, thyme, and/or chervil
¼ cup peeled and halved shallots
Salt and freshly ground black pepper to taste
3 tablespoons butter, softened
Minced fresh parsley for garnish

Preheat the oven to 450°F. Cut the belly flaps off the whiting and place it on its belly in a baking pan. Pour in the wine, add the herbs and shallots, and sprinkle with salt and pepper. Bake, uncovered, until the fish is just about done, about 15 minutes. (To check, run a thin-bladed knife down the middle of the fish's backbone, then peek inside; the fish should be barely pink.) Remove the fish to a serving platter and keep warm (the same oven, with the heat off and door open, will do nicely).

Strain the cooking juices into a small saucepan and reduce to about ½ cup over high heat. Lower the heat to a minimum and gently stir or swirl in the butter, 1 tablespoon at a time, until it melts.

Pour the sauce over the fish (make sure some gets in the cut you made to check for doneness), sprinkle with parsley, and serve.

ALTERNATIVE FISH FOR THIS RECIPE:

Same as for Whiting Baked in White Wine (page 345).

MERLUZA EN SALSA VERDE

Makes 6 servings
Time: 40 minutes

A typical preparation of Galicia—the northeasternmost area of Spain—where whiting is enormously popular.

6 whiting, about 1 pound each, gutted, scaled, and cut into halves or thirds as if making steaks
Juice of 1 lemon
¼ cup olive oil
4 cloves garlic, peeled but left whole
3 or 4 medium-size potatoes, peeled and sliced ¼ inch thick
1 cup any fish or chicken stock (pages 40–41) or water, more or less
½ cup chopped fresh parsley
½ bay leaf
Salt and freshly ground black pepper to taste

Sprinkle the whiting with the lemon juice and let stand. In a steep-sided skillet or casserole, heat the oil over medium-low heat. Add the garlic and cook, stirring, until lightly browned and puffy. Remove the garlic from the pan and set aside. Add the potato slices and about ½ cup of the stock to the pan. Cover the skillet and cook for about 5 minutes over medium-low heat; uncover and add more stock if necessary. Cover and cook until the potatoes are almost tender, 10 minutes or so.

Add the whiting and continue to cook, shaking

the pan occasionally. In a food processor or mortar and pestle, puree the garlic with the parsley and bay leaf; add this mixture, along with some salt and pepper, to the fish and potato mixture, and continue to cook until the whiting is tender and flakes easily, about 10 minutes. Serve immediately.

ALTERNATIVE FISH FOR THIS RECIPE:

Fillets or chunks of blackfish, carp, catfish, eel, grouper, monkfish, Atlantic pollock, rockfish, sea bass, red snapper, or wolffish; croaker or porgy. Adjust the cooking times accordingly.

PAN-FRIED WHITING WITH DILL AND SCALLIONS

Makes 4 servings
Time: 25 minutes

If you have large whiting, often called silver hake or kingfish, cut it into steaks or chunks before sautéing. You can also forget about the deglazing sauce and just serve the fried fish with lemon wedges.

8 small whiting, about ½ to ¾ pound each, scaled, gutted, and beheaded
⅓ cup olive oil
Salt and freshly ground black pepper to taste
1 cup cornmeal for dredging
2 tablespoons minced fresh dill
2 tablespoons minced scallions, green and white parts
¾ cup dry white wine
Lemon wedges

Dry the whiting with paper towels. Heat a 12-inch nonstick skillet over medium heat for 4 to 5 minutes. Add the olive oil and heat until the oil shimmers and becomes fragrant. One at a time, dredge the whiting well in the cornmeal and add to the pan. Cook until lightly browned; season with salt

and pepper, then turn, season, and brown the other side; total cooking time will be about 8 to 10 minutes, and the whiting will have no trace of redness in their cavities.

Remove the fish to a warm platter and add the dill and scallions to the pan. Cook, stirring, over medium heat, for about 1 minute. Add the wine and stir while you let most of it bubble away. Pour the sauce over the fish and serve immediately, with lemon quarters.

ALTERNATIVE FISH FOR THIS RECIPE:

Whole butterfish, croaker, flatfish, mackerel, pompano, porgy, sea bass, trout, or weakfish. Adjust the cooking times accordingly.

PAN-FRIED WHITING STEAKS WITH ONION COMPOTE

Makes 4 servings
Time: 40 minutes

Big whiting have the same Y-shaped bone as small ones; the advantage is that they're more difficult to overcook. When they're done, the tender meat remains moist but fairly tumbles from the bone.

3 tablespoons butter or olive oil
4 medium-size onions, sliced and separated into rings
Salt and freshly ground black pepper to taste
1 bay leaf
3 or 4 sprigs fresh marjoram, oregano, or thyme or a couple pinches dried
½ cup dry white or red wine
¼ cup red wine or balsamic vinegar
1 tablespoon honey
One 2- to 3-pound whiting, scaled, gutted, beheaded, and cut into 1-inch-thick steaks
Cornmeal for dredging
Olive or vegetable oil as needed

Heat the butter over medium heat in a large skillet; add the onions and cook briskly, stirring occasionally, until they begin to soften. Add the salt, pepper, bay leaf, and marjoram. Continue to cook without browning, lowering the heat if necessary, until the onions are mushy. Add the wine, vinegar, and honey, and allow to simmer until almost dry. Keep warm while you cook the fish.

Preheat a 12-inch nonstick skillet over medium-high heat for about 5 minutes. Trim the fish pieces of any belly flaps (the little pieces of almost meatless skin that hang loose from some of them) and place them in a colander. Toss them with cornmeal to cover. Coat the bottom of the skillet with a not too thin film of oil—about 1/8 inch is right. When the oil is hot (a pinch of cornmeal will sizzle), place the fish steaks, one at a time, in the skillet. Cook until golden brown and crisp on one side, then turn and cook the other side. (The total cooking time will be about 10 minutes, and the fish will easily come away from the bone when it is ready.) Garnish the whiting with a bit of the onion sauce and serve immediately, passing the remaining sauce at the table.

ALTERNATIVE FISH FOR THIS RECIPE:

Whole butterfish, croaker, flatfish, or porgy; steaks or chunks of blackfish, grouper, halibut, monkfish, or wolffish. Adjust the cooking times accordingly.

QUICK WHITING CHOWDER

Makes 4 servings
Time: 30 minutes
Big whiting can be filleted, and you may sometimes see it that way. When you do, take advantage of its tendency to flake when cooked to make a thick, creamy chowder.

4 medium-size potatoes (about 1 pound), peeled and diced
1/2 cup diced carrots
2 cups any fish or chicken stock (pages 40–41) or water
2 cups milk or half-and-half
Salt and freshly ground black pepper to taste
1/2 cup fresh or frozen green peas
1 pound skinless whiting fillet, cut into chunks
2 tablespoons butter (optional)

Place the potatoes, carrots, stock, and milk in a saucepan and bring to a boil. Simmer over medium heat until the potatoes are nearly tender, 10 to 15 minutes. Season with salt and pepper and add the peas and whiting; simmer until the fish flakes, 5 to 10 minutes. Add the butter and simmer until it melts. Check and adjust the seasoning and serve.

ALTERNATIVE FISH FOR THIS RECIPE:

Skinned fillets of cod, flatfish, haddock, Pacific pollock, or weakfish. Adjust the cooking times accordingly.

CURRIED WHITING CAKES

Makes 2 to 4 servings
Time: 30 minutes
A delicious fish cake, which can be made with leftovers of almost any fish. I like these with Worcestershire sauce.

1 whiting, about 1 1/2 pounds, gutted and beheaded
2 or 3 medium-size potatoes, peeled and quartered
1/2 cup milk
Salt and freshly ground black pepper to taste
Olive, peanut, or vegetable oil for frying
1 large egg
2 scallions or 1 small onion, minced

1 tablespoon curry powder or to taste
Unseasoned bread crumbs or cracker meal for
  dredging

Simmer the fish and potatoes over medium heat in water to cover. Both will be done in 10 to 15 minutes; remove the fish before it begins to fall from the bone. Strain the stock and reserve it for another use. Mash the potatoes with the milk, seasoning with salt and pepper. When the fish is cool enough to handle, remove the skin and bones.

Heat ⅛ inch of oil in a steep-sided skillet until shimmering and fragrant while you combine the fish, potatoes, egg, scallions, curry powder, salt, and pepper. Shape the fish mixture into hamburger-size cakes, dredge in the bread crumbs, and cook over medium-high heat until nicely browned on each side, 8 to 10 minutes total; drain on paper towels and serve.

ALTERNATIVE FISH FOR THIS RECIPE:

Cod or soaked salt cod, crabmeat (do not boil), haddock, halibut, ocean perch, pollock, salmon, or turbot. Adjust the cooking times accordingly.

DILLED FISH CAKES:

Omit the curry powder. Add 2 tablespoons chopped fresh dill (or 1 tablespoon dried) and 1 tablespoon fresh lemon juice to the mixture. Serve with lemon wedges.

WOLFFISH

Latin name(s): *Anarhichas lupus*.
Other common names: Ocean catfish, seacat.
Common forms: Whole, fillets.
General description: Fierce-looking fish with delicious firm white flesh; average market size is under ten pounds, although the fish can run to thirty or forty pounds. The gray skin is edible.
For other recipes see: Blackfish, catfish, cod, dogfish, flatfish, grouper, haddock, halibut, monkfish, ocean perch, pollock, rockfish, red snapper, tilefish, turbot, weakfish.
Buying tips: Flesh should be firm and pearly white with no evidence of graying or browning. Smell should be of seawater.

This is a wonderful fish of the North Atlantic, one which I would never pass up in a fish market. Although it remains hard to find, there are indications that it may become more common; the Norwegians have begun farming operations, and I've seen it in a few supermarkets.

With care, wolffish can be grilled, and it is good broiled or roasted; but it is really at its best when sautéed.

SAUTÉED WOLFFISH FILLETS WITH LIME SAUCE

Makes 2 or 3 servings
Time: About 30 minutes
Wolffish has the perfect texture for sautéing, and this fragrant lime sauce offsets its sweetness nicely.

3 tablespoons peanut oil
One 1-pound wolffish fillet
Flour for dredging
2 limes
1 clove garlic, minced

1 teaspoon peeled and minced fresh ginger
2 scallions, minced
½ cup dry white wine
2 tablespoons high-quality soy sauce

Preheat a 10 or 12-inch nonstick skillet over medium-high heat for 3 to 4 minutes. Add 2 tablespoons of the oil to the pan. A minute later, dredge the fish in the flour, shaking to remove the excess. Cook over medium-high to high heat until lightly browned and opaque and tender inside, about 4 minutes per side. While the fish is cooking, slice one lime in half and juice it; slice the other into four or five slices. When the fish is done, remove it to a warm platter, and decorate it with the lime slices.

Heat the remaining oil in the pan over high heat. Add the garlic, ginger, and scallions and cook, stirring, about 30 seconds. Add the wine and let it bubble away for 30 seconds to 1 minute or so. Add the soy sauce and half the lime juice, cook a few more seconds, and pour the sauce over the fish. Drizzle the remaining lime juice over the sauced fish at the table.

Blackfish, catfish, cod, dogfish, grouper, haddock, monkfish, ocean perch, pollock, rockfish, red snapper, or tilefish. Adjust the cooking times accordingly.

PAN-FRIED WOLFFISH
IN SPICY BROTH

Makes 4 servings
Time: 30 minutes

This is an unusual, lovely dish, as far from a fish chowder as you can get and yet equally warming and comforting. It cannot be beat for a winter lunch.

2 cups Full-flavored Chicken Stock (page 40)
1 teaspoon fresh or dried lemon grass, chopped (available in Asian markets)
1 tablespoon high-quality soy sauce
1 teaspoon distilled, rice, or white wine vinegar
1/4 teaspoon cayenne pepper, chili-garlic paste (available in Asian markets), or hot pepper sauce
Salt to taste
2 pounds wolffish fillets, cut into four 1/2-pound pieces
1/2 cup peanut oil, more or less
Flour for dredging
3 tablespoons minced scallions, both green and white parts
1 tablespoon peeled and minced fresh ginger
1 tablespoon minced cilantro (fresh coriander)
1 lime, quartered

Warm the stock gently in a small pot; add the lemon grass, soy sauce, vinegar, cayenne, and salt. Taste and adjust the seasonings; it should be flavorful but not overwhelmingly spicy. Keep hot.

Preheat a 12-inch nonstick skillet over medium-high heat for 3 to 4 minutes. Dry the wolffish well, using paper or cloth towels. Add enough oil to the pan so that, when you swirl it, it makes a not too thin layer. When a pinch of flour sizzles when dropped in the oil, begin to cook: Dredge one piece of fish at a time in the flour, shake off the excess, and put it in the pan. Do not hurry; it's not important to start each piece at the same time, and allowing 30 seconds or more between adding the pieces keeps the oil at a steady temperature.

When all four pieces are cooking, adjust the heat so that the oil is sizzling nicely but not burning. Tilt the pan occasionally so the oil "rinses" all the pieces equally. Turn each piece when it is nicely browned on the bottom, 5 minutes or so; then cook them all on the other side.

As each piece finishes cooking, remove it and place it in a soup bowl, the attractive side up. Top it with a quarter of the scallion and ginger, then ladle 1/2 cup of the broth over it. Sprinkle with the cilantro and top with a lime wedge. Serve immediately; have each diner squeeze the lime over their fish before eating.

ALTERNATIVE FISH FOR THIS RECIPE:

Cod, dogfish, haddock, halibut, pollock, sea bass, or tilefish. Adjust the cooking times accordingly.

INDEX

Note: Page numbers in *Italics* refer to illustrations.

Bean(s), Black (cont.)
  Stir-fried Salmon with Asparagus and, 234
  Stir-fried Squid with Tomatoes and, 299
Bean(s), Green, Stir-fried Shrimp with Garlic and, 264–265
Bean(s), White, Charred Tuna Salad with, 335–336
Beans and Shrimp, 267–268
Beard, James, 1, 280, 328
Beheading, 20, 21
  and boning anchovies or sardines, 239, 240
Beignets, Pollock, 207–208
Bisque:
  Lobster, 157–158
  Mussel, 185
Bitter Garlic Sauce, Monkfish Poached in, 179
Black Butter, Skate with, 274
Blackfish, 55–56
  Fillets en Papillote with Citrus, 56
  Grilled, with Cumin-Scented Red Pepper Relish, 55–56
  Provençal Style, 56
Bluefish, 57–63
  Broiled with Lime Mustard, 60
  with Cilantro and Lime, 62
  with Crisp Potatoes, 62
  Fillets in Sour Cream, 62–63
  Grilled Fillets, 58
  Grilled Whole, 58–59
  with Parsleyed Bread Crumbs, 62
  Pickled, Salad, 63
  removing dark meat from, 58
  Roasted Fillets with Eggplant Caponata, 60–61
  Roasted Fillets with Tomatoes, 62
  Roasted on Greens, 62
  Seviche, 60
  Simmered with Lemon Grass, 61
  Stir-fried with Scallops, 59
Boiled Fish Dinner, 323
Boning, 58, 229
  anchovies or sardines, 239, 240
Bonito, 64
Bouillabaisse, 46–47
  Even Simpler, 47–48
Braising, 36
Brandade de Morue, 98–99
Bread Crumbs:
  Cod Broiled with, 92
  Oysters with, 204

Parsleyed, Baked Shrimp with Tomatoes and, 270–271
  Roast Halibut with Butter and, 148
  Scallops with, 248
Broccoli:
  Red Snapper en Papillote with, 288
  Stir-fried Swordfish with, 318–319
Broiling, 28–29
Broth:
  Asian Seafood, 48–49
  Clams with Roasted Garlic in, 83–84
  Court Bouillon, 41, 286–287
  Sautéed Flatfish with Noodles and, 131–132
  Soy, Turbot Simmered in, 338
  Spicy, Pan-fried Wolffish in, 351
Butter(s):
  Anchovy, 44
  Balsamic, 45
  Black, Skate with, 274
  Compound, 44-45
  Cumin–Red Pepper, Grilled Mahi-mahi with, 168
  Dill, Broiled Dogfish with, 120–121
  drawn, 154
  Garlic, 44
  Garlic, Snails with, 281
  Garlic-Parsley, Swordfish with, 317
  Ginger, 45
  -grilled Crayfish, 116
  Herb, 44
  Herbed Smelts in, 278–279
  Horseradish, 44
  Jalapeño, 45
  Lime or Lemon, 45
  Mustard, 44
  Mustard, Broiled Mackerel Fillets with, 160–161
  Orange–Soy, Grilled Mahi-mahi with, 168
  Pernod, Broiled Mussels with, 187
  Roast Halibut with Bread Crumbs and, 148
  Sage, Cod with, 92–93
  Salmon Roasted in, 235
  Shad Fillets with, 259
  Steamed Littlenecks with Herbs and, 82–83
  Thyme, Pan-fried Sturgeon with, 310
  Toasted Pecan, Johnny Earles' Red Snapper Fillets with, 287–288
  Tomato-Herb, Broiled Red Snapper Fillets with Onion Confit and, 290
  Wasabi, 44

Wine, Broiled or Grilled Skate with, 275
Butterfish, 65–67
  Crispy Sautéed, 66
  Marinated, 66
  Pan-fried, with Spicy Tomato Puree, 65–66
  Roasted with Herbs, 66–67
  Sesame, 66
Buying fish, 5–12; see also specific fish

Cabbage:
  Gingered, "Blasted" Squid with, 296
  Napa, Stir-fried Catfish with Red Peppers and, 75
  Sautéed and Roasted, Roast Pollock with, 207
Cakes:
  Crab, 108–109
  Curried Whiting, 348–349
  Dilled Fish, 349
  Galette of Salmon and Potatoes, 232
  Salt Cod, 98
  Sartagnado, 344
  Spanish Mackerel, with Spicy Sauce, 164–165
Calamari, Deep-fried, with Three Dipping Sauces, 295–296
Caper(s):
  Flatfish with, 131
  Grilled Sturgeon with Tomatoes and, 312
  Sautéed Soft-shell Crabs with Shallots and, 112
  Shad Roe with Balsamic Vinegar and, 258
  Shrimp Salad with, 271–272
  -Tomato Sauce, Swordfish Sandwiches with, 317–318
Caponata, Eggplant:
  Roasted Bluefish Fillets with, 60–61
  Sautéed Soft-shell Crabs with, 111
Carp, 68–72
  Braised, 68–69
  Fillet with Smothered Onions, 70
  Helen Art's Gefilte Fish, 69
  Poached, 71–72
  Quenelles with Dill, 70–71
  with Sour Cream and Dill, 72
  Steamed, 71
Carrots, Red Snapper en Papillote with Zucchini and, 289
Cassoulet, Seafood, 267
Catfish, 73–76